Diagnosing and Managing Hashimoto's Disease:

Emerging Research and Opportunities

Mahmoud Sakr
Alexandria University, Egypt

A volume in the Advances in Medical Diagnosis, Treatment, and Care (AMDTC) Book Series

IGI Global
DISSEMINATOR OF KNOWLEDGE

Published in the United States of America by
IGI Global
Medical Information Science Reference (an imprint of IGI Global)
701 E. Chocolate Avenue
Hershey PA, USA 17033
Tel: 717-533-8845
Fax: 717-533-8661
E-mail: cust@igi-global.com
Web site: http://www.igi-global.com

Library of Congress Cataloging-in-Publication Data

Names: Sakr, Mahmoud, author.
Title: Diagnosing and managing Hashimoto's disease : emerging research and opportunities / by Mahmoud Sakr.
Description: Hershey PA : Medical Information Science Reference, [2020] | Includes bibliographical references.
Identifiers: LCCN 2019005237| ISBN 9781522596554 (hardcover) | ISBN 9781522596578 (ebook)
Subjects: | MESH: Hashimoto Disease
Classification: LCC RC657 | NLM WK 200 | DDC 616.4/44--dc23 LC record available at https://lccn.loc.gov/2019005237

This book is published in the IGI Global book series Advances in Medical Diagnosis, Treatment, and Care (AMDTC) (ISSN: 2475-6628; eISSN: 2475-6636)

British Cataloguing in Publication Data
A Cataloguing in Publication record for this book is available from the British Library.

For electronic access to this publication, please contact: eresources@igi-global.com.

Advances in Medical Diagnosis, Treatment, and Care (AMDTC) Book Series

ISSN:2475-6628
EISSN:2475-6636

MISSION

Advancements in medicine have prolonged the life expectancy of individuals all over the world. Once life-threatening conditions have become significantly easier to treat and even cure in many cases. Continued research in the medical field will further improve the quality of life, longevity, and wellbeing of individuals.

The **Advances in Medical Diagnosis, Treatment, and Care (AMDTC)** book series seeks to highlight publications on innovative treatment methodologies, diagnosis tools and techniques, and best practices for patient care. Comprised of comprehensive resources aimed to assist professionals in the medical field apply the latest innovations in the identification and management of medical conditions as well as patient care and interaction, the books within the AMDTC series are relevant to the research and practical needs of medical practitioners, researchers, students, and hospital administrators.

COVERAGE

- Experimental Medicine
- Patient Interaction
- Diagnostic Medicine
- Patient-Centered Care
- Internal Medicine
- Medical Procedures
- Critical Care
- Chronic Conditions
- Medical Testing
- Disease Management

IGI Global is currently accepting manuscripts for publication within this series. To submit a proposal for a volume in this series, please contact our Acquisition Editors at Acquisitions@igi-global.com or visit: http://www.igi-global.com/publish/.

The Advances in Medical Diagnosis, Treatment, and Care (AMDTC) Book Series (ISSN 2475-6628) is published by IGI Global, 701 E. Chocolate Avenue, Hershey, PA 17033-1240, USA, www.igi-global.com. This series is composed of titles available for purchase individually; each title is edited to be contextually exclusive from any other title within the series. For pricing and ordering information please visit http://www.igi-global.com/book-series/advances-medical-diagnosis-treatment-care/129618. Postmaster: Send all address changes to above address.

Titles in this Series

For a list of additional titles in this series, please visit:
https://www.igi-global.com/book-series/advances-medical-diagnosis-treatment-care/129618

Using Narrative Writing to Enhance Healing
Jennifer Lynne Bird (Oxbridge Academy, USA)
Medical Information Science Reference • copyright 2020 • 355pp • H/C (ISBN: 9781799819318) • US $275.00 (our price)

Strategies to Overcome Superbug Invasions Emerging Research and Opportunities
Dimple Sethi Chopra (Punjabi University, India)
Medical Information Science Reference • copyright 2020 • 284pp • H/C (ISBN: 9781799803072) • US $225.00 (our price)

Advanced Applications of Nanotechnology in Cancer Detection and Therapy
Alireza Heidari (Faculty of Chemistry, California South University, USA)
Medical Information Science Reference • copyright 2020 • 280pp • H/C (ISBN: 9781799801399) • US $275.00 (our price)

Developmental Challenges and Societal Issues for Individuals With Intellectual Disabilities
Rejani Thudalikunnil Gopalan (Mahatma Gandhi Medical College and Hospital, India)
Medical Information Science Reference • copyright 2020 • 416pp • H/C (ISBN: 9781799812234) • US $265.00 (our price)

Global Applications of One Health Practice and Care
Sandul Yasobant (Center for Development Research (ZEF), Germany) and Deepak Saxena (Indian Institute of Public Health Gandhinagar, India)
Medical Information Science Reference • copyright 2019 • 306pp • H/C (ISBN: 9781522563044) • US $245.00 (our price)

Pre-Screening Systems for Early Disease Prediction, Detection, and Prevention
Thierry Edoh (Technical University of Munich, Germany) Pravin Pawar (Philips Research, India) and Sagar Mohammad (Philips Research, India)

For an entire list of titles in this series, please visit:
https://www.igi-global.com/book-series/advances-medical-diagnosis-treatment-care/129618

IGI Global
DISSEMINATOR OF KNOWLEDGE

701 East Chocolate Avenue, Hershey, PA 17033, USA
Tel: 717-533-8845 x100 • Fax: 717-533-8661
E-Mail: cust@igi-global.com • www.igi-global.com

To my dear students and colleagues

Table of Contents

Preface

Thyroid surgery has now become a major specialty within the head and neck and endocrine surgical domain. We have endeavored to give some rein to the new developments, which are evidence-based and widely supported in the literature.

The purpose of this book is to provide a comprehensive review of the current and emerging knowledge of Hashimoto's thyroiditis. The disease was thought to be uncommon for many years, and diagnosis was usually made by the surgeon intra-operatively or by the pathologist after thyroidectomy. The increasing use of needle biopsy and serologic tests for antibodies have led to much more frequent recognition, and there is reason to believe that it may be increasing in frequency. Currently, it is one of the most common thyroid disorders and remains the most common cause of spontaneous hypothyroidism in areas of adequate iodine intake.

This book addresses a wide range of topics related to Hashimoto's thyroiditis starting with a historical review of the disease and including epidemiology, pathology, etiology, pathogenesis, clinical manifestations, diagnosis and differential diagnosis, association with papillary thyroid carcinoma, management including a separate Chapter on dietary management, as well as prognosis. Specific chapters discussing Hashimoto's encephalopathy, Hashimoto's ophthalmopathy, and relationship of Hashimoto's thyroiditis with anxiety and depression are also included.

This book has been structured in such a way to facilitate quick reference. We believe it will be a useful tool for clinicians to provide timely and up-to-date therapy of their patients suffering from this disease.

Acknowledgment

I would like to express my sincere gratitude to all those who provided support and help in the process of writing, editing, proof-reading, and producing this book. Last but not least, I would like to express my deepest gratitude to my family for their unlimited support and unconditioned love.

Chapter 1
Historical Review

ABSTRACT

Hashimoto thyroiditis (HT) is part of the spectrum of autoimmune thyroid diseases characterized by the destruction of thyroid cells by various cell- and antibody-mediated immune processes. It was first described by the Japanese surgeon Hakaru Hashimoto (1981-1934). It was not until 1956 when a link between antibodies to thyroid cells present in the serum of patients and HT was made. Over time, our understanding of the immunologic pathways involved in HT has evolved. We now recognize the association of this disease with other autoimmune diseases and thyroid cancer. The increasing use of the needle biopsy and serologic tests for antibodies have led to much more frequent recognition, and there is reason to believe that it may be increasing in frequency. It is now one of the most common thyroid disorders. This chapter gives a historical overview of Hashimoto's disease.

INTRODUCTION

Hashimoto thyroiditis is part of the spectrum of autoimmune thyroid diseases (AITDs), which include also the following variants; atrophic thyroiditis, juvenile thyroiditis, post-partum thyroiditis (PPT), silent thyroiditis, and focal thyroiditis (Fava et al., 2009).

Hashimoto disease (or Hashimoto's thyroiditis) is characterized by the destruction of thyroid cells by various cell- and antibody-mediated immune processes. It is the most common cause of hypothyroidism in the United States

DOI: 10.4018/978-1-5225-9655-4.ch001

after age 6 years. By strict criteria, Hashimoto thyroiditis is a histological diagnosis first described by the Japanese surgeon, *Hakaru Hashimoto.*

Hakaru Hashimoto (Figure 1) was born on May 5, 1881, in the village of Midai, Nishitsuge, in Mie Prefecture, Japan. He graduated from Kyushu University Medical School in 1907. He then entered the First Surgical Bureau and studied medicine under the direction of Professor Hayari Miyake (1867–1945), the first Japanese neurosurgeon. Several years after, he studied pathology under Professor Eduard Kaufmann at the Georg-August University of Göttingen.

Hakaru Hashimoto also studied in England, but with breaking out of World War I, he was forced to return home to Japan. In 1916, he came back to his hometown, Igamachi, and became the town doctor. Hashimoto was the surgeon who first described lymphocytic thyroiditis, which became known later as "Hashimoto's thyroiditis".

The year 2013 marked the centennial anniversary of his original description of "*struma lymphomatosa*;" his observation of unique histologic features, including lymphocytic infiltration, eosinophilic change to follicular cells, and interstitial fibrosis that were described in four women with goiters, were treated with thyroidectomy (Fava et al., 2009). His work was published in a German journal in 1912 and went unnoticed for over 40 years. At the time of his original description, Hashimoto realized that some stimulus was responsible for the reactive changes he noticed, but he admitted that he did not know the nature of that stimulus. Due to his sudden death in January 9, 1934 (at the age of 52) because of typhoid fever, he was never able to witness the impact of his discovery.

It was not until 1956 when a link between antibodies to thyroid cells present in the serum of patients and Hashimoto's disease was made. Hashimoto's disease was the *first organ* in which an immune etiology to a specific disease process was described. Over time, our understanding of the immunologic pathways involved in Hashimoto's thyroiditis has evolved. We now recognize the association of this disease with other autoimmune diseases and thyroid cancer (Nagar & Angelos, 2015).

The disease has been called Hashimoto's thyroiditis, chronic thyroiditis, lymphocytic thyroiditis, lymphadenoid goiter, and recently, autoimmune thyroiditis. Classically, it presents as a painless, diffuse enlargement of the thyroid gland in a young or middle-aged woman. It is often associated with hypothyroidism. The disease was thought to be uncommon for many years, and the diagnosis was usually made by the surgeon intra-operatively or by the pathologist after thyroidectomy. The increasing use of the needle biopsy

Figure 1. Hakaru Hashimoto (1881-1934)

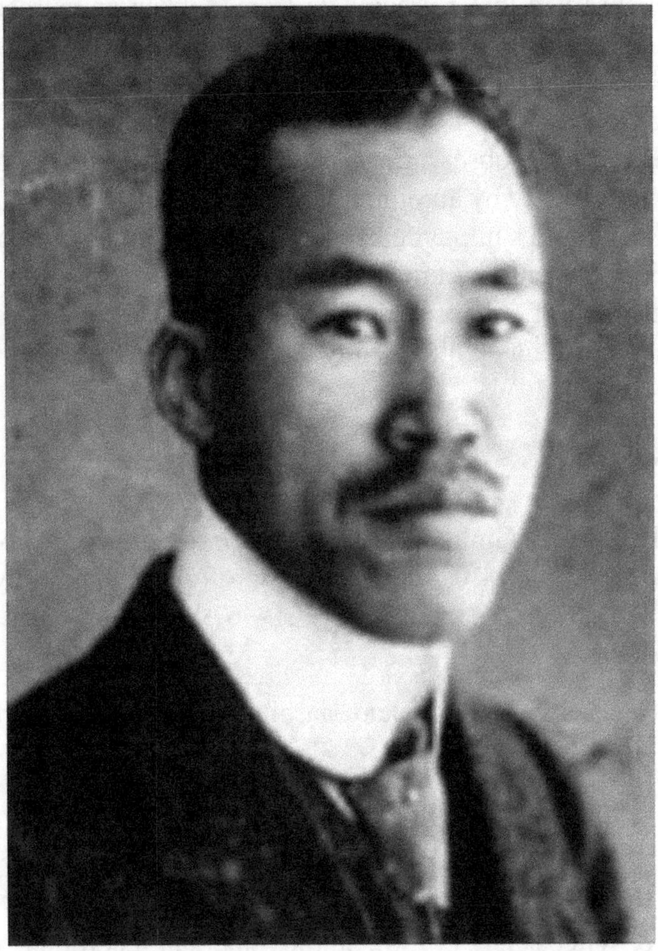

and serologic tests for antibodies have led to much more frequent recognition, and there is reason to believe that it may be increasing in frequency (Nagar & Angelos, 2015). It is now one of the most common thyroid disorders.

Rose and Witebsky (1956) reported that the first indication of an immunologic abnormality in this disease was an elevation of the plasma gamma globulin fraction. This finding, together with abnormalities in serum flocculation test results indicated that the disease might be related to a long-continued autoimmune reaction (Roitt, Doniach, Campbell, Hudson, 1956). Rose and Witebsky (1956) showed that immunization of rabbits with extracts of rabbit thyroids produced histologic changes in the thyroid glands resembling those seen in Hashimoto's thyroiditis. They also found anti-thyroglobulin antibodies in the blood of the animals. Subsequently, Roitt et al. (1956) observed that a precipitate formed when an extract of human thyroid gland was added to serum from a patient with Hashimoto's thyroiditis. Thus, it appeared that the serum contained antibodies to a constituent of the human thyroid and that these antibodies might be responsible for the disease process. These original observations led directly to entirely new concepts of the causation of disease by autoimmunization.

Hakaru Hashimoto's initial description of this disease was the necessary first step to our current-day understanding of Hashimoto's thyroiditis. His contributions to the fields of endocrinology and autoimmune disease are immense and unfortunately, frequently under-appreciated.

REFERENCES

Fava, A., Oliverio, R., Giuliano, S., Parlato, G., Michniewicz, A., Indrieri, A., ... Befiore, A. (2009). Clinical evolution of autoimmune thyroiditis in children and adolescents. *Thyroid, 19*(4), 361–367. doi:10.1089/thy.2008.0239 PMID:19226198

Nagar, S., & Angelos, P. (2015). Hakaru Hashimoto. *Surgical Endocrinopathies, 8*, 43–48.

Roitt, I. M., Doniach, D., Campbell, P. N., & Hudson, R. V. (1956). Autoantibodies in Hashimoto's thyroiditis (lymphadenoid goiter). *Lancet, 2*(6947), 820–823. doi:10.1016/S0140-6736(56)92249-8 PMID:13368530

Rose, N. R., & Witebsky, E. (1956). Studies on organ specificity. V. Changes in thyroid glands of rabbits following active immunization with rabbit thyroid extracts. *Journal of Immunology (Baltimore, Md.: 1950), 76*, 417–419. PMID:13332243

Chapter 2
Epidemiology

ABSTRACT

Hashimoto thyroiditis (HT) remains the most common cause of spontaneous hypothyroidism in areas of adequate iodine intake, such as North America. The incidence of HT is estimated to be 10-15 times higher in females. The most commonly affected age range is 30-50 years, with the peak incidence in men occurring 10-15 years later, but it may be seen in any age group, including children. Hashimoto's thyroiditis appears to occur in more than 10% of patients presenting with thyroid nodule and may be associated with other autoimmune disorders. The occurrence of papillary thyroid carcinoma in HT ranges widely from 0.5-30% of cases. The prevalence of thyroid antibodies is twice more common in women than in men, and higher in whites and Asians than Blacks or Mexicans. There is approximately a 30-fold increase in risk for developing HT in children and 20-fold increased risk in siblings of patients with HT, with females being significantly more often affected than males. This chapter explores the epidemiology of Hashimoto's disease.

INTRODUCTION

The most common cause of hypothyroidism Worldwide is ***iodine deficiency.*** However, Hashimoto thyroiditis remains the most common cause of spontaneous hypothyroidism in areas of adequate iodine intake, such as North America.

Iodine is a trace element (mineral) with the symbol "I" and atomic number 53. The heaviest of the stable halogens, it exists as a lustrous, purple-black

DOI: 10.4018/978-1-5225-9655-4.ch002

non-metallic solid at standard conditions that melts to form a deep violet liquid at 114 degrees Celsius, and boils to a violet gas at 184 degrees Celsius (Meija et al., 2016). Iodine is essential in the synthesis of thyroid hormones; thyroxine (T4) and triiodothyronine (T3). The two thyroid hormones regulate the metabolism in every cell of the body. This is required for the development of skeletal and nervous system. Iodine is is naturally present in some foods (Pennington, 1995; Teas, 2004; Dasgupta, 2008), added to others (iodized table salt) (World Health Organization, 2007; Food and Drug Administration, 2009), and available as a dietary supplement (Aquaron, Delange, Marchal, Lognoné, & Ninane, 2002).

Incidence

Worldwide Incidence

The annual *incidence* of Hashimoto's thyroiditis seen in practice Worldwide is unknown, but is approximately, 0.3-1.5 cases per 1,000 population per year) (Gordin, 1979; Ling, 1969; Tunbridge, 1977; Vanderpump, 1995; Vanderpump, 1998), which is roughly equal to that of Graves' disease (an autoimmune disease that affects the thyroid, frequently resulting in hyperthyroidism and an enlarged thyroid; also known as toxic diffuse goiter).

Incidence in United States

Hashimoto thyroiditis is the most common cause of hypothyroidism in the United States after the age of 6 years, with the incidence estimated to be 1.3% in a series of 5000 *children* aged 11-18 years. In *adults*, the incidence is estimated to be 3.5 per 1000 per year in women and 0.8 per 1000 per year in men. Incidence may be as high as 6% in the Appalachian region (Weetman, 2006).

Gender- and Age-Related Demographics

The incidence of Hashimoto's thyroiditis is estimated to be 10-15 times higher in *females*. The most commonly affected *age* range is 30-50 years, with the peak incidence in men occurring 10-15 years later, but it may be seen in any age group, including children. The overall incidence of hypothyroidism increases with age in men and women. It is certain that Hashimoto's disease exists with a much higher frequency than is diagnosed clinically, and its frequency seems to be increasing (Meng et al., 2015).

Prevalence

Prevalence of Hashimoto's Disease

Prevalence of Hashimoto's thyroiditis is 4.5% (4.2% subclinical and 0.3% clinical hypothyroid) based on biochemical analysis (Staii, Mirocha, Todorova-Koteva, Glinberg, & Jaum, 2010), but with cytological diagnosis prevalence increases to 13.4%. The annual risk of the subclinical hypothyroidism to overt hypothyroidism is 4%. In the Colorado Thyroid Disease Prevalence Study, involving 25,862 adults, the prevalence of elevated TSH in symptomatic and asymptomatic adults was 9.5%, with a greater percentage of those involved being *women*. The prevalence of hypothyroidism and of thyroid disease in general increases with *age* (Canaris, Manowitz, & Mayor, 2000).

Hashimoto's thyroiditis appears to occur in more than 10% of patients presenting with *thyroid nodule*. Hashimoto's thyroiditis is associated with *other autoimmune disorders* such as Addison's disease, diabetes mellitus type-1, rheumatoid arthritis, systemic lupus erythematosus or vitiligo. The occurrence of papillary thyroid carcinoma in Hashimoto's thyroiditis has been extensively studied and the association ranges from 0.5-30% of cases.

Prevalence of Thyroid Antibodies

For several decades a strong genetic predisposition to autoimmune thyroid disease has been recognized, predominantly on the basis of the family and twin studies. Family studies always bring to light a number of relatives with moderate enlargement of the thyroid gland suggestive of Hashimoto's thyroiditis. Many of these persons have thyroglobulin (Tg) and thyroid perioxidase (TPO) antibodies, and most are entirely asymptomatic.

More than 50 years ago, soon after the discovery of T-Abs, Hall and Stanbury (1967) reported the presence of T-Abs in 56% of siblings of patients with autoimmune thyroid disease (AITD). Early in 1975, Inoue et al. (1975) reported that 3% of Japanese children aged 6-18 years have thyroiditis. In most instances, biopsy revealed focal rather than diffuse thyroiditis.

This familial clustering of AITD and the presence of T-Abs in up to 60% of first-degree relatives of patients has been later confirmed by many authors

(Aho, 1983; Phillips, 1993; Desai, 1999; Segni, 2001; Marwaha, 2003). When both parents were affected, the prevalence of TPO-Abs and Tg-Abs was 42% in daughters and 33% in sons, compared with 28.9% and 16.7%, respectively, when only one parent was positive for T-Abs (Phillips et al., 1993). Among first-degree relatives of children with Hashimoto's thyroiditis, 34% were diagnosed TPO-Abs positive compared to only 13% first-degree relatives of children without AITD (Marwaha et al., 2003). In the National Health and Nutrition Examination Survey (NHANES) III, the prevalence of thyroid antibodies (T-Abs) was 18% regardless of age and gender. Moreover, the calculated sibling risk ratio for Hashimoto's thyroiditis was 28, thus confirming the highly significant contribution of genetic factors to the disease development (Villanueva, Greenberg, Davies, Tomer, 2003). The prevalence of T-Abs is twice more common in women than in men, and higher in whites and Asians than Blacks or Mexicans.

A recent German study also indicated a 32-fold increase in risk for developing Hashimoto's thyroiditis in children and 21-fold increased risk in siblings of patients with Hashimoto's thyroiditis, with females being significantly more often affected than males (Dittmar, Libich, Brenzel, & Kahaly, 2011).

Twin studies provided further valuable data on the genetic contribution to thyroid autoimmunity. In healthy twin siblings of patients with overt AITD, positive TPO-Abs and Tg-Abs in monozygotic twins were determined in 53% and 47%, respectively, in dizygotic twins in 22% and 13%, respectively, while in healthy control population only in 9% and 7%, respectively (Brix, Hansen, Kyvik, & Hegedüs, 2004). The concordance rates for TPO-Abs were 64% in monozygotic twins compared with 35% in dizygotic twins, while concordance rates for TgAbs were 74% and 32%, respectively (Phillips, Osmond, Baird, Huckle, & Rees-Smith, 2002). Moreover, the concordant rate for overt Hashimoto's hypothyroidism was 55% in monozygotic twins as compared to 0% in dizygotic twins (Brix, Kyvik, & Hegedüs, 2000)· indicating the importance of non-genetic influences on disease development. In a study of Danish twins, by Hansen et al (2006), 73% of the susceptibility to the development of T-Abs appeared to be attributable to genetic factors (Hansen, Brix, Iachine, Kyvik, & Hegedüs, 2006). In addition, a recent twin study by Brix and colleagues indicated that the liability to the production of antibodies directed against immunodominant region A of TPO is genetically determined (Brix, Hegedüs, Gardas, Banga, & Nielsen, 2011).

In addition to ***overt thyroiditis***, roughly 10% of most populations have positive Tg and TPO *antibody test results* in the apparent absence of thyroid disease by physical examination (Gordin, 1979; Ling, 1969; Tunbridge, 1977). Tunbridge et al (1977) reported that 1.9-2.7% of women had present or past thyrotoxicosis, 1.9% had overt hypothyroidism, 7.5% had elevated TSH levels, 10.3% had test results positive for TPO-Ab (microsomal antigen) measured by hemagglutination assay (MCHA), and about 15.0% had goiter. Men had 10- to 4-fold *lower* incidence of thyroid abnormalities. In a study of children whose parents had history of thyroid disease, Carey et al. (1980) found a 24% prevalence of thyroid "abnormalities", including a 6.9% of abnormal thyroids, and 9.3% with positive Tg-Ab measured by hemagglutination assay (TGHA) and 7.8% positive MCHA assays. Gordin et al. (1979) reported that 8% of adult Finns had positive TGHA results, and 26% had positive MCHA results; TSH levels were elevated in 30% of these persons.

On the basis of positive antibody titers and elevated TSH levels, 2-5% was believed to have ***asymptomatic thyroiditis***. These test results correlate with focal collection of lymphocytes on histological examination of the thyroid glands (Yoshida et al., 1978) that are frequently associated with elevated levels of TSH (Gordin A, Saarinen P, Pelkonen A, & Lamberg, 1974), and probably represent one end of a spectrum of thyroid damage. Women with both positive antibody test results and raised TSH levels become hypothyroid at the rate of 5%/year (Tunbridge et al., 1981). A reasonable approximation of the prevalence of positive antibody tests in women is >10%, and of clinical disease is at least 2%. Men have only 10% of this prevalence.

Several epidemiological studies showed that women present with positive T-Abs up to three times more often than men (Aghini-Lombardi, 1999; Hollowell, 2002; Spencer, 2007; Lucas, 2010; Knudsen, 1999; Pedersen, 2003; Hoogendoom, 2006; Simmonds, 2014). The largest National Health and Nutrition Examination Survery (NHANES) III study indicated also that women were positive for TPO-Abs and Tg-Abs in 17% and 15.2%, respectively, as compared to only in 8.7% and 7.6%, respectively in men (Hollowell et al., 2002). The study of Hansen et al. (2006) on Danish twins, showed that the genetic contribution to TPO-Ab and Tg-Ab susceptibility in females was 72% and 75%, respectively, while in males it was only 61% and 39%, respectively.

A number of small datasets have suggested a potential role for *skewed X-chromosome activation (XCI)*, away from the expected 50:50 parent of origin ratio, as an explanation for the strong female preponderance seen in the common autoimmune thyroid diseases, Graves' disease and Hashimoto's thyroiditis (Simmonds et al., 2014).

A possible role for fetal cell micro-*chimerism* in triggering an autoimmune process has been repeatedly proposed, based on the evidence that autoimmune diseases have a higher prevalence in females, with peak incidence in women of child-bearing age. Fetal micro-chimeric cells have been found to be significantly more represented within the thyroid gland of women with Hashimoto's thyroiditis and Graves' disease compared to those without thyroid autoimmunity, suggesting a pathogenic role (Klintschar, 2001; Klintschar, 2006).

REFERENCES

Aghini-Lombardi, F., Antonangeli, L., Martino, E., Vitti, P., Maccherini, D., Leoli, F., ... Pinchera, A. (1999). The spectrum of thyroid disorders in an iodine-deficient community: The Pescopagano survey. *The Journal of Clinical Endocrinology and Metabolism*, *84*, 561–566. PMID:10022416

Aho, K., Gordin, A., Sievers, K., & Takala, J. (1983). Thyroid autoimmunity in siblings: A population study. *Acta Endocrinologica. Supplementum*, *251*, 11–15. PMID:6573098

Aquaron, R., Delange, F., Marchal, P., Lognoné, V., & Ninane, L. (2002). Bioavailability of seaweed iodine in human beings. *Cellular and Molecular Biology*, *48*(5), 563–569. PMID:12146713

Brix, T. H., Hansen, P. S., Kyvik, K. O., & Hegedüs, L. (2004). Aggregation of thyroid autoantibodies in first-degree relatives of patients with autoimmune thyroid disease is mainly due to genes: A twin study. *Horumon To Rinsho*, *60*(3), 329–334. doi:10.1111/j.1365-2265.2004.01983.x PMID:15008998

Brix, T. H., Hegedüs, L., Gardas, A., Banga, J. P., & Nielsen, C. H. (2011). Monozygotic twin pairs discordant for Hashimoto's thyroiditis share a high proportion of thyroid peroxidase autoantibodies to the immunodominant region A. Further evidence for genetic transmission of epitopic "fingerprints". *Autoimmunit*, *44*(3), 188–194. doi:10.3109/08916934.2010.518575 PMID:20883148

Brix, T. H., Kyvik, K. O., & Hegedüs, L. (2000). A population-based study of chronic autoimmune hypothyroidism in Danish twins. *Horumon To Rinsho*, *53*, 171–176. doi:10.1046/j.1365-2265.2000.01025.x PMID:10931097

Canaris, G. J., Manowitz, N. R., Mayor, G., & Ridgway, E. C. (2000). The Colorado Thyroid Disease Prevalence Study. *Archives of Internal Medicine*, *160*(4), 526–534. doi:10.1001/archinte.160.4.526 PMID:10695693

Carey, C., Skosey, C., Pinnamaneni, K. M., Barsano, C. P., & DeGroot, L. J. (1980). Thyroid abnormalities in children of parents who have Graves' disease. Possible pre-Graves' disease. *Metabolism: Clinical and Experimental*, *29*(4), 369–374. doi:10.1016/0026-0495(80)90012-8 PMID:6892833

Dasgupta, P. K., Liu, Y., & Dyke, J. V. (2008). Iodine nutrition: Iodine content of iodized salt in the United States. *Environmental Science & Technology*, *42*(4), 1315–1323. doi:10.1021/es0719071 PMID:18351111

Desai, M. P., & Karandikar, S. (1999). Autoimmune thyroid disease in childhood: A study of children and their families. *Indian Pediatrics*, *36*, 659–668. PMID:10740302

Dittmar, M., Libich, C., Brenzel, T., & Kahaly, G. J. (2011, March). Increased familial clustering of autoimmune thyroid diseases. *Hormone and Metabolic Research. Hormon- und Stoffwechselforschung. Hormones et Metabolisme*, *43*(3), 200–204. doi:10.1055-0031-1271619 PMID:21287436

Gordin, A., Maatela, J., Miettinen, A., Helenius, T., & Lamberg, A. (1979). Serum thyrotrophin and circulating thyroglobulin and thyroid microsomal antibodies in a Finnish population. *Acta Endocrinologica*, *90*(1), 33–39. doi:10.1530/acta.0.0900033 PMID:760358

Gordin, A., Saarinen, P., Pelkonen, A., & Lamberg, A. (1974). Serum thyroglobulin and the response to thyrotropin releasing hormone in symptomless autoimmune thyroiditis and in borderline and overt hypothyroidism. *Acta Endocrinologica*, *75*(2), 274–277. doi:10.1530/acta.0.0750274 PMID:4133483

Hall, R., & Stanbury, J. B. (1967). Familial studies of autoimmune thyroiditis. *Clinical and Experimental Immunology*, *2*, 719–725. PMID:5590107

Hansen, P. S., Brix, T. H., Iachine, I., Kyvik, K. O., & Hegedüs, L. (2006). The relative importance of genetic and environmental effects for the early stages of thyroid autoimmunity: A study of healthy Danish twins. *European Journal of Endocrinology*, *154*(1), 29–38. doi:10.1530/eje.1.02060 PMID:16381988

Hollowell, J. G., Staehling, N. W., Flanders, W. D., Hannon, W. H., Gunter, E. W., Spencer, C. A., & Braverman, L. E. (2002). Serum TSH, T(4), and thyroid antibodies in the United States population (1988 to 1994): National Health and Nutrition Examination Survey (NHANES III). *The Journal of Clinical Endocrinology and Metabolism*, *87*(2), 489–499. doi:10.1210/jcem.87.2.8182 PMID:11836274

Hoogendoorn, E. H., Hermus, A. R., de Vegt, F., Ross, H. A., Verbeek, A. L., Kiemeney, L. A., & den Heijer, M. (2006). Thyroid function and prevalence of anti-thyroperoxidase antibodies in a population with borderline sufficient iodine intake: Influences of age and sex. *Clinical Chemistry, 52*(1), 104–111. doi:10.1373/clinchem.2005.055194 PMID:16254196

Inoue, M., Taketani, N., Sato, T., & Nakajima, H. (1975). High incidence of chronic lymphocytic thyroiditis in apparently healthy school children: Epidemiological and clinical study. *Endocrinologia Japonica, 22*(6), 483–487. doi:10.1507/endocrj1954.22.483 PMID:1243913

Klintschar, M., Immel, U. D., Kehlen, A., Schwaiger, P., Mustafa, T., Mannweiler, S., ... Hoang-Vu, C. (2006). Fetal microchimerism in Hashimoto's thyroiditis: A quantitative approach. *European Journal of Endocrinology, 154*(2), 237–241. doi:10.1530/eje.1.02080 PMID:16452536

Klintschar, M., Schwaiger, P., Mannweiler, S., Regauer, S., & Kleiber, M. (n.d.). Evidence of fetal microchimerism in Hashimoto's thyroiditis. *The Journal of Clinical Endocrinology and Metabolism, 86*, 2494–2498. PMID:11397845

Knudsen, N., Jorgensen, T., Rasmussen, S., Christiansen, E., & Perrild, H. (1999). The prevalence of thyroid dysfunction in a population with borderline iodine deficiency. *Horumon To Rinsho, 51*, 361–367. PMID:10469017

Ling, S. M., Kaplan, S. A., Weitzman, J. J., Reed, G. B., Costin, G., & Landing, B. H. (1969). Euthyroid goiters in children. Correlation of needle biopsy with other clinical and laboratory findings in chronic lymphocytic thyroiditis and simple goiter. *Pediatrics, 44*, 695–699. PMID:4911917

Lucas, A., Julián, M. T., Cantón, A., Castell, C., Casamitjana, R., Martínez-Cáceres, E. M., & Granada, M. L. (2010). Undiagnosed thyroid dysfunction, thyroid antibodies, and iodine excretion in a Mediterranean population. *Endocrine, 38*(3), 391–396. doi:10.100712020-010-9397-2 PMID:20972723

Marwaha, R. K., Sen, S., Tandon, N., Sahoo, M., Walia, R. P., Singh, S., ... Jain, S. K. (2003). Familial aggregation of autoimmune thyroiditis in first-degree relatives of patients with juvenile autoimmune thyroid disease. *Thyroid, 13*(3), 297–300. doi:10.1089/105072503321582114 PMID:12729480

Meija, J., Coplen, T. B., Berglund, M., Brand, W. A., De Bièvre, P., Gröning, M., ... Prohaska, T. (2016). Atomic weights of the elements 2013 (IUPAC Technical Report). *Pure and Applied Chemistry, 88*(3), 265–291. doi:10.1515/pac-2015-0305

Meng, Z., Liu, M., Zhang, Q., Liu, L., Song, K., Tan, J., ... Zhang, J. (2015). Gender and Age Impacts on the Association Between Thyroid Function and Metabolic Syndrome in Chinese. *Medicine; Analytical Reviews of General Medicine, Neurology, Psychiatry, Dermatology, and Pediatries*, *94*(50), e2193. doi:10.1097/MD.0000000000002193 PMID:26683929

Pedersen, I. B., Knudsen, N., Jørgensen, T., Perrild, H., Ovesen, L., & Laurberg, P. (2003). Thyroid peroxidase and thyroglobulin autoantibodies in a large survey of populations with mild and moderate iodine deficiency. *Horumon To Rinsho*, *58*, 36–42. PMID:12519410

Pennington, J. A., Schoen, S. A., Salmon, G. D., Young, B., Johnson, R. D., & Marts, R. W. (1995). Composition of Core Foods of the U.S. Food Supply, 1982-1991. III. Copper, Manganese, Selenium, and Iodine. *Journal of Food Composition and Analysis*, *8*(2), 171–217. doi:10.1006/jfca.1995.1014

Phillips, D. I., Osmond, C., Baird, J., Huckle, A., & Rees-Smith, B. (2002). Is birthweight associated with thyroid autoimmunity? A study in twins. *Thyroid*, *12*(5), 377–380. doi:10.1089/105072502760043440 PMID:12097197

Phillips, D. I., Shields, D. C., Dugoujon, J. M., Prentice, L., McGuffin, P., & Ree, S. (1993). Complex segregation analysis of thyroid autoantibodies: Are they inherited as an autosomal dominant trait? *Human Heredity*, *43*(3), 141–146. doi:10.1159/000154169 PMID:8330876

Renno, C., Ramos-Lopez, E., Steimle-Grauer, S. A., Ziolkowski, P., Pani, M. A., & Luther, C. (2004). Thyroid fetal male micro-chimerism in mothers with thyroid disorders: Presence of Y-chromosomal immuno-fluorescence in thyroid infiltrating lymphocytes is more prevalent in Hashimoto's thyroiditis and Graves' disease than in follicular adenomas. *The Journal of Clinical Endocrinology and Metabolism*, *89*(11), 5810–5814. doi:10.1210/jc.2004-1049 PMID:15531546

Segni, M., Wood, J., Pucarelli, I., Toscano, V., Toscano, R., & Pasquino, A. M. (2001). Clustering of autoimmune thyroid diseases in children and adolescents: A study of 66 families. *Journal of Pediatric Endocrinology & Metabolism*, *14*, 1271–1275. PMID:11964022

Simmonds, M. J., Kavvoura, F. K., Brand, O. J., Newby, P. R., Jackson, L. E., Hargreaves, C. E., ... Gough, S. C. (2014). Skewed X chromosome inactivation and female preponderance in autoimmune thyroid disease: An association study and meta-analysis. *The Journal of Clinical Endocrinology and Metabolism*, *99*(1), 27–31. doi:10.1210/jc.2013-2667 PMID:24187400

Spencer, C. A., Hollowell, J. G., Kazarosyan, M., & Braverman, L. E. (2007). National Health and Nutrition Examination Survey III thyroid-stimulating hormone (TSH)-thyroperoxidase antibody relationships demonstrate that TSH upper reference limits may be skewed by occult thyroid dysfunction. *The Journal of Clinical Endocrinology and Metabolism*, *92*(11), 4236–4240. doi:10.1210/jc.2007-0287 PMID:17684054

Staii, A., Mirocha, S., Todorova-Koteva, K., Glinberg, S., & Jaum, J. (2010). Hashimoto thyroiditis is more frequent than expected when diagnosed by cytology which uncovers a pre-clinical state. *Thyroid Research*, *3*(1), 11–16. doi:10.1186/1756-6614-3-11 PMID:21172028

Teas, J., Pino, S., Critchley, A., & Braverman, L. E. (2004). Variability of iodine content in common commercially available edible seaweeds. *Thyroid*, *14*(10), 836–841. doi:10.1089/thy.2004.14.836 PMID:15588380

Tunbridge, W. G., Brewis, M., French, J. M., Appleton, D., Bird, T., Clark, F., ... Young, E. (1981). Natural history of autoimmune thyroiditis. *British Medical Journal*, *282*(6260), 258–263. doi:10.1136/bmj.282.6260.258 PMID:6779977

Tunbridge, W. M., Evered, D. C., Hall, R., Appleton, D., Brewis, M., Clark, F., ... Smith, P. A. (1977). The spectrum of thyroid disease in a community. The Whickham Survey. *Horumon To Rinsho*, *7*, 481–486. doi:10.1111/j.1365-2265.1977.tb01340.x PMID:598014

U.S. Food and Drug Administration. (2009). Code of Federal Regulations, CFR 21, Sections 184.1634 and 184.1265. Silver Spring, MD: Food and Drug Administration.

Vanderpump, M. P., French, J. M., Appleton, D., Tunbridge, & Kendall-Taylor. (1998). The prevalence of hyperprolactinaemia and association with markers of autoimmune thyroid disease in survivors of the Whickham Survey cohort. *Horumon To Rinsho*, *48*(1), 39–44. doi:10.1046/j.1365-2265.1998.00343.x PMID:9509066

Vanderpump, M. P., Tunbridge, W. M., & French, J. M. (1995). The incidence of thyroid disorders in the community: A twenty-year follow-up of the Whickham Survey. *Horumon To Rinsho*, *43*(1), 55–68. doi:10.1111/j.1365-2265.1995.tb01894.x PMID:7641412

Villanueva, R., Greenberg, D. A., Davies, T. F., & Tomer, Y. (2003). Sibling recurrence risk in autoimmune thyroid disease. *Thyroid*, *13*(8), 761–764. doi:10.1089/105072503768499653 PMID:14558919

Weetman, A. P. (2006). Thyroid disease. In The Autoimmune Disease. Elsevier.

World Health Organization. (2007). *United Nations Children's Fund & International Council for the Control of Iodine Deficiency Disorders. In Assessment of iodine deficiency disorders and monitoring their elimination* (3rd ed.). Geneva, Switzerland: World Health Organization.

Yoshida, H., Amino, N., Yagawa, K., Uemura, K., Satoh, M., Miyai, K., & Kumahara, Y. (1978). Association of serum antithyroid antibodies with lymphocytic infiltration of the thyroid gland: Studies of seventy autopsied cases. *The Journal of Clinical Endocrinology and Metabolism*, *46*(6), 859–864. doi:10.1210/jcem-46-6-859 PMID:263468

Chapter 3
Pathology

ABSTRACT

Grossly, thyroid enlargement in Hashimoto's thyroiditis (HT) is generally symmetrical, often with a characteristic conspicuous pyramidal lobe. The tissue involved by HT is pinkish-tan to frankly yellowish in color and tends to have a rubbery firmness. There is no necrosis or calcification. The capsule is intact and non-adherent to peri-thyroid structures. Microscopically, there is a diffuse process consisting of a combination of epithelial cell destruction, lymphoid cellular infiltration, and fibrosis. Lymphocytes are predominantly T-cells and plasma cells. Most infiltrating T-cells have α/β T-cell receptors. Gamma/delta T-cells are rare. Hashimoto's thyroiditis has been graded based on lymphocytic infiltration seen on cytology, into Grades 0-III, where Grade 0 means no lymphoid cells and Grade III severe lymphoid cell infiltration. Deposits of dense material representing IgG are found along the basement membrane on electron microscopy. This chapter explores the pathology of Hashimoto's disease.

INTRODUCTION

Gross Appearance

In Hashimoto's disease, thyroid enlargement is symmetrical, often with a characteristic conspicuous pyramidal lobe. Although the gland is symmetrically enlarged, the accentuation of lobulations may make the gland appear lobular on gross examination.

DOI: 10.4018/978-1-5225-9655-4.ch003

The tissue involved by Hashimoto's thyroiditis is pinkish-tan (Figure 1) to frankly yellowish (Figure 2) in color and tends to have a rubbery firmness. There is no necrosis or calcification.

The capsule is intact and the capsular surface is gently lobulated and non-adherent to peri-thyroid structures i.e. the gland itself is still distinct from surrounding tissue. It may have adhesions but thyroid gland is easily separated from other structures

Microscopic Picture

In Hashimoto's thyroiditis, there is a diffuse process consisting of a combination of epithelial cell destruction, lymphoid cellular infiltration, and fibrosis. Lymphocytes are predominantly T cells and plasma cells (polyclonal).

The thyroid cells tend to be slightly larger in size and assume an acidophilic staining character; they are then called *Hurthle* or *Askanazy* cells and are packed with mitochondria. The follicular spaces shrink, and colloid is absent or sparse.

Fibrosis may be completely absent or present in degrees ranging from slight to moderate; it may be severe, as observed in subacute or Riedel's thyroiditis but does not extend beyond capsule.

Foreign body giant cells and granulomas are *not* features of Hashimoto's thyroiditis, in contrast to subacute thyroiditis. In children, oxyphilia and fibrosis are less prominent, and hyperplasia of epithelial cells may be marked.

Figure 1. Hashimoto's thyroiditis. Note the symmetrical enlargement of the gland and the pinkish-tan

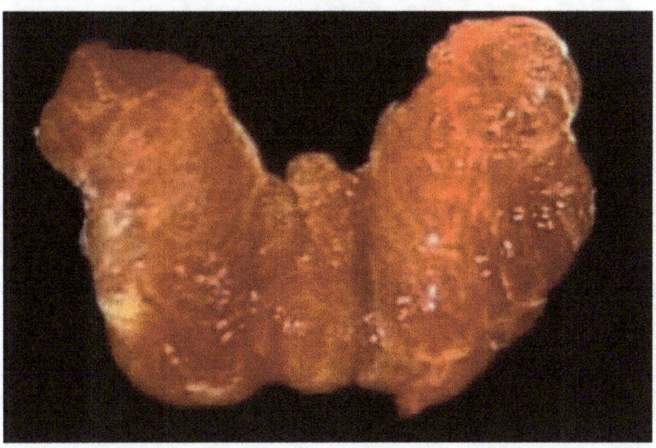

Figure 2. Hashimoto's thyroiditis. Note the symmetrical enlargement of the gland and the yellowish discoloration.

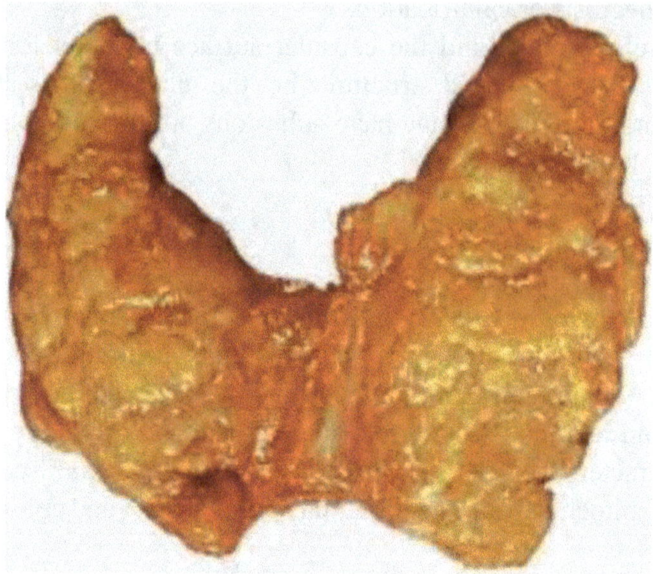

Deposits of dense material representing IgG are found along the basement membrane on electron microscopy (Figure 3).

Clusters of macrophage-like cells may be seen within the follicles. The lymphoid infiltration in the interstitial tissue is accompanied by actual follicles and germinal centers (Figure 4). Plasma B-cells are prominent and can often be seen as secondary lymphoid follicles (germinal centers, not to be confused with the normally present colloid-filled follicles that constitute the thyroid). Totterman et al. (1977) studied the characteristics of the lymphocytes in the thyroid and reported that they are made up of equal proportions of T- and B-cells.

Most infiltrating T-cells have α/β T-cell receptors. Gamma/delta T-cells are rare (Paolieri et al., 1995) although their proportion in intra-thyroidal lymphocytes is higher than that in peripheral lymphocytes (Iwatani et. al, 1993). CD4+/CD8+ cells and CD3lo-TCRα/β-lo/CD4-CD8- cells also are present in the infiltrate in the thyroid (Iwatani et al., 1993). Infiltrating T-cells are considered to be a highly restricted population, based on the study of T-cell receptor Vα- (Davies et al., 1991) and β- (Davies et al., 1993) gene expression. Heuer et al. (1996) studied cytokine mRNA expression in intra-

Figure 3. Electron microscopy image of thyroid tissue of a patient with Hashimoto's autoimmune thyroiditis showing anti-body deposited basement membrane (white arrow)

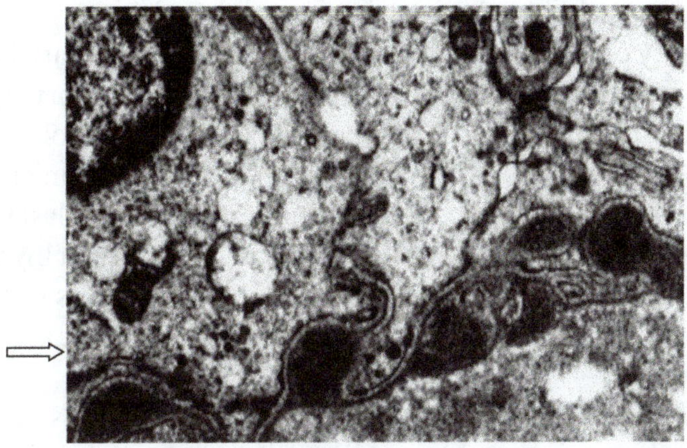

Figure 4. Microscopic picture of Hashimoto's thyroiditis. The dominant feature is a profuse mononuclear lymphocytic infiltrate (arrow) accompanied by actual follicles and germinal centers (Hematoxylin-eosin stain)

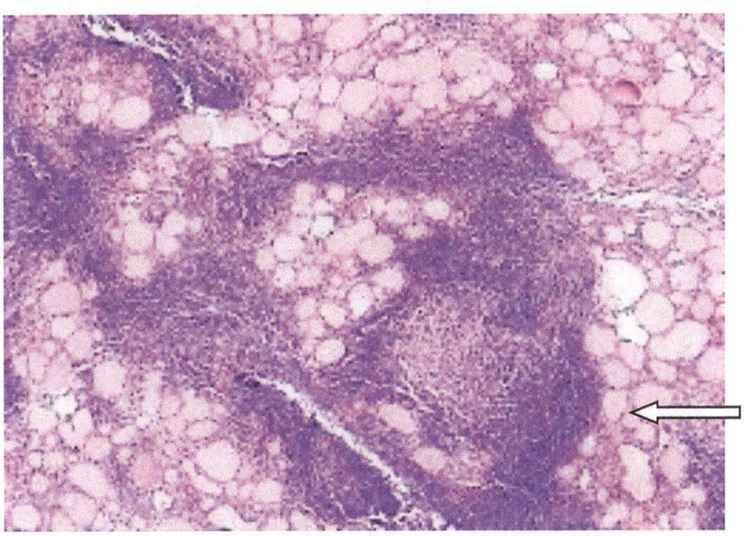

thyroidal T-cells and reported increased expression of IFN-gamma, IL-2 and CD25 cytokines in Hashimoto's thyroiditis.

Thyroglobulin-binding lymphocytes were increased in a percentage relative to their occurrence in blood.

The quantity of parenchymal tissue left in the thyroid is variable. In some instances it is actually increased, perhaps as a compensatory hyperplastic response to inefficient iodide metabolism. Typically, the pathological process involves the entire lobe or gland. *Focal thyroiditis*, which is microscopically similar, may be found in thyroid glands with diffuse hyperplasia of *Graves' disease*, in association with thyroid tumors, or in multinodular thyroid glands.

The thymus, which is frequently enlarged in thyroiditis as it is in Graves' disease, does not present the picture of enhanced immunologic activity (Gunn, 1964; Michie, 1967).

The histological feature in *painless (or silent) thyroiditis* is almost similar to that of Hashimoto's thyroiditis. All specimens show chronic thyroiditis, focal or diffuse type, and lymphoid follicles were present in about half of the specimen (Mizukami et al., 1988).

The follicular disruption is characteristic and a common histological feature at the time of destructive thyrotoxicosis but disappears during the late recovery phase of disease. Thus, painless thyroiditis may be induced by the activation of autoimmune reaction within the thyroid gland in patients with Hashimoto's thyroiditis. As seen in Table 1, Bhatia et al. (2007) graded Hashimoto's thyroiditis based on lymphocytic infiltration seen on cytology, into Grades 0-III, where "Grade 0" means no lymphoid cells, Grade I is mild (Figure 5), Grade II moderate (Figure 6) and Grade III severe lymphoid cell infiltration (Figure 7).

Figure 5. Grade I thyroiditis with mild lymphocytic inflammatory infiltrate (arrows) (May Grünwald Giemsa)

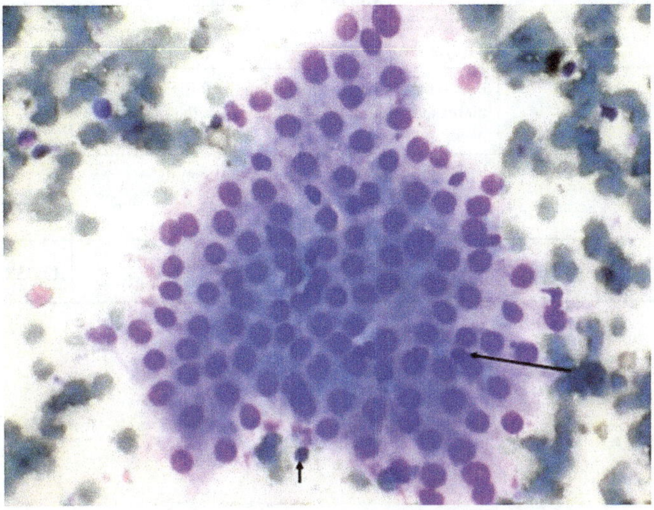

Figure 6. Grade II thyroiditis with moderate lympho-cytic inflammation (May Grünwald

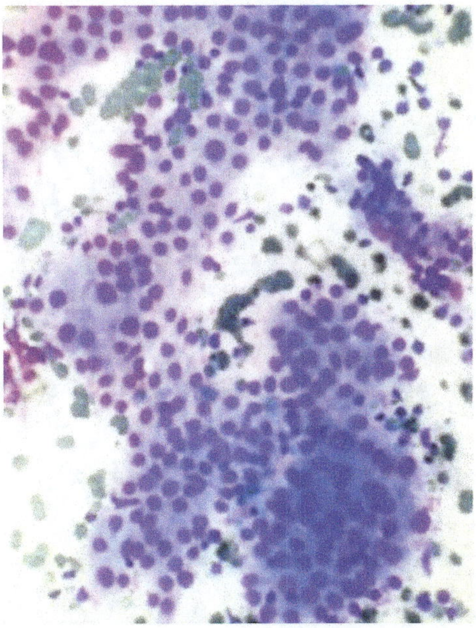

Table 1. Grading of thyroiditis on cytological material

Grade	Morphological Features	% in Study of Bhatia et al. (2007)
Grade 0	No lymphoid cells.	0
Grade I (Mild)	Few lymphoid cells infiltrating the follicles/ increased number of lymphocytes in the background.	38.67%
Grade II (Moderate)	Moderate lymphocytic infiltration or mild lymphocytic infiltration with Hurthle cell change/ giant cells/anisonucleosis.	44%
Grade III (Severe)	Florid lymphocytic inflammation with germinal center formation, very few follicular cells left	17.33%

Figure 7. Grade III thyroiditis, marked inflammation, and germinal center formation. Note polymorphic population of lymphoid cells in contrast to lymphoma (May Grünwald Giemsa)

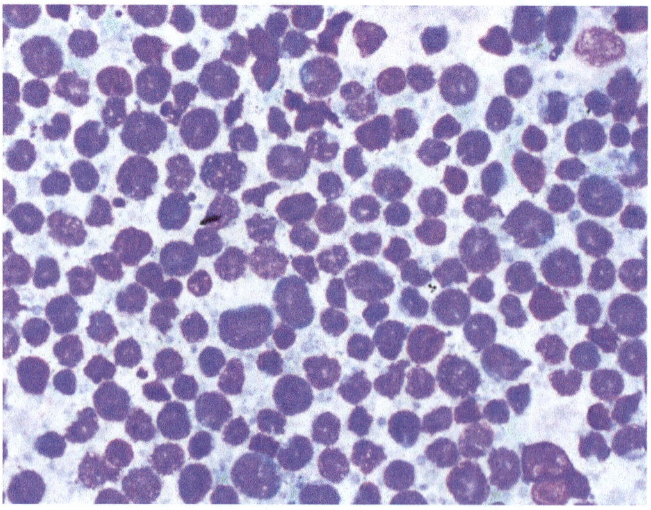

REFERENCES

Bhatia, A., Rajwanshi, A., Dash, R. J., Mittal, B. R., & Saxena, A. K. (2007). Lymphocytic Thyroiditis – is cytological grading significant? a correlation of grades with clinical, biochemical, trasonographic and radionuclide parameters. *CytoJournal*, *4*(1), 10. doi:10.1186/1742-6413-4-10 PMID:17470291

Davies, T. F., Concepcion, E. S., Ben-Nun, A., Graves, P. N., & Tarjan, G. (1993). T-cell receptor V gene use in autoimmune thyroid disease: Direct assessment by thyroid aspiration. *The Journal of Clinical Endocrinology and Metabolism*, *76*, 660–666. PMID:8445022

Davies, T. F., Martin, A., Concepcion, E. S., Graves, P., Cohen, L., & Ben-Nun, A. (1991). Evidence of limited variability of antigen receptors on intra-thyroidal T cells in autoimmune thyroid disease. *The New England Journal of Medicine*, *325*(4), 238–244. doi:10.1056/NEJM199107253250404 PMID:1829139

Gunn, A., Michie, W., & Irvine, W. J. (1964). The thymus in thyroid disease. *Lancet*, *2*(7363), 776–779. doi:10.1016/S0140-6736(64)90558-6 PMID:14187463

Heuer, M., Aust, G., Ode-Hakim, S., & Scherbaum, W. A. (1996). Different cytokine mRNA profiles in Graves' disease, Hashimoto's thyroiditis, and non-autoimmune thyroid disorders determined by quantitative reverse transcriptase polymerase chain reaction (RT-PCR). *Thyroid*, *6*(2), 97–106. doi:10.1089/thy.1996.6.97 PMID:8733879

Iwatani, Y., Hidaka, Y., Matsuzuka, F., Kuma, K., & Amino, N. (1993). Intrathyroidal lymphocyte subsets, including unusual CD4+ CD8+ cells and CD3loTCR alpha beta lo/-CD4-CD8- cells, in autoimmune thyroid disease. *Clinical and Experimental Immunology*, *93*(3), 430–436. doi:10.1111/j.1365-2249.1993.tb08196.x PMID:8370171

Michie, W., Beck, J. S., Mahaffy, R. G., Honein, E. F., & Fowler, G. B. (1967). Quantitative radiological and histological studies of the thymus in thyroid disease. *Lancet*, *1*(7492), 691–694. doi:10.1016/S0140-6736(67)92177-0 PMID:4163941

Mizukami, Y., Michigishi, T., Hashimoto, T., Tonami, N., Hisada, K., Matsubara, F., & Takazakura, E. (1988). Silent thyroiditis: A histologic and immunohistochemical study. *Human Pathology*, *19*(4), 423–431. doi:10.1016/S0046-8177(88)80492-1 PMID:3284807

Paolieri, F., Pronzato, C., Battifora, M., Fiorino, N., Canonica, G. W., & Bagnasco, M. (1995). Infiltrating gamma/delta T-cell receptor-positive lymphocytes in Hashimoto's thyroiditis, Graves' disease and papillary thyroid cancer. *Journal of Endocrinological Investigation*, *18*(4), 295–298. doi:10.1007/BF03347816 PMID:7560812

Totterman, T. H., Maenpaa, J., Gordin, A., Makinen, T., & Andersson, A. C. (1977). Blood and thyroid-infiltrating lymphocyte subclasses in juvenile autoimmune thyroiditis. *Clinical and Experimental Immunology*, *30*, 193–197. PMID:304781

Chapter 4
Iodide Metabolism and Effects

ABSTRACT

Iodine (I2) is essential in the synthesis of thyroid hormones T4 and T3 and functioning of the thyroid gland. Both T3 and T4 are metabolically active, but T3 is four times more potent than T4. Our body contains 20-30 mg of I2, which is mainly stored in the thyroid gland. Iodine is naturally present in some foods, added to others, and available as a dietary supplement. Serum thyroid stimulating hormone (TSH) level is a sensitive marker of thyroid function. Serum TSH is increased in hypothyroidism as in Hashimoto's thyroiditis. In addition to regulation of thyroid function, TSH promotes thyroid growth. If thyroid hormone synthesis is chronically impaired, TSH stimulation eventually may lead to the development of a goiter. This chapter explores the iodide metabolism and effects of Hashimoto's disease.

INTRODUCTION

Thyroid function is controlled by the anterior pituitary gland, which is influenced by the hypothalamus that releases the "thyrotropin releasing hormone" (TRH). The TRH stimulates the pituitary to release the "thyroid-stimulating hormone" (TSH), which causes the thyroid to release the thyroxin (T4) and tri-iodothyronin (T3). If the serum levels of thyroid hormones are high, TSH release is inhibited (*feedback mechanism*). Iodine is essential in the synthesis of thyroid hormones; T4 and T3 and functioning of the thyroid gland. It plays an important role in preventing breast fibrocystic diseases,

DOI: 10.4018/978-1-5225-9655-4.ch004

cognitive impairment, cretinism, hypothyroidism, hyperthyroidism, and multiple miscarriages.

Sources of Iodine (I_2)

Our body contains 20-30 mg of iodine (I_2), which is stored in the thyroid gland. Some amounts of iodine are also found in the lactating mammary glands, salivary glands, stomach lining and blood.

Iodine is is naturally present in some foods, added to others, and available as a dietary supplement. Details will be discussed further in chapter 15.

- *Foods*: Iodine-rich food sources that can help prevent a deficiency include the following: seaweed, cod (a versatile white fish), milk and dairy products, shrimp, Tuna, eggs (mainly egg yolk), dried prunes and plums, and Lima beans (Pennington, 1995; Teas, 2004; Dasgupta, 2008).
- *Iodized salt:* More than 70 countries, including the United States (US) and Canada, have salt iodization programs. As a result, approximately 70% of house-holds worldwide use iodized salt (World Health Organization, 2007). The US Food and Drug Administration (2009) has approved potassium iodide and cuprous iodide for salt iodization, while the World Health Organization (2007) recommends the use of potassium iodate due to its greater stability, particularly in tropical climates.
- *Dietary supplements:* Many multi-vitamin/mineral supplements contain iodine in the forms of potassium iodide or sodium iodide. Dietary supplements of iodine or iodine-containing kelp (a type of seaweed) are also available. A small study found that potassium iodide is almost completely (96.4%) absorbed in humans (Aquaron, Delange, Marchal, Lognoné, & Ninane, 2002).

Biosynthesis, Secretion and Metabolism of Thyroid Hormones (Figure 1)

Dietary inorganic iodide is *absorbed* by the intestine and then *trapped and stored* by the follicular cells of the thyroid gland (*trapping enzyme*) through an active transport system (*iodide pump*) by a transporter (*pendrin*) located on the surface of the follicular cell. In the follicle, iodide is *oxidized* by the enzymes oxidase and thyroid perioxidase (TPO) to form iodine (I_2).

Iodine combines with tyrosine *(iodination of tyrosine)* in the thyroglobulin to form mono-iodotyrosine (MIT) and di-iodotyrosine (DIT) by the organic binding enzyme (*tyrosinase*) (De la Vieja, Dohan, Levy, & Carrasco, 2000). Subsequently, the iodotyrosines are *coupled*, with the formation of T4 and T3. The coupling reaction is also mediated by *peroxidase*. These are stored in the colloid linked to *thyroglobulin* (Tg) (thyroid binding globulin, TBG) and thyroid binding pre-albumin (TBPA).

In response to TSH, a small amount of colloid is engulfed by the epithelial cell and proteolyzed (*protease enzyme*), with release of T3 and T4, which diffuse into the circulation according to body needs. The Tg not undergoing proteolysis also enters the circulation in small quantities. Serum Tg has been used as a tumor marker in differentiated thyroid cancer; it becomes undetectable following thyroidectomy and Iodine-131 (^{131}I) ablation, and its subsequent rise indicates a recurrence. Stimulation of TSH, by promoting colloid endocytosis, increases the amount of thyroglobulin released. Thus, serum thyroglobulin is considered a more reliable tumor marker at high TSH levels (Sarkar & Savitch, 2004).

The most abundant thyroid hormone is thyroxin with a ratio of 10:1 for T4 and T3, respectively. Both T_3 and T_4 are metabolically active, but T_3 is four times more potent than T_4. Most T_3 is produced by extra-thyroidal conversion of T_4 to T_3 (by peripheral non-iodination of T_4 in the liver, kidneys and muscles).

Most of the circulating thyroid hormones are bound to plasma proteins, the free fraction comprising about 0.05% of T4 and 0.2% of T3. Only the free hormone has metabolic effects, and it is a more accurate measure of thyroid function than the total hormone, which varies with plasma proteins levels. The active hormone is T3. About 20-30% of the circulating T3 is secreted by the thyroid gland and the remainder is produced by monodeiodination (MDI) of T4 in extra-thyroid tissues, notably the liver, kidney, brain and pituitary gland.

Synthetic forms of thyroid hormones are commonly used for replacement and/or suppressive therapy, T4 is preferred for this purpose because it has a longer biological half-life (6-7 days) compared with T3 (1-2 days); however, T3 has a more rapid onset of action and may be useful in selected clinical situations (Sarkar, 1996).

Mechanism of Action of TSH (Thyrotropine)

Thyrotopine (TSH) binds to TSH-receptors on the thyroid plasma membrane, which results in ↑ cyclic AMP production via production of adenylate cyclase enzyme that stimulates the thyroid cellular function.

Thyrotropin-releasing hormone (TRH), a tripeptide originating from the hypothalamic median eminence, stimulates the secretion and synthesis of TSH by the anterior pituitary. The TSH comprises an alpha unit, also present in other anterior pituitary hormones (Follicle stimulating hormone and Leutinizimg hormone), and a beta unit responsible for its specific actions. The production and release of TSH are influenced by the concentration of T3 within the pituitary. When the T3 concentration falls below a "set point", TSH secretion increases, and synthesis and release of thyroid hormones are accelerated. Conversely, when the T3 level rises above the set point, TSH release is inhibited. In addition to its pituitary effect, T3 inhibits hypothalamic TRH release. Other mechanisms reported more recently include the inhibitory actions of the released TSH on TRH secretion, and on TSH receptors in the

Figure 1. Physiology of the thyroid gland (biosynthesis, secretion and metabolism) (Hypothalamic-pituitary-thyroid axis)

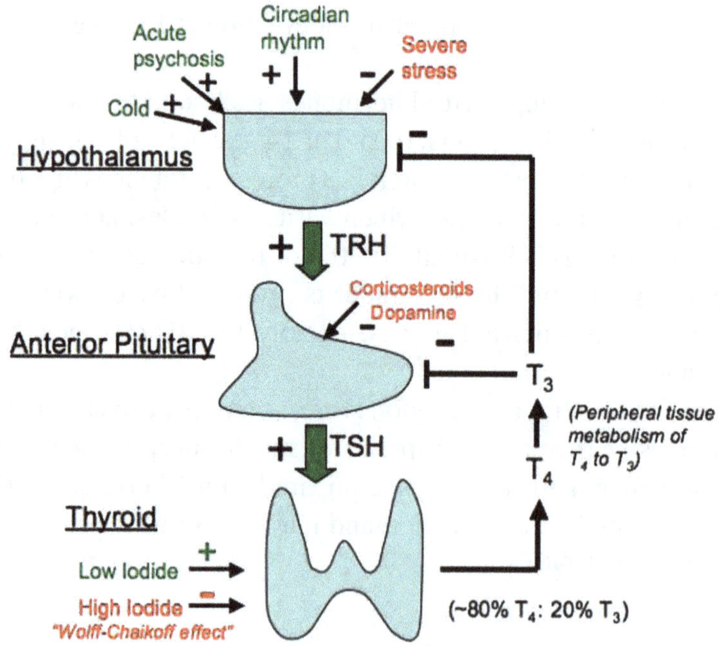

pituitary itself. In conclusion, TSH secretion is influenced by thyroid to pituitary, thyroid to hypothalamus, pituitary to hypothalamus and pituitary to pituitary feedback control mechanisms, which combine to reduce fluctuations in circulating T3 and T4 (Prummel, 2004; Refetoff, 1993).

Serum TSH level is a sensitive marker of thyroid function. Normal serum TSH is approximately 0.45-4.5 μ units/ml and levels upto 20 μU/ml are considered normal in newborns because of the contribution of maternal TSH. During early gestation, TSH tends to be at low normal levels, which coincide with a surge in human chorionic gonadotropin release. Serum TSH is increased in primary hypothyroidism and is decreased in hyperthyroxinemia of all etiologies except for the uncommon entity of thyrotropin induced hyperthyroidism. In the rare condition of partial tissue resistance to thyroid hormone, the pituitary fails to respond to increasing T3 levels, so that TSH continues to be secreted and serum TSH and thyroid hormones are both elevated. Individuals with this condition may become hyperthyroid if tissue resistance is limited to the pituitary or remain euthyroid if resistance is generalized (Refetoff, Weiss, & Usala, 1993).

In addition to regulation of thyroid function, TSH promotes thyroid growth. If thyroid hormone synthesis is chronically impaired, as in I_2 deficiency and autoimmune thyroid disease, chronic TSH stimulation eventually may lead to the development of a goiter.

Effects of Hashimoto's Thyroiditis

Many patients with Hashimoto's thyroiditis do not respond to injected TSH with the expected increase in radio-active iodine uptake (RAIU) or release of thyroxin from the gland (Skillern et al., 1956). It is conceivable that the gland is partially destroyed by the autoimmune attack and is unable to augment iodine metabolism further. Moreover, the thyroid gland of the patient with Hashimoto's disease does not undergo normal organification (Paris, McConahey, Tausie, Woolner, & Bahn, 1961). Administration of 400 mg potassium perchlorate one hour after giving a tracer iodide releases 20%-60% of the glandular radioactivity. In addition, a fraction of the iodinated compounds in the serum of patients with Hashimoto's thyroiditis is not soluble in butanol, as are the thyroid hormones, but is an abnormal peptide-linked iodinated component. This low-weight iodo-protein is probably serum albumin that has been iodinated in the thyroid gland. A similar iodo-protein is also found in several other thyroid diseases, including carcinoma, Graves' disease, and one form of goitrous cretinism. It may be formed as part of the hyperplastic response. Thyroglobulin (Tg) is also detectable in their serum.

Iodide is actively transported from blood to thyrocytes and recently the sodium / iodide symporter (NIS) has been cloned. Antibodies against NIS were found in autoimmune thyroid disease (Endo et al., 1996). This antibody has an inhibitory activity on iodide transport and may modulate the thyroid function in Hashimoto's thyroiditis. More recent studies reported rather low prevalence (<10%) of anti-NIS antibodies in Hashimoto's disease and clinical relevance is still unknown (Chin, 2000; Seissler, 2000).

In experimental animals, iodine depletion prevents the development of autoimmune thyroiditis (Brown, Zhao, Palmer, & Sundick, 1998). Though controversial, it has been suggested that mild iodine deficiency protects against autoimmune thyroid disease at least partly (Laurberg, 1998; Nagata, 1998). In a region where iodine-containing food (such as seaweed) is common, as in Japan, excessive dietary iodine intake (1000 μg/day or more) may cause transient hypothyroidism in patients with subclinical autoimmune thyroiditis. This condition is easily reversible with a reduction in iodine intake (Tajiri, Higashi, Morita, Umeda, & Sato, 1986).

Iodine is important not only for thyroid hormone synthesis but also for induction and modulation of thyroid autoimmunity. In general, iodine deficiency attenuates, while iodine excess accelerates autoimmune thyroiditis in autoimmune-prone individuals (Ruwhof & Drexhage, 2001). In animal experiments, it is revealed that enhanced iodination of Tg facilitates the selective processing and presentation of a cryptic phatogenic peptide in-vivo or in-vitro. Moreover, it is suggested that iodine excess stimulates thymus development and effects function of various immune cells (Dai, Rao, & Carayanniois, 2002).

REFERENCES

Aquaron, R., Delange, F., Marchal, P., Lognoné, V., & Ninane, L. (2002). Bioavailability of seaweed iodine in human beings. *Cellular and Molecular Biology*, *48*(5), 563–569. PMID:12146713

Brown, T. R., Zhao, G., Palmer, K. C., & Sundick, R. S. (1998). Thyroid injury, autoantigen availability, and the initiation of autoimmune thyroiditis. *Autoimmunity*, *27*, 1–12. PMID:9482203

Chin, H. S., Chin, D. K., Morgenthaler, N. G., Vassart, G., & Costagliola, S. (2000). Rarity of anti- Na+/I-symporter (NIS) antibody with iodide uptake inhibiting activity in autoimmune thyroid diseases (AITD). *The Journal of Clinical Endocrinology and Metabolism*, *85*, 3937–3940. PMID:11061560

Dai, Y. D., Rao, V. P., & Carayanniois, G. (2002). Enhanced iodination of thyroglobulin facilitates processing and presentation of a cryptic pathogenic peptide. *Journal of Immunology (Baltimore, Md.: 1950)*, *168*(11), 5907–5911. doi:10.4049/jimmunol.168.11.5907 PMID:12023396

Dasgupta, P. K., Liu, Y., & Dyke, J. V. (2008). Iodine nutrition: Iodine content of iodized salt in the United States. *Environmental Science & Technology*, *42*(4), 1315–1323. doi:10.1021/es0719071 PMID:18351111

De la Vieja, A., Dohan, O., Levy, O., & Carrasco, N. (2000). Molecular analysis of the sodium/iodide symporter: Impact on thyroid and extrathyroid pathophysiology. *Physiological Reviews*, *80*(3), 1083–1105. doi:10.1152/physrev.2000.80.3.1083 PMID:10893432

Endo, T., Kaneshige, M., Nakazato, M., Kohgai, T., Saito, T., & Onaya, T. (1996). Autoantibody against thyroid iodide transporter in the sera from patients with Hashimoto's thyroiditis possesses iodide transport inhibitory activity. *Biochemical and Biophysical Research Communications*, *228*(1), 199–204. doi:10.1006/bbrc.1996.1639 PMID:8912659

Freitas, J., Gross, M. D., & Sarkar, S. D. (2003). Laboratory (in vitro) assessment of thyroid function. In M. P. Sandler & ... (Eds.), *Diagnostic nuclear medicine* (4th ed.; pp. 591–606). Philadelphia, PA: Lippincott Williams and Wilkins.

Laurberg, P., Pedersen, K. M., Hreidarsson, A., Sigfusson, N., Iversen, E., & Knudsen, P. R. (1998). Iodine intake and the pattern of thyroid disorders: A comparative epidemiological study of thyroid abnormalities in the elderly in Iceland and in Jutland, Denmark. *The Journal of Clinical Endocrinology and Metabolism*, *83*(3), 765–769. doi:10.1210/jcem.83.3.4624 PMID:9506723

Nagata, K., Takasu, N., Akamine, H., Ohshiro, C., Komiya, I., Murakami, K., ... Nomura, T. (1998). Urinary iodine and thyroid antibodies in Okinawa, Yamgata, Hyogo, and Nagano, Japan: The differences in iodine intake do not affect thyroid antibody positivity. *Endocrine Journal*, *45*(6), 797–803. doi:10.1507/endocrj.45.797 PMID:10395237

Paris, J., McConahey, W. M., Tausie, W. N., Woolner, L. B., & Bahn, R. C. (1961). The effect of iodides on Hashimoto's thyroiditis. *The Journal of Clinical Endocrinology and Metabolism*, *21*(9), 1037–1042. doi:10.1210/jcem-21-9-1037 PMID:13732794

Pennington, J. T., Schoen, S. A., Salmon, G. D., Young, B., Johnson, R. D., & Marts, R. W. (1995). Composition of Core Foods of the U.S. Food Supply, 1982-1991. III. Copper, Manganese, Selenium, and Iodine. *Journal of Food Composition and Analysis*, *8*(2), 171–217. doi:10.1006/jfca.1995.1014

Prummel, M. F., Brokken, L. S., & Wiersinga, W. M. (2004). Ultra short-loop feedback control of thyrotropin secretion. *Thyroid*, *14*(10), 825–829. doi:10.1089/thy.2004.14.825 PMID:15588378

Refetoff, S., Weiss, R. E., & Usala, S. J. (1993). The syndromes of resistance to thyroid hormone. *Endocrine Reviews*, *14*, 348–399. PMID:8319599

Ruwhof, C., & Drexhage, H. A. (2001). Iodine and thyroid autoimmune disease in animal models. *Thyroid*, *11*(5), 427–436. doi:10.1089/105072501300176381 PMID:11396701

Sarkar, S. D. (1996). Thyroid pathophysiology. In M. P. Sandler, R. E. Coleman, & F. J. Wackers (Eds.), *Diagnostic nuclear medicine* (pp. 899–909). Baltimore, MD: Williams and Wilkins.

Sarkar, S. D., & Savitch, I. (2004). Management of thyroid cancer. *Applied Radiology*, *11*, 34–45.

Seissler, J., Wagner, S., Schott, M., Feldkamp, J., Scherbaum, W. A., & Morgenthaler, N. G. (2000). Low frequency of autoantibodies to the human Na+/I -symporter (NIS) in patients with autoimmune thyroid disease. *The Journal of Clinical Endocrinology and Metabolism*, *85*, 4630–4634. PMID:11134119

Skillern, P. G., Crile, G. Jr, McCullaugh, E. P., Hazard, J. B., Lewis, L. A., & Brown, H. (1956). Struma lymphomatosa: Primary thyroid failure with compensatory thyroid enlargement. *The Journal of Clinical Endocrinology and Metabolism*, *16*(1), 35–39. doi:10.1210/jcem-16-1-35 PMID:13278381

Tajiri, J., Higashi, K., Morita, M., Umeda, T., & Sato, T. (1986). Studies of hypothyroidism in patients with high iodine intake. *The Journal of Clinical Endocrinology and Metabolism*, *63*(2), 412–417. doi:10.1210/jcem-63-2-412 PMID:3722332

Teas, J., Pino, S., Critchley, A., & Braverman, L. E. (2004). Variability of iodine content in common commercially available edible seaweeds. *Thyroid*, *14*(10), 836–841. doi:10.1089/thy.2004.14.836 PMID:15588380

U.S. Food and Drug Administration. (2009). Code of Federal Regulations, CFR 21, Sections 184.1634 and 184.1265. Silver Spring, MD: Food and Drug Administration.

World Health Organization. (2007). *United Nations Children's Fund & International Council for the Control of Iodine Deficiency Disorders. In Assessment of iodine deficiency disorders and monitoring their elimination* (3rd ed.). Geneva, Switzerland: World Health Organization.

Chapter 5
Etiology and Risk Factors

ABSTRACT

The etiology of Hashimoto's thyroiditis (HT) arises from an interaction between genetic and non-genetic factors. The genes implicated vary in different ethnic groups and the incidence is increased in people with chromosomal disorders. HT is usually associated with auto-antibodies against thyroglobulin (Tg) and thyro-perioxidase (TPO) leading to primary hypothyroidism. Having other autoimmune diseases is a risk factor to develop HT. First-degree relatives of persons with HT have greater risk of developing the disease. Female gender is associated with an eight-fold increased risk for HT possibly due to the effects of sex hormones, X-chromosome-encoded susceptibility, skewed X-chromosome inactivation, pregnancy, and fetal micro-chimerism. In genetically susceptible individuals, environmental factors, including high iodine intake, selenium deficiency, infectious diseases, stress, and certain drugs, have been implicated in initiating the autoimmune process. This chapter explores the etiology and risk factors of Hashimoto's disease.

DOI: 10.4018/978-1-5225-9655-4.ch005

INTRODUCTION

The etiology of HT is multifactorial arising from interaction between *genetic* and *non-genetic factors* (environmental, dietary and demographic).

Genetic Factors

The strong genetic component is borne out in studies on *monozygotic twins*, with a concordance of 38-55%, with an even higher concordance of circulating thyroid antibodies not in relation to clinical presentation (up to 80% in monozygotic twins). Neither result was seen to a similar degree in *dizygotic twins*, offering strong favor for high genetic etiology.

The *genetic polymorphisms* of the Human leukocyte antigens (HLA) mainly, HLA-DR3 and HLA-DR5, T-cell immune response genes such as cytotoxic T-lymphocyte-associated antigen-4 (CTLA-4) and protein tyrosine phosphate-22 (PTPN-22), vitamin D receptor (VDR) and thyroid specific genes play a major role in the development of Hashimoto's thyroiditis. Single neucleotide polymorphism at the thyroglobulin promotor site leads to activation of T-cell response, and polymorphism at CD-40 gene leads to proliferation of B-cells, antibody secretion and generation of memory cells. CTLA-4 down-regulates, i.e. transmits an inhibitory signal to T-cells, so reduced functioning is associated with increased T-lymphocyte activity. Both, CTLA-4 and PTPN-22 are major negative regulators of cell-mediated immunity. Thus, depletion of regulatory T-cell (Treg) leads to autoimmunity (Zaletel & Gaberek, 2011).

The genes implicated vary in different ethnic groups and the incidence is increased in people with chromosomal disorders, including Turner, Down, and Klinefelter syndromes usually associated with auto- antibodies against thyroglobulin (Tg) and thyro-perioxidase (TPO). Progressive depletion of these cells as the cytotoxic immune response leads to higher degrees of primary hypothyroidism, presenting with low thyroxine (T4) and triiodothyronine (T3), and compensatory elevations of TSH.

The initiating process in Hashimoto thyroiditis is not well understood (Hadj-Kacem, 2009; Duntas, 2008; tomer, 2009; Jorgesen, 2010). The thyroid gland is typically *goitrous* but may be *atrophic* or *normal* in size. Antibodies binding to and blocking the thyroid-stimulating hormone (TSH) receptor, thyrotropin receptor blocking antibodies (TBII) have also been described and may contribute to impairment in thyroid function. The result is inadequate thyroid hormone production and secretion, although initially, preformed T4 and T3 may "leak" into the circulation from damaged cells.

Patients with Hashimoto thyroiditis have *antibodies* to various thyroid antigens, most frequently anti-thyroid peroxidase (anti-TPO), anti-thyroglobulin (anti-Tg), and to a lesser extent, TSH receptor-blocking antibodies (TBII). Nevertheless, a small percentage (approximately 10%-15%) of patients with Hashimoto thyroiditis may be serum antibody negative. Other antithyroid antibodies found in autoimmune thyroid disease (AITD) (including Hashimoto thyroiditis) include thyroid-stimulating antibody and cytotoxic antibody.

Having *other autoimmune diseases* is a risk factor to develop Hashimoto's thyroiditis, and the opposite is also true. Hashimoto thyroiditis has a markedly higher clustering of other autoimmune diseases, including pernicious anemia, adrenal insufficiency, celiac disease, and type 1-diabetes mellitus, vitiligo, and alopecia (Wiebolt, 2011; Vestgaard, 2008). A study by Ruggeri et al indicated that Hashimoto's thyroiditis is associated with different non-thyroidal autoimmune diseases (NTADs) at different ages. Associated NTADs were significantly more prevalent in adults than children/adolescents in that study, and more adults than children/adolescents suffered from two or more associated NTADs, with the frequency of arthropathies and connective tissue diseases being greater in adults and the frequency of type 1 diabetes mellitus and celiac disease being higher in children/adolescents (Ruggeri et al., 2017).

- *Family History:* A study by Bothra et al reported that, compared with the general population, *first-degree relatives* of persons with Hashimoto's thyroiditis have a nine-fold greater risk of developing the disease (Bothra et al., 2017).
- *Patient Gender: Female gender* is associated with an 8-fold increased risk for Hashimoto's thyroiditis than male gender; the possible mechanisms being the effects of sex hormones, X-chromosome-encoded susceptibility, skewed X-chromosome inactivation, pregnancy, and fetal micro-chimerism.

Thus, a possible explanation for the high female predominance in AITD might be associated with the *X chromosome* containing a number of sex and immune-related genes, which are important for preservation of immune tolerance (McCombe, Greer, & Mackay, 2009). Thus, increased immuno-reactivity might be related to genetic defects of the X chromosome, such as structural abnormalities or monosomy. Accordingly, a higher incidence of AITD was reported in patients with a higher rate of X chromosome monosomy in peripheral white blood cells (Invernizzi et al., 2005) or in patients with Turner's syndrome (Larizza, Calcaterra, & Martinetti, 2009).

Another potential mechanism of impaired immuno-tolerance in females is *skewed X-chromosome inactivation* (XCI) leading to the escape of X-linked self-antigens from presentation in thymus with subsequent loss of T-cell tolerance. Skewed XCI was associated with a higher risk of developing AITD. Recently reported frequencies of skewed XCI in Hashimoto's thyroiditis were 31%, 34.3%, 25.6% and 20%, respectively, which is significantly higher than in healthy controls, where the prevalences were only 8%, 8%, 8.6% and 11.2%, respectively (Brix,2005; Ozxelik, 2006; Yin, 2007; Chabchoub, 2009). Furthermore, a study of Danish twins demonstrated a significant association of skewed XCI with TPO-Ab serum concentrations in dizygotic but not in monozygotic twin pairs, indicating that shared genetic determinants of XCI pattern and TPO-Ab production are more likely than causal relationship (Brix, Hansen, Kyvik, & Hegedüs, 2010).

The tolerance of the fetal semi-allograft during *pregnancy* is enabled by the state of immunosuppression which result from hormonal changes and trophoblast expression of key immuno-modulatory molecules. The pivotal players in regulation of the immune response are the regulatory T-cells (Tregs), which rapidly increase during pregnancy. Consequently, both cell-mediated and humoral immune responses are attenuated with a shift towards humoral immune response, resulting in immune tolerance of the conceptus tissues and suppression of autoimmunity (Gwerin, 2009; Weetman, 2010). Accordingly, the decrease of both TPO-Ab and Tg-Ab concentrations during pregnancy has been reported, reaching the lowest values in the third trimester (Kampe, 1990, Kuijpens, 1998; Smyth, 2005; Lazarus, 2011).

In the *post-partum period*, the rapid decrease of Tregs and re-establishment of the immune response to the pre-pregnancy state may cause or aggravate thyroid autoimmunity (Weetman, 2010). The increase of TPO-Ab concentrations occurred as soon as 6 weeks after delivery (Smyth et al., 2005), reaching the baseline level at approximately 12 weeks and the maximum level at about 20 weeks after delivery (Kampe, 1990; Kuijpens, 1998). In up to 50% of women with positive TPO-Abs in early pregnancy, thyroid autoimmunity, in the form of postpartum thyroiditis may occur within the first year after delivery, usually presenting clinically with transient thyrotoxicosis and/or transient hypothyroidism. In about one-third of women permanent hypothyroidism may even develop (Lazarus, 2011). Interestingly, a significantly higher secretion of IFN-γ and IL-4 together with a lower median plasma cortisol concentration in 36th week of gestation has been reported in women with postpartum thyroiditis than in euthyroid females, indicating that weaker immunosupression in the former group of women in late pregnancy could contribute to the postpartum thyroid dysfunction (Kokandi, Parkes, Premawardhana, John, & Lazarus, 2003).

Fetal micro-chimerism is defined by the "presence of fetal cells in maternal tissues being transferred in the maternal circulation during pregnancy". Several years after the delivery, the chimeric male cells can be detected in the maternal peripheral blood (Bianchi, 1996; Evans, 1999) and in maternal tissues, such as thyroid, lung, skin, or lymph nodes (Koopmans et al., 2008). The fetal immune cells, settled in the maternal thyroid gland, may become activated in the post-partum period when the immuno-tolerance ceases, representing a possible trigger that may initiate or exaggerate AITD. In Hashimoto's thyroiditis, fetal micro-chimeric cells were detected in the thyroid gland in 28% to 83%,(Srivtsa, 2001; Klintschar, 2001; Renne, 2004; Klintschar, 2006), which is significantly higher than that reported in the absence of AITD. Furthermore, a recent study of twins supported the putative role of micro-chimerism in triggering thyroid autoimmunity, showing a significantly higher prevalence of T-Abs in opposite sex twins compared to monozygotic twins (Brix, Hansen, Kyvik, & Hegedüs, 2009). In addition, euthyroid women with previous pregnancy presented significantly more often with positive TPO-Ab as compared to women with no history of pregnancy (Strieder, Prummel, Tijssen, Endert, & Wiersinga, 2003). However, the relation between parity and AITD was not confirmed by large population-based studies, advocating against the essential contribution of fetal micro-chimerism to the pathogenesis of AITD including Hashimoto's thyroiditis (Walsh, 2005; Bulow, 2006; Friedrich, 2008; Sgerbi, 2010).

Non-Genetic (Environmental) Factors

In genetically-susceptible individuals, preventable environmental factors, including high iodine intake, selenium deficiency, infectious diseases and certain drugs, have been implicated in the development of autoimmune thyroid disease (may initiate the autoimmune process). These factors may act through epigenetic modifications, like DNA methylation and histone modification at the tissue level, which is evidenced by twin studies.

Iodine-Intake

The association between *iodine-intake* and Hashimoto's thyroiditis has been extensively studied. More than adequate intake of I_2 induces autoimmunity by various mechanisms including a) increasing the immunogenicity of thyroglobulin (Tg) molecules exposing cryptic epitopes that facilitate presentation by antigen presenting cell (APC) and subsequent T-cell activation, b) release of free radicals, which induce elevated expression of intra-cellular adhesion molecule-1 that attracts immuno-competent cells, c) free radicals damaging thyrocytes and exposing auto-antigens, d) promoting follicular cell apoptosis by abnormal expression of tumor necrosis factor-related apoptosis-inducing ligand (TRAIL) and its death receptor e) increased maturation of APC, B-cells and T-cells. A country wide screening program done by All India Institute of Medical Science (AIIMS), Delhi revealed that there is increased incidence of *juvenile autoimmune thyroiditis* including Hashimoto's thyroiditis among the goitrous young girls in post-iodinization phase in India (Strieder, Prummel, Tijssen, Endert, & Wiersinga, (2003).

Selenium Deficiency

There is some evidence supporting the role of selenium deficiency in development of thyroid autoimmunity. *Selenium deficiency* decreases the activity of seleno-proteins leading to raised concentrations of hydrogen peroxide, thus promoting inflammation and disease (Brown & Arthur, 2001).

Vitamin D Deficiency

Recently, Mazokopakis et al., (2015) reported that *Vitamin D deficiency* has has an association with the development of Hashimoto thyroiditis. The study, which included 218 patients with Hashimoto thyroiditis, found serum 25-hydroxy vitamin D levels to be negatively correlated with anti-TPO levels in all patients, with the anti-TPO levels being significantly greater in the 186 patients who were vitamin D deficient. After receiving oral vitamin D3 supplementation of 1200-4000 IU daily for 4 months, serum anti-TPO levels in the vitamin D-deficient patients were significantly reduced.

Drugs, Infections and Chemicals

Drugs such as Interferon-alpha (INF-α), lithium, amiodarone, *infections* due to hepatitis C, Rubella, Herpes simplex virus, Epistein-Bell virus, Human T-cell lympho-trophic viruses, and exposure to *chemicals* such as poly-aromatic hydrocarbons, poly-halogenated biphenyls as well as heavy metals like mercury and lead, which can be found in body care products, amalgam fillings, as well as some water and food supplies can also trigger autoimmune thyroid disease. There is evidence that mercury, in particular, accumulates in the thyroid gland and is one cause of autoimmune thyroid response (Blum, 2013). Drugs will be discussed further in details in chapter 6.

Lipid Profile

Levels of TSH positively correlate with serum levels of total cholesterol, triglycerides, low-density lipoprotein (LDL), high-density lipoprotein (HDL), and non-HDL, as well as with the ratio of LDL to HDL. Free T4 levels, on the other hand, are negatively correlated with these lipid parameters (Blum, 2013).

Demographic Factors

Age: The risk of Hashimoto's thyroiditis and development of hypothyroidism are known to increase with age of the patient. In a study of 830 patients with Hashimoto thyroiditis, Tagami et al., (2010) reported a slight, but significant increase in TSH serum levels and decrease in free T4 levels with increasing patient age.

Gender: Women are associated with an 8-fold increased risk for Hashimoto's thyroiditis than men. Several putative mechanisms have been proposed including the effects of sex hormones, X-chromosome-encoded susceptibility, skewed X-chromosome inactivation, pregnancy, as well as fetal micro-chimerism as mentioned before.

The overall increased occurrence of autoimmune disease among women is believed by some authors to be influenced by the fluctuations in hormones that women experience. Alterations in the immune system can profoundly affect a woman's hormone balance. Autoimmunity is characterized by inflammation, which can affect the hormonal systems including the thyroid and female sex hormones and affecting also the balance between estrogen and progesterone. There is also some new evidence to suggest that autoimmunity can even disrupt the male hormones in a woman's body, resulting in premature menopause. In polycystic ovarian syndrome (PCOS), the most common hormonal disorder in women, there is a higher than normal rate of autoimmune processes. Menopause makes the symptoms of Hashimoto's worse and vice versa. Sometimes, it is during menopause when a woman initially discovers that she also has autoimmune thyroid disease. Remission of Hashimoto's thyroiditis, with disappearance of goiter, hypothyroidism, and serum thyroid auto-antibodies, has been reported during pregnancy, with relapse after delivery (Amino et al., 1976). Antibody levels usually fall during pregnancy (Amino et al., 1978). These phenomena may reflect the immunosuppressive effects of pregnancy. After delivery thyroid auto-antibody levels rise, and after 2-6 months there may be sudden development of goiter and hypothyroidism (Amino et al., 1977).

Stress

Stress, physical or emotional, is a known risk factor of auto-immunity. Stress makes it harder for the body to heal itself and perform the necessary immune functions. Stressful situations cause changes in the adrenal system resulting in release of hormones stimulated by the pituitary gland; cortisol, aldosterone, and dehydro-epiandrosterone. In the event of adrenal fatigue, the pituitary gland could perhaps not be functioning properly. With the thyroid being a part of the endocrine system, understanding the link between various hormones is important to understand autoimmune thyroid disease.

REFERENCES

Amino, N., Kuro, R., Tanizawa, O., Tanaka, F., Hayashi, C., Kotani, K., ... Kumahar.a, Y. (1978). Changes. of serum antithyroid antibodies during and after pregnancy in autoimmune thyroid diseases. *Clinical and Experimental Immunology*, *31*, 30–35. PMID:639347

Amino, N., Miyai, K., Kuro, R., Tanizawa, O., Azukizawa, M., Takai, S., & Kumahara, Y. (1977). Transient postpartum hypothyroidism. Fourteen cases with autoimmune thyroiditis. *Annals of Internal Medicine*, *87*(2), 155–159. doi:10.7326/0003-4819-87-2-155 PMID:889196

Amino, N., Miyai, K., Onishi, T., Hashimoto, T., Arai, K., Ishibashi, K., & Kumahara, Y. (1976). Transient hypothyroidism after delivery in autoimmune thyroiditis. *The Journal of Clinical Endocrinology and Metabolism*, *42*(2), 296–301. doi:10.1210/jcem-42-2-296 PMID:946603

Bianchi, D. W., Zickwolf, G. K., Weil, G. J., Sylvester, S., & DeMaria, M. A. (1996). Male fetal progenitor cells persist in maternal blood for as long as 27 years postpartum. *Proceedings of the National Academy of Sciences of the United States of America*, *93*(2), 705–708. doi:10.1073/pnas.93.2.705 PMID:8570620

Blum, S. (2013). *The Immune System Recovery Plan*. New York: Scribner.

Bothra, N., Shah, N., Goroshi, M., Jadhav, S., Padalkar, S., Thakkar, H., ... Bandgar, T. (2017). Hashimo.to's thyroiditis: Relative recurrence risk ratio and implications for screening of first degree relatives. *Horumon To Rinsho*, *87*(2), 201–206. doi:10.1111/cen.13323 PMID:28273382

Brix, T. H., Hansen, P. S., Kyvik, K. O., & Hegedüs, L. (2009). Aggregation of thyroid autoantibodies in twins from opposite-sex pairs suggests that microchimerism may play a role in the early stages of thyroid autoimmunity. *The Journal of Clinical Endocrinology and Metabolism*, *94*(11), 4439–4443. doi:10.1210/jc.2009-0813 PMID:19808849

Brix, T. H., Hansen, P. S., Kyvik, K. O., & Hegedüs, L. (2010). Preliminary evidence of a noncausal association between the X-chromosome inactivation pattern and thyroid autoimmunity: A twin study. *European Journal of Human Genetics*, *18*(2), 54–257. doi:10.1038/ejhg.2009.156 PMID:19789576

Brix, T. H., Knudsen, G. P., Kristiansen, M., Kyvik, K. O., Orstavik, K. H., & Hegedüs, L. (2005). High frequency of skewed X-chromosome inactivation in females with autoimmune thyroid disease: A possible explanation for the female predisposition to thyroid auto-immunity. *The Journal of Clinical Endocrinology and Metabolism*, *90*(11), 5949–5953. doi:10.1210/jc.2005-1366 PMID:16105963

Brown, K. M., & Arthur, J. R. (2001). Selenium, selenoproteins and human health: A review. *Public Health Nutrition*, *4*(2b), 593–599. doi:10.1079/PHN2001143 PMID:11683552

Bülow, P. I., Laurberg, P., Knudsen, N., Jørgensen, T., Perrild, H., Ovesen, L., & Rasmussen, L. B. (2006). Lack of association between thyroid autoantibodies and parity in a population study argues against microchimerism as a trigger of thyroid autoimmunity. *European Journal of Endocrinology*, *154*(1), 39–45. doi:10.1530/eje.1.02070 PMID:16381989

Chabchoub, G., Uz, E., Maalej, A., Mustafa, C. A., Rebai, A., Mnif, M., ... Ayadi, H. (2009). Analysis of skewed X-chromosome inactivation in females with rheumatoid arthritis and autoimmune thyroid diseases. *Arthritis Research & Therapy*, *11*(4), R106. doi:10.1186/ar2759 PMID:19589151

Duntas, L. H. (2008). Environmental factors and autoimmune thyroiditis. *Nature Clinical Practice. Endocrinology & Metabolism*, *4*(8), 454–460. doi:10.1038/ncpendmet0896 PMID:18607401

Evans, P. C., Lambert, N., Maloney, S., Furst, D. E., Moore, J. M., & Nelson, J. L. (1999). Long-term fetal microchimerism in peripheral blood mononuclear cell subsets in healthy women and women with scleroderma. *Blood*, *93*(6), 2033–2037. doi:10.1182/blood.V93.6.2033.406k18_2033_2037 PMID:10068676

Friedrich, N., Schwarz, S., Thonack, J., John, U., Wallaschofski, H., & Völzke, H. (2008). Association between parity and autoimmune thyroiditis in a general female population. *Autoimmunity*, *41*(2), 174–180. doi:10.1080/08916930701777629 PMID:18324487

Guerin, L. R., Prins, J. R., & Robertson, S. A. (2009). Regulatory T-cells and immune tolerance in pregnancy: A new target for infertility treatment? *Human Reproduction Update*, *15*(5), 517–535. doi:10.1093/humupd/dmp004 PMID:19279047

Hadj-Kacem, H., Rebuffat, S., Mnif-Feki, M., Belguith-Maalej, S., Ayadi, H., & Péraldi-Roux, S. (2009). Autoimmune thyroid diseases: Genetic susceptibility of thyroid-specific genes and thyroid autoantigens contributions. *International Journal of Immunogenetics*, *36*(2), 85–96. doi:10.1111/j.1744-313X.2009.00830.x PMID:19284442

Invernizzi, P., Miozzo, M., Selmi, C., Persani, L., Battezzati, P. M., Zuin, M., ... Podda, M. (2005). X chrom.osome monosomy: A common mechanism for autoimmune diseases. *Journal of Immunology (Baltimore, Md.: 1950)*, *175*(1), 575–578. doi:10.4049/jimmunol.175.1.575 PMID:15972694

Jørgensen, K. T., Rostgaard, K., Bache, I., Biggar, R. J., Nielsen, N. M., Tommerup, N., & Frisch, M. (2010). Autoimmune diseases in women with Turner's syndrome. *Arthritis & Rheumatology (Hoboken, N.J.)*, *62*(3), 658–666. doi:10.1002/art.27270 PMID:20187158

Kämpe, O., Jansson, R., & Karlsson, F. A. (1990). Effects of L-thyroxine and iodide on the development of autoimmune postpartum thyroiditis. *The Journal of Clinical Endocrinology and Metabolism*, *70*(4), 1014–1018. doi:10.1210/jcem-70-4-1014 PMID:2318931

Klintschar, M., Immel, U. D., Kehlen, A., Schwaiger, P., Mustafa, T., Mannweiler, S., ... Hoang-Vu, C. (2006). Fetal microchimerism in Hashimoto's thyroiditis: A quantitative approach. *European Journal of Endocrinology*, *154*(2), 237–241. doi:10.1530/eje.1.02080 PMID:16452536

Klintschar, M., Schwaiger, P., Mannweiler, S., Regauer, S., & Kleiber, M. (2001). Evidence of fetal microchimerism in Hashimoto's thyroiditis. *The Journal of Clinical Endocrinology and Metabolism*, *86*, 2494–2498. PMID:11397845

Kokandi, A. A., Parkes, A. B., Premawardhana, L. D., John, R., & Lazarus, J. H. (2003). Association of postpartum thyroid dysfunction with antepartum hormonal and immunological changes. *The Journal of Clinical Endocrinology and Metabolism*, *88*(3), 1126–1132. doi:10.1210/jc.2002-021219 PMID:12629095

Koopmans, M., Kremer, I. C., Baelde, H. J., Harvey, M. S., de Heer, E., Bruijn, J. A., & Bajema, I. M. (2008). Chimerism occurs in thyroid, lung, skin and lymph nodes of women with sons. *Journal of Reproductive Immunology*, *78*(1), 68–75. doi:10.1016/j.jri.2008.01.002 PMID:18329105

Kuijpens, J. L., Pop, V. J., Vader, H. L., Drexhage, H. A., & Wiersinga, W. M. (1998). Prediction of post partum thyroid dysfunction: Can it be improved? *European Journal of Endocrinology*, *139*, 36–43. doi:10.1530/eje.0.1390036 PMID:9703376

Larizza, D., Calcaterra, V., & Martinetti, M. (2009). Increased prevalence of autoimmunity in Turner syndrome--influence of age. *Journal of Autoimmunity*, *33*, 25–30. doi:10.1016/j.jaut.2009.03.002 PMID:19349146

Lazarus, J. H. (2011). The continuing saga of postpartum thyroiditis. *The Journal of Clinical Endocrinology and Metabolism*, *96*(3), 614–616. doi:10.1210/jc.2011-0091 PMID:21378224

Marwaha, R. K., Tandon, N., Karak, A. K., Gupta, N., Verma, K., & Kochupillai, N. (2000). *Hashimoto's Thyroiditis: Countrywide Screening of Goitrous Healthy Young Girls in Post-iodization Phase in India*. New Delhi, India: All India Institute of Medical Sciences.

Mazokopakis, E. E., Papadomanolaki, M. G., Tsekouras, K. C., Evangelopoulos, A. D., Kotsiris, D. A., & Tzortzinis, A. A. (2015). Is vitamin D related to pathogenesis and treatment of Hashimoto's thyroiditis? *Hellenic Journal of Nuclear Medicine*, *18*(3), 222–227. PMID:26637501

McCombe, P. A., Greer, J. M., & Mackay, I. R. (2009). Sexual dimorphism in autoimmune disease. *Current Molecular Medicine*, *9*(9), 1058–1079. doi:10.2174/156652409789839116 PMID:19747114

Ozcelik, T., Uz, E., Akyerli, C. B., Bagislar, S., Mustafa, C. A., Gursoy, A., ... Gullu, S. (2006). Evidence from autoimmune thyroiditis of skewed X-chromosome inactivation in female predisposition to autoimmunity. *European Journal of Human Genetics*, *14*(6), 791–797. doi:10.1038j.ejhg.5201614 PMID:16596118

Renne, C., Ramos-Lopez, E., Steimle-Grauer, S. A., Ziolkowski, P., Pani, M. A., Luther, C., ... Badenhoop, K. (2004). Thyroid fetal male microchimerisms in mothers with thyroid disorders: Presence of Y-chromosomal immunofluorescence in thyroid-infiltrating lymphocytes is more prevalent in Hashimoto's thyroiditis and Graves' disease than in follicular adenomas. *The Journal of Clinical Endocrinology and Metabolism*, *89*(11), 5810–5814. doi:10.1210/jc.2004-1049 PMID:15531546

Ruggeri, R. M., Trimarchi, F., Giuffrida, G., Certo, R., Cama, F., Campini, A., ... Wasniews.ka, M. (2017). Autoimm.une co-morbidities in Hashimoto's thyroiditis: Different patterns of association in adulthood and childhood/adolescence E*uropea.n. The Journal of Endocrinology*, *176*(2), 133–141. PMID:27913607

Sgarbi, J. A., Kasamatsu, T. S., Matsumura, L. K., & Maciel, R. M. (2010). Parity is not related to autoimmune thyroid disease in a population-based study of Japanese-Brazilians. *Thyroid*, *20*(10), 1151–1156. doi:10.1089/thy.2009.0424 PMID:20883173

Smyth, P. P., Wijeyaratne, C. N., Kaluarachi, W. N., Smith, D. F., Premawardhana, L. D., Parkes, A. B., ... Lazarus, J. H. (2005). Sequential studies on thyroid antibodies during pregnancy. *Thyroid*, *15*(5), 474–477. doi:10.1089/thy.2005.15.474 PMID:15929669

Srivatsa, B., Srivatsa, S., Johnson, K. L., Samura, O., Lee, S. L., & Bianchi, D. W. (2001). Microchimerism of presumed fetal origin in thyroid specimens from women: A case-control study. *Lancet*, *358*(9298), 2034–2038. doi:10.1016/S0140-6736(01)07099-4 PMID:11755610

Strieder, T. G., Prummel, M. F., Tijssen, J. G., Endert, E., & Wiersinga, W. M. (2003). Risk factors for and prevalence of thyroid disorders in a cross-sectional study among healthy female relatives of patients with autoimmune thyroid disease. *Horumon To Rinsho*, *59*(3), 396–401. doi:10.1046/j.1365-2265.2003.01862.x PMID:12919165

Tagami, T., Tamanaha, T., Shimazu, S., Honda, K., Nanba, K., Nomura, H., ... Naruse, M. (2010). Lipid Profiles in the Untreated Patients with Hashimoto Thyroiditis and the Effects of Thyroxine Treatment on Subclinical Hypothyroidism with Hashimoto Thyroiditis. *Endocrine Journal*, *57*(3), 253–258. doi:10.1507/endocrj.K09E-315 PMID:20032565

Tomer, Y., & Huber, A. (2009). The etiology of autoimmune thyroid disease: A story of genes and environment. *Journal of Autoimmunity*, *32*(3-4), 231–239. doi:10.1016/j.jaut.2009.02.007 PMID:19307103

Vestgaard, M., Nielsen, L. R., Rasmussen, A. K., Damm, P., & Mathiesen, E. R. (2008). Thyroid peroxidase antibodies in pregnant women with type 1 diabetes: Impact on thyroid function, metabolic control and pregnancy outcome. *Acta Obstetricia et Gynecologica Scandinavica*, *87*(12), 1336–1342. doi:10.1080/00016340802499261 PMID:18972269

Walsh, J. P., Bremner, A. P., Bulsara, M. K., O'Leary, P., Leedman, P. J., Feddema, P., & Michelangeli, V. (2005). Parity and the risk of autoimmune thyroid disease: A community-based study. *The Journal of Clinical Endocrinology and Metabolism*, *90*(9), 5309–5312. doi:10.1210/jc.2005-0771 PMID:15956077

Weetman, A. P. (2010). Immunity, thyroid function and pregnancy: Molecular mechanisms. *Nature Reviews. Endocrinology*, *6*(6), 311–318. doi:10.1038/nrendo.2010.46 PMID:20421883

Wiebolt, J., Achterbergh, R., den Boer, A., van der Leij, S., Marsch, E., Suelmann, B., ... van Haeften, T. W. (2011). Clustering of additional autoimmunity behaves differently in Hashimoto's patients compared with Graves' patients. *European Journal of Endocrinology*, *164*(5), 789–794. doi:10.1530/EJE-10-1172 PMID:21378091

Yin, X., Latif, R., Tomer, Y., & Davies, T. F. (2007). Thyroid epigenetics: X chromosome inactivation in patients with autoimmune thyroid disease. *Annals of the New York Academy of Sciences*, *1110*(1), 193–200. doi:10.1196/annals.1423.021 PMID:17911434

Zaletel, K., & Gaberek, S. (2011). Hashimoto's Thyroiditis: From Genes to the Disease. *Current Genomics*, *12*(8), 576–588. doi:10.2174/138920211798120763 PMID:22654557

Chapter 6
Pathogenesis

ABSTRACT

Hashimoto's thyroiditis (HT) is one of the most prevalent autoimmune diseases provoked in genetically susceptible individuals by several triggers. Immune-regulatory genes such as HLA, CTLA-4, and PTPN22 play a major role in the pathogenesis of autoimmune thyroiditis. The thyroid-specific gene currently showing the association with HT (and also Graves' disease) is the gene for thyroglobulin (Tg). The VDR gene is another HT predisposing gene, common for other organ-specific autoimmune diseases such as type-I diabetes or Addison's disease. Furthermore, cytokine genes such as IFN-γ, IL-4, or TGF-β indicate the association with the development and severity of HT. A complex interaction between genetic and non-genetic factors results in enhanced thyroid antigen presentation and reduced immune tolerance leading to predominantly Th1-type autoimmunity, thyroid destruction, and clinical disease. The exact mechanisms of initiation and progression of HT are yet to be clarified. This chapter explores the pathogenesis of Hashimoto's disease.

INTRODUCTION

Hashimoto's thyroiditis is the most prevalent autoimmune thyroid disorder, where lymphocytic infiltration of the thyroid gland may be followed by a gradual destruction and fibrous replacement of the thyroid parenchymal tissue. The thyroid gland may or may not be enlarged. There are multiple suggested mechanisms, though not fully understood, by which the pathology of Hashimoto's thyroiditis develops.

DOI: 10.4018/978-1-5225-9655-4.ch006

Various *auto-antibodies* may be present against thyroid peroxidase (TPO), thyroglobulin (Tg) and thyroid stimulating hormone (TSH) receptors, although a small percentage of people may have none of these antibodies present. At the same time, as indicated in various twin studies, a percentage of the population may also have these antibodies without developing Hashimoto's thyroiditis. Nevertheless, *antibody-dependent cell-mediated cytotoxicity* is a substantial factor behind the apoptotic fall-out of Hashimoto's thyroiditis. Activation of *cytotoxic T-lymphocytes* (CD8+ T-cells) in response to cell-mediated immune response affected by helper T-lymphocytes (CD4+ T-cells) is central to thyrocyte destruction. As is characteristic of *type IV hyper-sensitivity,* recruitment of macrophages is another effect of the helper T-lymphocyte activation, with Th1 axis lymphocytes producing certain inflammatory cytokines within the thyroid tissue for further macrophage activation and migration into the thyroid gland for direct effect.

In Hashimoto's thyroiditis, the immunological attack appears to be typically aggressive and destructive, rather than stimulatory, as in Graves' disease, and the difference is most likely due to the characteristics of the immune response. Hashimoto's thyroiditis is reported to occur in two varieties, an *atrophic variety*, perhaps associated with human leukocytic antigen-DR3 (HLA-DR3) gene inheritance, and a *goitrous form* associated with HLA-DR5 (Zeitlin et al., 2008).

Many of the genes associated with autoimmune thyroid disease (AITD) are also associated with *other autoimmune diseases*, which highlights a key role for disrupted T-cell central tolerance, antigen monitoring and peripheral immune tolerance in autoimmune onset. In studies of autoimmune hypothyroidism in *monozygotic twins*, the concordance rate is below 1 and thus, *environmental factors* are also etiologically important (Brix et al., 2008).

Susceptibility Genes

Human Leukocyte Antigen (HLA) Genes

The first gene locus identified in association with the autoimmune thyroid disease (AITD) was major histocompatibility complex (MHC) region on the *chromosome 6p21*, which encodes human leukocyte antigens (HLAs). The HLA region, which is highly polymorphic, comprises several immune response genes. The HLA molecule, located on antigen presenting cells

(APCs), binds and presents an antigenic peptide enabling T-cell recognition and response to an antigen. Presumably, specific HLA alleles have a higher affinity for autoantigenic thyroidal peptides and are thus likely to contribute to the development of the AITD. However, in order to initiate thyroid autoimmunity, autoantigen occurrence within the thyroid gland or its draining lymph nodes is needed, being followed by HLA presentation. In Hashimoto's thyroiditis, aberrant expression of HLA class II molecules on thyrocytes has been demonstrated. Presumably, such thyrocytes may act as APCs capable of presenting the thyroid autoantigens and initiating AITD (Jacobson et al., 2008).

While in Graves' disease, HLA-DR3 was reported by several studies as the primary susceptibility allele, no consistent associations were observed in Hashimoto's thyroiditis. The large United Kingdom (UK) Caucasian Hashimoto's Thyroiditis Case Control Cohort Study demonstrated clear differences in association within the HLA class II region between Hashimoto's thyroiditis and Graves' disease. Differences in HLA class II genotype may, in part, contribute to the different immuno-pathological processes and clinical presentation of these related diseases (Zeitlin et al., 2008). Major histocompatibility complex (MHC) class-II molecules expressed on the thyroid follicles of Hashimoto's thyroiditis patients are induced by viral infections or inflammatory cytokines. They act as non-professional (APCs) and present self as foreign antigens initiating an autoimmune response. The activated T-helper cell stimulates B-cells and plasma cells to produce antithyroid antibodies. Interferon-gamma (INF-γ), tumor necrosis factor–alpha (TNF-α), and interleukin-1 (IL-1) produced by Th1 cells activate macrophages that destroy thyroid follicles.

In *Caucasians*, different forms of Hashimoto's thyroiditis were repored to be associated with various HLA alleles, including DR3, DR5, DQ7, *DQB1*03* (Hunt et al., 2001), *DQw7* (Badenhoop et al., 1990), or DRB1*04-DQB1*0301 Haplo-type (Petrone et al., 2001). In *Japanese* patients, associations with *DRB4*0101*, *HLA-A2* (Wan et al., 1989) and *DRw53* (Honda et al., 1989) were shown while in *Chinese* patients association with *DRw9* was observed (Hawkins et al., 1987).

Cytotoxic T-Lymphocyte Antigen-4 (CTLA-4) Gene

Cytotoxic T-cell antigen-4 (CTLA-4*)* gene locus, which lies on *chromosome 2q33,* was reported by Jacobson et al (2007) to be associated with various autoimmune diseases, including type-1 diabetes (T1D), myasthenia gravis, systemic lupus erythematosus (SLE), systemic sclerosis, Graves' disease, and Hashimoto's thyroiditis (Jacobson, & Tomer, 2007).

Cytotoxic T-cell antigen-4 is the second major negative regulator of T-cell-mediated immune functions. The expression of CTLA-4 on the surface of T-cells induced by the activation of the T-cell receptor results in suppression of T-cell activation. CTLA-4 gene polymorphisms may reduce expression or function of the CTLA-4 antigen and may therefore contribute to the reduced inhibition of T-cell proliferation and subsequently increase susceptibility to an autoimmune response. Studies on several polymorphisms of the CTLA-4 gene in patients with Hashimoto's thyroiditis showed that (AT)n microsatellite CTLA-4 polymorphism in the 3' untranslated region (UTR) was associated with Hashimoto's thyroiditis in *Caucasian* (Kosta et al., 1997) and *Japanese* patients (Akamizu et al., 2000), but not in *Italian* population (Petrone et al., 2001). In the exon 1 located 49A/G single nucleotide polymorphism (SNP), resulting in threonine to alanine substitution, was associated with Hashimoto's thyroiditis (Donner, 1997; Nithiyananthan, 2002; Terauchi, 2003); however, this observation was not confirmed by other studies (Park, 2000; Sahin, 2009; Bicek, 2009). A large meta-analysis of 866 patients with Hashimoto's thyroiditis showed a significant association with 49A/G (Kavvoura et al., 2007). The initial observations of the association with Hashimoto's thyroiditis (Ueda, 2003; Ban, 2005) were not confirmed by later studies (Bicek, 2009; Ikegani, 2006); however, the results of the meta-analysis indicated a significant association with CT60 SNP (Kavvoura et al., 2007). Nevertheless, further studies are still needed to determine which CTLA-4 polymorphism is causative.

Apart from being associated with Hashimoto's thyroiditis, CTLA-4 seems to be the major thyroid antibody (T-Ab) susceptibility gene. In 2001, Tomer and colleagues demonstrated a link of the CTLA-4 region to the presence of T-Abs by a whole genome linkage analysis (Tomer, Greenberg, Barbesino, Concepcion, & Davies, 2001). Later, CTLA-4 was confirmed as a main locus for T-Ab status by other researchers (Ban, 2003; Ban, 2008). In 2011, the studies by Zaletel and Gaberšček (2011) of Slovenian Hashimoto's thyroiditis patients indicated a strong association between T-Ab production and the three CTLA-4 SNPs, including -318C/T in the promoter, 49A/G and CT60. In patients carrying one of those three SNPs, evidently higher TPO-Ab concentrations were demonstrated in relation to the polymorphous CTLA-4 gene, while the association with the Tg-Ab concentrations was weaker (Zaletel, 2006, Zaletel, 2010).

Protein Tyrosine Phosphatase Nonreceptor-Type 22 (PTPN22) Gene

Functional polymorphism of PTPN22, C1858T (R620W), is associated with susceptibility to several autoimmune disorders including AITD (Graves' disease and Hashimoto's thyroiditis), type-1 diabetes (T1D), rheumatoid arthritis (RA), and systemic lupus erythematosis (SLE) (Begovich, 2004; Bottini, 2004; Criswell, 2005; Kyogoku, 2004; Smyth, 2004; Velaga, 2004).

PTPN22 was recently identified as an immune-regulatory gene, located on *chromosome 1p13*. Similar to CTLA-4, PTPN22, which is predominantly expressed in lymphocytes, acts as a negative regulator of T-cell activation. 1858C/T SNP of the PTPN22 gene, causing arginine to tryptophan substitution at codon 620 (R620W), was shown to be a risk factor for many autoimmune diseases though the mechanism is still not clear (Burn et al., 2011). Criswell et al. (2005) reported a significant association of Hashimoto's thyroiditis with 1858C/T SNP. However, this observation was not confirmed in *German*, *Tunisian*, or *Japanese* populations (Kahles, 2005; Chabchoub, 2009; Ban, 2005). In a small group of patients with both Hashimoto's thyroiditis and autoimmune diabetes, Dultz et al. (2009) reported that T allele was determined in 50% of patients as compared to only 14% in healthy controls; however, one year later, Kordonouri et al., (2010) estimating the same polymorphism, did not confirm this association. Five other PTPN22 SNPs have been tested by Ban et al (2010) in Japanese patients and showed no relation with Hashimoto's thyroiditis, but a novel protective haplotype containing those SNPs has been observed (Ban et al., 2010).

Thyroglobulin Gene

Thyroglobulin (Tg) is an important thyroid-specific antigen, also present in the circulation, which makes it an easy target of autoimmune response. The gene for Tg is located on the *chromosome 8q24* and the link of this region with Hashimoto's thyroiditis and AITD was first identified by a Japanese and an American whole genome studies (Sakai, 2001; Tomer, 2003). A subsequent fine mapping of this region by Tomer et al. (2002), exposed Tg gene as one of the major thyroid-specific susceptibility genes, linked and associated with the AITD. Later, different alleles of various microsatellite markers and different SNPs of Tg gene were related to Hashimoto's thyroiditis, possibly affecting its expression, antigenicity, iodination, or binding to HLA. The association of Tgms2 microsatellite marker in intron 27 with Hashimoto's thyroiditis was confirmed in both Japanese (Ban et al., 2004) and Caucasian populations (Collins et al., 2003). Sequencing of human Tg revealed 14 SNPs among which four SNPs, including exon 10-12 SNP cluster and exon 33 SNP, were reported by Ban et al (2003) to be associated with Hashimoto's thyroiditis (Ban et al., 2003). However, this observation was neither confirmed in the United Kingdom Caucasian patients (Collins, 2004) nor in *Chinese* population, although in a later study by Maierhaba et al. (2008), one haplotype was significantly associated with Hashimoto's thyroiditis and Tg-Ab positivity.

Vitamin D Receptor Gene

Vitamin D, which acts *via* vitamin D receptor (VDR), possesses immuno-modulatory properties and its deficiency has been implicated in the development of autoimmune diseases. Many immune cells express VDR, particularly dendritic cells, where VDR stimulation has been shown to enhance their tolerogenicity (Toubi and Shoenfeld, 2010). The VDR gene is located on the *chromosome 12q12* and its polymorphisms have been related to different autoimmune disorders such as type I diabetes or Addison's disease. In 2001, the association between *VDR-FokI* SNP in exon 2 and Hashimoto's thyroiditis was identified by Ban et al. (2001) and confirmed later by Lin et al. (2006) in *Taiwanese Chinese* patients. In the *Croatian* population VDR gene 3' region polymorphisms were related to Hashimoto's thyroiditis, possibly affecting VDR mRNA expression (Stefani et al., 2008). A significant relation has also been discovered between Hashimoto's thyroiditis and both promoter and intron 6 gene polymorphisms of CYP27B1 hydroxylase, which is located on chromosome 12q13, catalysing the conversion of 25 hydroxyvitamin D_3 to its active form (Lopez et al., 2004).

FCRL3 Gene

The FCRL3 affects B-cell receptor signaling and results in the incomplete induction of anergy to autoreactive B-cells (Kochi et al., 2009), causing an elevated expression of FCRL3 to induce the generation of these cells. The C allele of the -169C/T polymorphism (rs7528684) in the FCRL3 promoter region, which was more closely related to a higher expression of FCRL3 than the -169T allele (Gibson et al., 2009), was found to be associated with the susceptibility to autoimmune diseases, such as rheumatoid arthritis, type-1 diabetes, systemic lupus erythematosis, multiple sclerosis (MS), and AITDs (Graves' disease and Hashimoto's thyroiditis) (Duchatelet, 2008; Ikari, 2006; Mao, 2010; Matesanz, 2008).

ZFAT Gene (Zinc Finger And AT-Hook Domain Containing)

ZFAT is expressed on B- and T-lymphocytes and has been shown to be a critical transcriptional regulator (Koyanagi et al, 2009) and as an anti-apoptotic molecule in lymphocytes (fujimoto et al., 2009). The Ex9b-SNP10 (rs16905194) polymorphism in ZFAT was associated with the susceptibility to AITDs (Shinasawa et al., 2004). The T allele of Ex9b-SNP10 was associated with a lower expression of small antisense transcription of ZFAT (SAS-ZFAT) than its A allele. SAS-ZFAT suppresses the expression of 3′UTR of truncated-ZFAT (TR-ZFAT), which is strongly expressed on B-cells and monocytes (Shinasawa et al., 2004). However, the functions of TR-ZFAT and SAS-ZFAT remain to be determined. The G allele of Ex9b-SNP2 (rs1036819) was also associated with the development of AITD among the Japanese, although the function of Ex9b-SNP2 was not determined (Shinasawa et al., 2004).

Cytokine Genes and Other Immune-Related Genes

Recently, several genes encoding different inflammatory cytokines have been shown to influence the severity of Hashimoto's thyroiditis. *Interferon-gamma* (IFN-γ), produced by T-helper type 1 (Th1) cells, promotes cell-mediated cytotoxicity, which underlies thyroid destruction in Hashimoto's thyroiditis. Ito et al. (2006) reported that T allele of the +874A/T IFN-γ SNP, causing increased IFN-γ production, was associated with severity of hypothyroidism in Hashimoto's thyroiditis patients (Ito et al., 2006). A higher frequency of severe hypothyroidism was also observed in patients carrying CC genotype of -590C/T *interleukin 4* (IL-4) SNP, leading to a lower production of IL-4, one of the key Th2 cytokines, which suppresses cell-mediated autoimmunity (Nanba, Watanabe, Akamizu, & Iwatani, 2008). Gene polymorphism of *transforming growth factor* (TGF)-β, inhibitor of cytokine production, was also associated with Hashimoto's thyroiditis. T allele of +369T/C SNP, leading to a lower secretion of TGF-β, was more frequent in severe hypothyroidism than in mild hypothyroidism (Yamada, Watanabe, Nanba, Akamizu, & Iwatani, 2008). Moreover, reported in 2010 that more severe forms of Hashimoto's thyroiditis were associated with -2383C/T SNP of gene for forkhead box P3

(FoxP3), an essential regulatory factor for the development of Tregs (Inoue et al., 2010). Unlike the severity of hypothyroidism, the development of Hashimoto's thyroiditis itself was associated with C allele of *tumor necrosis factor* (TNF)-α -1031T/C SNP. C-allele carriers had higher concentration of TNF-α, which acts as the stimulator of the IFN-γ production as demonstrated also by Inoue et al. (2009).

Genome-wide association studies (GWAS) detected other susceptibility genes of AITD (tomer, 2010) including *FOXE1* and *IL-2RA* (Simmonds, 2013). Association of polymorphisms in *micro-RNA* genes (miR499A and miR125A) with autoimmune thyroid diseases has been reported (Cai et al., 2017). There is a report that micro-RNAs (miRNAs) miR-146a1, miR-155-2, and miR-200a1 are altered in autoimmune thyroid diseases (AITD). Accumulating data suggest that miRNAs crucially control innate and adaptive immune responses, and implicate some miRNAs as having an important role in the pathophysiology of immunity and autoimmunity (Xiao and Rajewsky, 2009). For example, miR-155-2 was previously shown to possess important functions in the mammalian immune system. MicroRNA-142-5p may contribute to Hashimoto's thyroiditis by targeting CLDN1 (Zhu et al., 2016).

Environmental Factors

Regarding environmental factors, high iodine (I_2) intake, selenium deficiency, pollutants such as tobacco smoke, infectious diseases such as chronic hepatitis C, and certain drugs are implicated in the development of autoimmune thyroiditis (Duntas, 2010; Pacini, 1998). Environmental factors have not yet, however, been sufficiently investigated to clarify their roles in the pathogenesis of Hashimoto's disease, and there is a need to assess their effects on development of the autoimmune process and the mechanisms of their interactions with susceptibility genes.

Iodine-Intake

Increased iodine intake is well-established environmental factor for triggering thyroid autoimmunity. Prevalence of T-Abs was 13% in iodine-deficiency areas (Aghini-Lombardi et al., 1999), approximately18% with sufficient iodine intake (Hollowell et al., 200) and about 25% in areas with excessive iodine intake (Kasagi et al., 2009). Moreover, up to four-fold increase in prevalence of T-Abs was shown after higher iodine intake as iodine prophylaxis in previously iodine-deficient areas (Heydarian, 2007; Gokowski, 2007; Fountoulakis, 2007). In an interventional study by Kahaly et al (1998), deliberate exposure to 500 μg of iodine provoked thyroid autoimmunity in 20% of previously healthy individuals (Kahly et al., 1998). Rose et al. (2002), using experimental animal models of autoimmune thyroiditis, reported that the prevalence and severity of thyroid autoimmunity significantly increased when the dietary iodine was added.

Several putative mechanisms by which iodine may promote thyroid autoimmunity have been proposed. *Firstly*, long-term I_2 exposure leads to increased iodination of thyroglobulin (Tg), which increases its antigenicity by creating novel iodine-containing epitopes or exposing cryptic epitopes, and thus initiates the autoimmune process in genetically-susceptible individuals by facilitating presentation by APC and enhancing the binding affinity of the T-cell receptor leading to specific T-cell activation (Rose, Bonita, & Burek, 2002). *Secondly*, iodine exposure increases the level of reactive oxygen species in the thyrocyte, which is generated during TPO oxidation of excessive amounts of iodine. They enhance the expression of the intra-cellular adhesion molecule-1 (ICAM-1) on the thyroid follicular cells, which could attract the immuno-competent cells into the thyroid gland (Burek, & Talor, 2009). *Thirdly*, iodine toxicity to thyrocytes has been reported by Fountoulakis et al. (2007). Highly reactive oxygen species may bind to membrane lipids and proteins, causing release of auto-antigens and thyrocyte damage. *Fourthly*, Yu et al. (2011) reported that iodine excess promotes follicular cell apoptosis by inducing an abnormal expression of tumor necrosis factor-related apoptosis-inducing ligand (TRAIL) and its death receptor (DR)-5 in thyroid. *Fifthly*, in-vitro evidence also suggests an enhancing influence of iodine on the cells of the immune system, including augmented maturation of dendritic cells, increased number of T-cells and stimulated B-cell immunoglobulin production (Fountoulakis, Philippou, & Tsatsoulis, 2007).

Selenium Deficiency

Selenium deficiency decreases the activity of seleno-proteins, including glutathione peroxidases, which can lead to raised concentrations of hydrogen peroxide and thus promote inflammation and disease.

In animal models, selenium has been shown to exert protective effects in cases of excessive iodine ingestion (Xu et al., 2006). Similarly, human studies have demonstrated that when addressing iodine deficiency through supplementation, co-administration of selenium is important to maintain adequate GPx function (Thomson, Campbell, Miller, & Skeaff, 2011).

Drugs

Certain drugs were reported to initiate or exacerbate thyroid autoimmunity in susceptible individuals. Interferon-alpha (IFN-α), used to treat chronic hepatitis, is frequently associated with AITD since T-Abs were observed in up to 40% and clinical disease in 5-10% of patients treated with IFN-α. Presumably, IFN-α has toxic effects on the thyroid gland with consequent auto-antigen presentation and immune effects, such as switching to Th1 immune response, suppression of Treg function, activation of immune cells, stimulation of cytokine release and expression of MHC class I on thyroid cells (Tomer, 2010). Similarly, interleukin-2 (IL-2) used for treatment of melanoma and renal carcinoma, seems to act through immune and toxic mechanisms, leading to both T-Ab positivity and hypothyroidism (Barbesino, 2010). In patients with known AITD, *lithium* may increase the risk of hypothyroidism. Some studies reported that treatment with lithium increases T-Ab titers and the prevalence of thyroid autoimmunity, although this observation was not confirmed by other reports (Barbesino, 2010; Baethge, 2005). Among putative mechanisms, direct toxicity of lithium on the thyroid gland or toxicity of increased intra-thyroidal iodine resulting from lithium treatment were reported by Barbesino et al. (2010). Similarly, *amiodarone* may be cytotoxic leading to thyroid auto-antigen presentation and provoke thyroid autoimmunity (Martino, Bartalena, Bogazzi, & Braverman, 2001).

Infections

Not only the IFN-α treatment, but also *hepatitis C* infection itself has been reported to be associated with thyroid autoimmunity and hypothyroidism. Possible mechanisms include the molecular mimicry between viral and self-antigens, and activation of auto-reactive T-cells by the release of pro-inflammatory mediators caused by the viral infection (Thomson, Campbell, Miller, & Skeaff, 2011). Moreover, in Hashimoto's thyroiditis, several other putative triggering viruses have been implicated such as parvovirus, rubella, herpes simplex virus, Epstein Barr virus, and human T-lymphotropic virus type 1 (Desailloud, & Hober, 2009). A recent study of sera in pregnant women has also indicated an association between a prior infection with Toxoplasma gondii and an increase of TPO-Abs (Wasserman et al., 2009). Nevertheless, the evidences are scarce and further studies are required in order to confirm the role of infections as causative agents.

Chemicals

The exposure to environmental toxicants such as polyaromatic hydrocarbons or polyhalogenated biphenyls, both commonly used in a variety of industrial applications, has been shown to provoke thyroid auto-immunity in both, experimental animals and humans. Recently, a significantly higher prevalence of Hashimoto's thyroiditis and T-Ab (9.3% and 17.6%, respectively) has been demonstrated in residents living in the area of petrochemical complex of Sao Paolo (*Brasil*) compared to the control area (3.9% and 10.3%, respectively) (de Freitas et al., 2010). In Slovakia, the exposure to polychlorinated biphenyls was associated with T-Ab and hypothyroidism (Langer et al., 2007). Although there is strong evidence attesting the contribution of chemicals to thyroid autoimmunity, the exact mechanisms of their action are yet to be established.

Radiation Exposure

An increase in the prevalence of thyroid auto-antibodies (AT-Abs) was reported 6-8 years after the *Chernobyl* accident in *radiation-exposed* children and adolescents (Agate et al., 2008). TPO-Ab prevalence in adolescents exposed to radioactive fallout was still increased in Belarus 13-15 years after the Chernobyl accident. (Elfstrom et al., 2008). This increase was less evident than previously reported and was not accompanied by thyroid dysfunction. These data suggest that radioactive fallout elicited a transient autoimmune reaction, without triggering full-blown thyroid autoimmune disease. Longer observation periods are needed to exclude later effects.

Protection Against Thyroid Autoimmunity

Two mechanisms enable the maintenance of self-tolerance. *Central tolerance* refers to thymic deletion of auto-reactive T-cells during fetal life. Cells that escape central tolerance are prevented from triggering autoimmunity by mechanisms of *peripheral tolerance* where the pivotal role is played by Tregs (Shevach, 2006). They have a suppressive effect on the effector T-cells, APCs and B-cells, therefore maintaining the immunological unresponsiveness to self-antigens and suppressing the excessive immune response (Sakaguchi, Yamaguchi, Nomura, & Onol, 2008). They may directly suppress target cells or act through secreted suppressor cytokines.

Tregs derive from thymus as a sub-population of T- cells or from naive T-cells in the periphery and express CD25 (α-chain of IL-2 receptor) and FoxP3. Thus, the critical role in the immune system is played by $CD4^{+}CD25^{+}Foxp3^{+}$ Tregs (Shevach, 2006). Cells with the highest CD25 expression (CD4+CD25 high) are responsible for regulatory suppressive effects (Baecher-Allan, Wolf, & Hafler, 2005). The role of Tregs in self-tolerance was extensively studied in murine experimental autoimmune thyroiditis, where protection against autoimmunity was mediated by thymically-derived $CD4^{+}CD25^{+}Foxp3^{+}$ Tregs (Kong et al., 2009). In humans, CD25 expression was higher in patients with Hashimoto's thyroiditis than in healthy controls (Watanabe et al., 2002). In patients with AITD, the proportion of Tregs was lower intra-thyroidally than in peripheral blood (Nakano et al., 2007). When compared to controls, a higher proportion of special Tregs with high levels of FoxP3 (termed CD4+CD25 high HLA-DR+ cells) in patients with Hashimoto's thyroiditis was found by three-color flow cytometry (Baecher-Allan, Wolf, & Hafler, 2006). This indicates a compensatory expansion of Tregs sub-population in order to diminish the immune response (fountoulakis et al., 2008).

The expression of Foxp3 and generation of Treg cells are both induced by TGF-β produced in Tregs, fibroblasts, macrophages, endothelial cells in inflammatory thyroid tissue and in thyrocytes (toda, 1999; Betteli, 2007). Transforming growth factor- beta (TGF-β) is a key regulator of immune tolerance, which stimulates suppressive Tregs and inhibits T-cell differentiation (Betteli, Korn, & Kuchroo, 2007). Accordingly, in patients with Hashimoto's thyroiditis, serum levels of TGF-β were lower than in controls, which did not change after the treatment with levothyroxine. Thus, TGF-β levels seem to be associated with Hashimoto's thyroiditis and not thyroid dysfunction (Akinci et al., 2008). Suppressive effect of TGF-β was established in the development of experimental autoimmune thyroiditis Guimaraes et al., 196). At the later stage of the thyroiditis TGF-β may trigger the development of fibrosis (Chen, Wei, Sharp, & Braley-Mullen, 2003).

Development of Thyroid Gland Autoimmunity

The exact mechanisms of initiation and progression of thyroid autoimmunity have not been completely clarified yet. Nevertheless, proper interaction of thyroid cells, APCs, and T-cells is essential for the initiation of thyroid autoimmunity. The result is a secretion of different cytokines leading to Th1 response, a characteristic of Hashimoto's thyroiditis. Cytokines have an important role in AITD and are secreted by the immune cells, thyroid follicular cells and inflammatory cells (Ajjan, Watson, & Weetman, 2009).

T-lymphocytes proliferate and secrete cytokines after being stimulated by two signals. The ***first signal*** is the activation of T-cell receptor induced by binding of antigen peptide presented on HLA molecule on the surface of APC. The ***second signal*** is ligation of CD28 on the surface of the T-cell to B7 ligands (B7.1 and B7.2) expressed on APC, including dendritic cells, activated macrophages and activated B-cells. Activation of T-cells induces the expression of CTLA-4, which suppresses further T-cell activation by binding and blocking of B7 ligands. In patients with Hashimoto's thyroiditis, but not in Graves' disease or goitrous patients, thyroid follicular cells were positive for B7.1 (Battifora et al., 1998) and may also express MHC class II molecules induced by interferon-gamma (IFN-γ), which is secreted by intrathyroidal lymphocytes (Weetman, 2004). Colocalization of MHC class II and B7.1 antigens on the same thyroid follicular cell indicates that in the pathogenesis of Hashimoto's thyroiditis, follicular cells may act also as APCs and may be capable of inducing or maintaining the autoimmune process (Weetman, 2004).

Autoimmune response is predominantly determined by the antigen, nature of APC, and several genetic, endogenous, and environmental triggers (Weetman, 2004). In Hashimoto's thyroiditis, autoimmune response is mediated predominantly by Th1-type cytokines such as tumor necrosis factor-alpha (TNF-α), IFN-γ and interleukin-2 (IL-2) (Ajjan, Watson, Mcintosh, & Weetman, 1996). When exposed to a thyroid self-antigen such as human Tg, peripheral blood mononuclear cells from patients with Hashimoto's thyroiditis produced more TNF-α, IL-2, IL-10, IFN-γ, and less IL-5 than controls. Since higher production was observed with autologous sera than with pooled normal sera, the importance of serum elements, such as the complement and serum anti-Tg activity, was proposed. It was postulated that these two serum elements accelerate Th1/Th2 cell cytokine reaction by increasing the uptake of autoantigens by APCs (Nielsen et al., 2006). Patients with more severe hypothyroidism presented with a higher Th1/Th2 ratio compared with those with mild hypothyroidism. (Nanba, Watanabe, Inoue, & Iwatani, 2009). Furthermore, the correlation between the TPO-Ab levels and the production of TNF-α and IFN-γ has been demonstrated by Karanikas et al. (2005) and later confirmed by Nielsen et al. (2009). In their study, they indicated that TPO-Abs seem to promote TPO-elicited cytokine production, including IFN-γ, TNF-α, and IL-6 (Nielsen et al., 2009).

High titers of antibody against thyroglobulin (Tg) and thyroid peroxidase (TPO) are present in most patients with Hashimoto's thyroiditis (Kawakami, Fisfalen, & DeGroot, 1992), and TPO antibodies are complement fixing and may be cytotoxic. However, the evidence of cytotoxicity is scant, especially since normal trans-placental antibody passage of anti-TPO Ab to the human fetus does *not* usually induce thyroid damage. Thus, it is conceivable that cytotoxic T-cells, or killer (K) or natural killer (NK) cells, or regulatory T (Treg) or suppressor T-cells, may play an important role. A few reports do show T-cell line or clone cytotoxicity toward isologous thyroid epithelial cells, and experimental thyroiditis can be transferred by lymphocytes. T-cells from patients with Hashimoto's disease proliferate when exposed to Tg and TPO. These responses are known to be directed to specific sequences in the TPO molecule, including epitopes at aa 110-129, 210-230, 420-439, and 842-861 (Ng, & Kung, 2006). T-cells from mice immunized to TPO react strongly to TPO sequence 540-559, and when immunized with this peptide, develop hypothyroidism and thyroiditis. This peptide may be a central factor in immunity to TPO (Hikada et al., 1992). Muixí et al. (2008) identified natural HLA-DR-associated peptides in autoimmune organs that will allow finding peptide-specific T-cells in-situ.

In-vitro binding identified HLA-DR3 as the allele to which one of these peptides likely associates in-vivo. Computer modeling and bioinformatics analysis suggested other HLA-DR alleles for binding of other thyroglobulin peptides. Increased K- and NK-cell function has been reported in Hashimoto's thyroiditis (Itoh et al., 1999). Dysfunction of regulatory (or suppressor) CD4+ T-cell populations may lead to the development of various organ-specific autoimmune diseases including Hashimoto's thyroiditis (McLachlan et al., 2007).

In the past few years, a new subset of (T-helper) Th cells, designated Th17 (T-helper type 17), has been studied. Th17 cells have also been proved highly pro-inflammatory by producing the pro-inflammatory cytokine IL-17, and may lead to autoimmunity in animal models and potentially also in human autoimmune diseases. The possible importance of Th17 in the pathogenesis of Hashimoto's thyroiditis has been indicated by a recent study showing increased levels of Th17 lymphocytes and Th17 cytokines compared with healthy controls (Figueroa-Vega et al., 2010). Similarly, when estimating the expression in peripheral blood mononuclear cells, Th17 cells rather than Th1 cells predominated in Hashimoto's thyroiditis patients (Shi et al., 2010). Imbalance of Th17/Treg is reported in different subtypes of autoimmune thyroid diseases. Increased Th17 lymphocytes may play a more important role in the pathogenesis of HT and GO while decreased Treg may be involved in Graves' disease (Li et al., 2016). In contrast, a significant decrease in the ratios of CD4 + IL17+/CD4 + CD25 + CD127 - ($p < 0.0001$) and CD4 + IL17+/CD4 + CD25 + CD127 - FoxP3 + ($p < 0.0001$) T-cells was observed in Hashimoto's thyroiditis in comparison to healthy children (Hamano et al., 2001).

Destruction of the Thyroid Gland

Despite the lack of understanding of the primary cause(s), it is certain that thyroid autoimmunity drives the lymphocyte collection in the thyroid and is responsible for thyroid epithelial cell damage. Progressive thyroid cell damage can change the apparent clinical picture from goitrous hypothyroidism to that of primary hypothyroidism, or "atrophic" thyroiditis. Primary hypothyroidism is considered to be the end-stage of Hashimoto's thyroiditis. In the TSHR-immunized murine model of Graves' disease, Treg depletion (particularly CD25)-induced thyroid lymphocytic infiltrates with transient or permanent hypothyroidism (Kosugi, Ban, Akamizu, & Kohn, 1992). Lymphocytic infiltration was associated with inter-molecular spreading of the TSHR antibody response to other self-thyroid antigens, murine thyroid peroxidase and Tg. These data suggest a role for (regulatory T-cells) Tregs in the natural progression of hyperthyroid Graves' disease to Hashimoto's thyroiditis and hypothyroidism in humans.

An alternative cause of "*atrophic" hypothyroidism* is the development of thyroid stimulation blocking antibodies (TSB-Ab), which, as the name implies, prevent TSH binding to TSH-R, but do not stimulate thyroid cells and cause hypothyroidism. It has been proposed that TSB-Ab bind to epitopes near the carboxyl end of the TSH-R extra-cellular domain, in contrast to thyroid stimulating antibodies (TS-Ab), which bind to epitopes near aa 40 at the amino terminus (Tamaki et al., 1990). This syndrome occurs in neonates, children and adults. The prevalence of TSB-Ab in adult hypothyroid patients has been reported to be 10% (Okamura et al., 1990). However, in contrast to the usual progressive and irreversible thyroid damage occurring in the usual setting, these blocking antibodies tend to follow the course of TSAb--that is, they decrease or disappear over time, and the patient may become euthyroid again (Okamura et al., 1990). A change from a predominant TSAb response to a predominant TSB-Ab response can cause patients to have sequential episodes of hyper- and hypothyroid function (Takasu et al., 1992). HLA antigens of hypothyroid patients with TSB-Ab were found to be different from patients with idiopathic myxedema or Hashimoto's thyroiditis, and rather similar to patients with Graves' disease (Mori et al., 1994).

Thyroid destruction in Hashimoto's thyroiditis is mostly a consequence of the *apoptotic processes* combined with CD8+ cell-mediated cytotoxicity, changes in cell junctions, and complement activation.

Apoptosis is characterized by cytoskeletal disruption, cell shrinkage, chromatin condensation, nuclear fragmentation, membrane blebbing and DNA fragmentation (Thompson, 1995). In general, apoptosis enables adult healthy tissue homeostasis, while excessive cell death causes a loss of active tissue and an impaired function (Thompson, 1995). Two major apoptotic signal pathways have been thoroughly investigated (Mitsiades, 2001). The ***first pathway*** consists of Fas receptor (Apo-1 or CD95), a type I trans-membrane protein and a member of TNF receptor superfamily, and Fas ligand (Fas-L), a type II trans-membrane protein, which binds to Fas receptor and activates apoptotic process (Nagata & Golstein, 1995). The ligand for Fas (Fas-L) was shown to be constitutively expressed on thyrocytes and lL-1α, abundantly produced in the thyroid gland of Hashimoto's thyroiditis, induced Fas expression on thyrocytes. Thus Fas-FasL interaction on thyrocytes may induce apoptosis and thyroid cell destruction (Giordano et al., 1997).

Furthermore, in relation to the Fas-Fas-L system, Dong et al. (2002) reported that mutations of Fas, which induce loss of function, were found in thyroid lymphocytes in 38.1% of patients with Hashimoto's thyroiditis. These mutations are found in 65.4% of patients with lymphoma (Takakuwa et al., 2001), which usually develops from Hashimoto's thyroiditis. These changes are possibly important for progression of Hashimoto's thyroiditis.

The ***second pathway*** includes tumour necrosis factor (TNF)-related apoptosis-inducing ligand (TRAIL) (Apo2L), a member of TNF receptor family, which activates apoptosis by binding to its receptors TRAIL-R1 (DR4) and TRAIL-R2 (DR5) (Pan, 2001; Pan, 1997). Both pathways lead to the activation of proteolytic enzymes caspases, which destroy thyroid cells. In normal conditions, the Fas pathway is inhibited, whereas in inflammation, it is activated by cytokines (Wang et al., 2002). *In-vitro* studies have shown that TSH inhibited Fas-mediated apoptosis, while the absence of TSH induced apoptosis (Kawakami et al., 1996). A combination of IFN-γ with TNF-α or IL-1β stimulated the Fas-activated apoptosis in cultured thyroid follicular cells (Bretz et al., 1999). TRAIL receptors are also expressed in thyroid cells by cytokines (Bretz et al., 2001) and TRAIL could mediate the programmed cell death under appropriate conditions (Bretz, Arscott, Myc, & Baker, Jr., 1999). Thyroid follicular cells were able to express TRAIL in the presence of IFN-γ, TNF-α, and IL-1β *in-vitro*. Thus, such inflammatory cytokines can influence immune-mediated apoptosis (Bretz, Arscott, Myc, & Baker, Jr., 1999). Additional inductor of programmed cell death is TGF-β (Bursch et al., 1993). Its release from thyroid cells is stimulated by the epidermal growth factor (EGF) (Gartner et al., 1997). Thus, the mechanism of apoptosis in Hashimoto's thyroiditis seems to be induced by cytokines secreted from local lymphocytes (Bechtner, 1999; Giordano, 1997).

The main apoptotic mechanism in Hashimoto's thyroiditis represents Fas-mediated apoptosis together with down-regulation of Bcl-2, which is an inhibitor of apoptosis highly expressed in normal thyrocytes (Arscott, 1998; Mitsiades, 1998; Fountoulakis, 2008; Wang, 2007). Immuno-histochemically, patients with Hashimoto's thyroiditis had a lower percentage of Bcl-2 stainings and a higher percentage of caspase-3 reactions than control subjects (Kaczmarek, Lacka, Jarmolowska-Jurczyszyn, Sidor, & Majewski, 2011). In thyroid glands with Hashimoto's thyroiditis, a strong staining for Fas and Fas-L and a high percentage of apoptosis were observed in thyroid follicles adjacent to lymphocytes when compared with healthy thyroid tissue.

In addition to apoptosis, CD8+ cell-mediated cytotoxicity contributes to thyroid destruction mediated by intracellular circulating adhesion molecule-1 (ICAM-1) (CR 54), which is expressed by thyroid follicular cells and increases CD8+ cell binding (Weetmn, 2004). Levels of ICAM-1, vascular cell adhesion molecule-1 (VCAM-1), and tissue inhibitor of metallo-proteinases 1 (TIMP-1) were significantly higher in patients with functional abnormality due to the AITD than in euthyroid subjects. Authors postulated that the autoimmune process itself may have an impact on vascular inflammation, endothelial dysfunction, and tissue remodeling (Joblanc et al., 2010).

Finally, changes in gap junctions consequently leading to cell-to-cell communication changes may contribute to the thyroid destruction. In Hashimoto's thyroiditis, decreased levels of connexin 43 (Cx43) were observed immunohistochemically when compared with the normal thyroid tissue (Jiang, Feng, Li, Zhao, & Yin, 2010). Cx43 is a part of connexons, which constitute a gap junction channel in organized tissues and in thyroid tissues. Similarly, reduced proteins Cx43, Cx32, and Cx26 were established in animal models of AITD (Green, Lazarus, LaBue, & Shah, 1995). Mitasíková et al. (2009) also showed that T_3 increased the level of Cx43. Therefore, the number of gap junctions may be increased in Graves' disease and decreased in Hashimoto's thyroiditis (Jiang, Feng, Li, Zhao, & Yin, 2010). Disruption of thyroid integrity may allow TPO-Abs to bind to TPO and activate complement (Weetman, 2004).

IgG4-Related Disease (IgG4-RD)

The *IgG4-related disease (IgG4-RD)* is a new disease entity first proposed in relation to autoimmune pancreatitis (AIP) by Hamano et al. (2001). A high prevalence of hypothyroidism has been reported in patients with AIP (Komatuso et al., 2005). In 2009, it was reported that on the basis of the immunohistochemistry (IHC) of IgG4, Hashimoto's thyroiditis can be divided into two groups, which were proposed as IgG4 thyroiditis (IgG4-positive plasma cell-rich group) and non-IgG4 thyroiditis (IgG4-positive plasma cell poor group) (Li et al., 2009). The IgG4 thyroiditis group shows indistinguishable histological features and may have a close relationship with IgG4-RD in other organs. In 2010, it was demonstrated that IgG4 thyroiditis is clinically associated with a lower female-to-male ratio, more rapid progress, subclinical hypothyroidism, diffuse low echogenicity, and a higher level of circulating thyroid auto-antibodies than non-IgG4 thyroiditis (Dahlgren et al., 2010).

Riedel thyroiditis is another candidate for IgG4-RD. It is a rare form of chronic thyroiditis, characterized by inflammatory proliferative fibrosis which involves the thyroid parenchyma and surrounding tissue structures. In 2010, Dahlgren and colleagues reported that IgG4-RD was the underlying condition in a part of the cases of Riedel thyroiditis (Kakudo et al., 2012). When IgG4-RD occurs in a systemic pattern, the thyroid involvement may present as Riedel thyroiditis rather than Hashimoto's thyroiditis (Nystrom, Bengtsson, Lapidus, Petersen, & Lindstedt, 1993).

REFERENCES

Agate, L., Mariotti, S., Elisei, R., Mossa, P., Pacini, F., Molinaro, E., ... Pinchera, A. (2008). Thyroid Autoantibodies and Thyroid Function in Subjects Exposed to Chernobyl Fallout during Childhood: Evidence for a Transient Radiation-Induced Elevation of Serum Thyroid Antibodies without an Increase in Thyroid Autoimmune Disease. *The Journal of Clinical Endocrinology and Metabolism*, *93*(7), 2729–2736. doi:10.1210/jc.2008-0060 PMID:18430771

Aghini-Lombardi, F., Antonangeli, L., Martino, E., Vitti, P., Maccherini, D., Leoli, F., ... Pincher.a, A. (1999). The spe.ctrum of thyroid disorders in an iodine-deficient community: The Pescopagano survey. *The Journal of Clinical Endocrinology and Metabolism*, *84*, 561–566. PMID:10022416

Ajjan, R. A., Watson, P. F., Mcintosh, R. S., & Weetman, A. P. (1996). Intrathyroidal cytokine gene expression in Hashimoto's thyroiditis. *Clinical and Experimental Immunology*, *105*(3), 523–528. doi:10.1046/j.1365-2249.1996.d01-784.x PMID:8809144

Ajjan, R. A., Watson, P. F., & Weetman, A. P. (2009). Cytokines and thyroid function. *Advances in Neuroimmunology*, *6*(4), 359–386. doi:10.1016/S0960-5428(97)00027-7 PMID:9183517

Akamizu, T., Sale, M. M., Rich, S. S., Hiratani, H., Noh, J. Y., Kanamoto, N., ... Bowden, D. W. (2000). Associa.tion of autoimmune thyroid disease with microsatellite markers for the thyrotropin receptor gene and CTLA-4 in Japanese patients. *Thyroid*, *10*(10), 851–858. doi:10.1089/thy.2000.10.851 PMID:11081251

Akinci, B., Comlekci, A., Yener, S., Bayraktar, F., Demir, T., Ali-Ozcan, M., ... Yesil, S. (2008). Hashimoto's thyroiditis, but not treatment of hypothyroidism, is associated with altered TGF-β1 levels. *Archives of Medical Research*, *39*(4), 397–401. doi:10.1016/j.arcmed.2007.12.001 PMID:18375250

Arscott, P. L., & Baker, J. R. Jr. (1998). Short analytical review. Apoptosis and thyroiditis. *Clinical Immunology and Immunopathology*, *87*(3), 207–217. doi:10.1006/clin.1998.4526 PMID:9646829

Badenhoop, K., Schwartz, G., Walfish, P. G., Drummond, V., Usadel, K. H., & Bottazzo, G. F. (1990). Susceptibility to thyroid autoimmune disease: Molecular analysis of HLA-D region genes identifies new markers for goitrous Hashimoto's thyroiditis. *The Journal of Clinical Endocrinology and Metabolism*, *71*(5), 1131–1137. doi:10.1210/jcem-71-5-1131 PMID:1977755

Baecher-Allan, C., Wolf, E., & Hafler, D. A. (2005). Functional analysis of highly defined, FACS-isolated populations of human regulatory CD4+CD25+T cells. *Clinical Immunology (Orlando, Fla.)*, *115*(1), 10–18. doi:10.1016/j.clim.2005.02.018 PMID:15870015

Baecher-Allan, C., Wolf, E., & Hafler, D. A. (2006). Class II expression identifies functionally distinct human regulatory T cells. *Journal of Immunology (Baltimore, Md.: 1950)*, *176*(8), 4622–4631. doi:10.4049/jimmunol.176.8.4622 PMID:16585553

Baethge, C., Blumentritt, H., Berghöfer, A., Bschor, T., Glenn, T., Adli, M., ... Finke, R. (2005). Long-term lithium treatment and thyroid antibodies: A controlled study. *Journal of Psychiatry & Neuroscience*, *30*, 23–427. PMID:16327876

Ban, Y., Davies, T. F., Greenberg, D. A., Kissin, A., Marder, B., Murphy, B., ... Tomer, Y. (2003). Analysis of the CTLA-4, CD28, and inducible costimulator (ICOS) genes in autoimmune thyroid disease. *Genes and Immunity*, *4*(8), 586–593. doi:10.1038j.gene.6364018 PMID:14647199

Ban, Y., Greenberg, D. A., Concepcion, E., Skrabanek, L., Villanueva, R., & Tomer, Y. (2003). Amino acid substitutions in the thyroglobulin gene are associated with susceptibility to human and murine autoimmune thyroid disease. *Proceedings of the National Academy of Sciences of the United States of America*, *100*(25), 15119–15124. doi:10.1073/pnas.2434175100 PMID:14657345

Ban, Y., Greenberg, D. A., Davies, T. F., Jacobson, E., Concepcion, E., & Tomer, Y. (2008). Linkage analysis of thyroid antibody production: Evidence for shared susceptibility to clinical autoimmune thyroid disease. *The Journal of Clinical Endocrinology and Metabolism*, *93*(9), 3589–3596. doi:10.1210/jc.2008-0364 PMID:18559906

Ban, Y., Taniyama, M., & Ban, Y. (2001). Vitamin D receptor gene polymorphisms in Hashimoto's thyroiditis. *Thyroid*, *11*(6), 607–608. doi:10.1089/105072501750302967 PMID:11442012

Ban, Y., Tozaki, T., Taniyama, M., Nakano, Y., Ban, Y., & Hirano, T. (2010). Association of the protein tyrosine phosphatase nonreceptor 22 haplotypes with autoimmune thyroid disease in the Japanese population. *Thyroid, 20*(8), 893–899. doi:10.1089/thy.2010.0104 PMID:20615141

Ban, Y., Tozaki, T., Taniyama, M., Tomita, M., & Ban, Y. (2004). Association of a thyroglobulin gene polymorphism with Hashimoto's thyroiditis in the Japanese population. *Horumon To Rinsho, 61*(2), 263–268. doi:10.1111/j.1365-2265.2004.02096.x PMID:15272924

Ban, Y., Tozaki, T., Taniyama, M., Tomita, M., & Ban, Y. (2005). Association of a CTLA-4 3′ untranslated region (CT60) single nucleotide polymorphism with autoimmune thyroid disease in the Japanese population. *Autoimmunity, 38*(2), 151–153. doi:10.1080/08916930500050319 PMID:16040335

Ban, Y., Tozaki, T., Taniyama, M., Tomita, M., & Ban, Y. (2005). The codon 620 single nucleotide polymorphism of the protein tyrosine phosphatase-22 gene does not contribute to autoimmune thyroid disease susceptibility in the Japanese. *Thyroid, 15*(10), 1115–1118. doi:10.1089/thy.2005.15.1115 PMID:16279843

Barbesino, G. (2010). Drugs affecting thyroid function. *Thyroid, 20*(7), 763–770. doi:10.1089/thy.2010.1635 PMID:20578900

Battifora, M., Pesce, G., Paolieri, F., Fiorino, N., Giordano, C., Riccio, A. M., ... Bagnasco, M. (1998). B7.1 costimulatory molecule is expressed on thyroid follicular cells in Hashimoto's thyroiditis, but not in Graves' disease. *The Journal of Clinical Endocrinology and Metabolism, 83*, 4130–4139. PMID:9814503

Bechtner, G., Fröschl, H., Sachse, A., Schopohl, D., & Gärtner, R. (1999). Induction of apoptosis in porcine thyroid follicles by transforming growth factor β1 and epidermal growth factor. *Biochimie, 81*(4), 315–320. doi:10.1016/S0300-9084(99)80076-5 PMID:10401664

Begovich, A. B., Carlton, V. E., Honigberg, L. A., Schrodi, S. J., Chokkalingam, A. P., Alexander, H. C., ... Gregersen, P. (2004). A missense single-nucleotide polymorphism in a gene encoding a protein tyrosine phosphatase (PTPN22) is associated with rheumatoid arthritis. *American Journal of Human Genetics, 75*(2), 330–337. doi:10.1086/422827 PMID:15208781

Betteli, E., Korn, T., & Kuchroo, V. K. (2007). Th17: The third member of the effector T cell trilogy. *Current Opinion in Immunology*, *19*(6), 652–657. doi:10.1016/j.coi.2007.07.020 PMID:17766098

Bicek, A., Zaletel, K., Gaberscek, S., Pirnat, E., Krhin, B., Stopar, T. G., & Hojker, S. (2009). 49A/G and CT60 polymorphisms of the cytotoxic T-lymphocyte-associated antigen 4-gene associated with autoimmune thyroid disease. *Human Immunology*, *70*(10), 820–824. doi:10.1016/j.humimm.2009.06.016 PMID:19559744

Bottini, N., Musumeci, L., Alonso, A., Rahmouni, S., Nika, K., Rostamkhani, M., ... Musteli.n, T. (2004). A funct.ional variant of lymphoid tyrosine phosphatase is associated with type I diabetes N*ature. Genetics*, *36*, 337–338. PMID:15004560

Bretz, J. D., Arscott, P. L., Myc, A., & Baker, J. R. Jr. (1999). Inflammatory cytokine regulation of Fas-mediated apoptosis in thyroid follicular cells. *The Journal of Biological Chemistry*, *274*(36), 25433–25438. doi:10.1074/jbc.274.36.25433 PMID:10464273

Bretz, J. D., & Baker, J. R. Jr. (2001). Apoptosis and autoimmune thyroid disease: Following a TRAIL to thyroid destruction? *Horumon To Rinsho*, *55*, 1–11. PMID:11453945

Bretz, J. D., Rymaszewski, M., Arscott, P. L., Myc, A., Ain, K. B., Thompson, N. W., & Baker, J. R. Jr. (1999). TRAIL death pathway expression and induction in thyroid follicular cells. *The Journal of Biological Chemistry*, *274*(33), 23627–23632. doi:10.1074/jbc.274.33.23627 PMID:10438545

Brix, T. H., Kyvik, K. O., & Hegedus, L. (2008). A population-based study of chronic autoimmune hypothyroidism in Danish twins. *The Journal of Clinical Endocrinology and Metabolism*, *85*, 536–539. PMID:10690851

Burek, C. L., & Talor, M. V. (2009). Environmental triggers of autoimmune thyroiditis. *Journal of Autoimmunity*, *33*(3-4), 183–189. doi:10.1016/j.jaut.2009.09.001 PMID:19818584

Burn, G. L., Svensson, L., Sanchez-Blanco, C., Saini, M., & Cope, A. P. (2011). Why is PTPN22 a good candidate susceptibility gene for autoimmune disease? *FEBS Letters*, *585*(23), 3689–3698. doi:10.1016/j.febslet.2011.04.032 PMID:21515266

Bursch, W., Oberhammer, F., Jirtle, R. L., Askari, M., Sedivy, R., Grasl-Kraupp, B., ... Schulte-Hermann, R. (1993). Transforming growth factor-beta 1 as a signal for induction of cell death by apoptosis. *British Journal of Cancer*, *67*(3), 531–536. doi:10.1038/bjc.1993.98 PMID:8439503

Cai, T., Li, J., An, X., Yan, N., Li, D., Jiang, Y., ... Zhang, J. A. (2017). Polymorphisms in MIR499A and MIR125A gene are associated with autoimmune thyroid diseases. *Molecular and Cellular Endocrinology*, *15*, 106–115. doi:10.1016/j.mce.2016.11.017 PMID:27888002

Chabchoub, G., Teixiera, E. P., Maalej, A., Ben-Hamad, M., Bahloul, Z., Cornelis, F., & Ayadi, H. (2009). The R620W polymorphism of the protein tyrosine phosphatase 22 gene in autoimmune thyroid diseases and rheumatoid arthritis in the Tunisian population. *Annals of Human Biology*, *36*(3), 342–349. doi:10.1080/03014460902817968 PMID:19343596

Chen, K., Wei, Y., Sharp, G. C., & Braley-Mullen, H. (2003). Mechanism of spontaneous resolution versus fibrosis in granulomatous experimental autoimmune thyroiditis. *Journal of Immunology (Baltimore, Md.: 1950)*, *171*(11), 6236–6243. doi:10.4049/jimmunol.171.11.6236 PMID:14634140

Collins, J., Heward, J. M., Carr-Smith, J., Daykin, J., Franklyn, J. A., & Gough, S. C. (2003). Association of a rare thyroglobulin gene microsatellite variant with autoimmune thyroid disease. *The Journal of Clinical Endocrinology and Metabolism*, *88*(10), 5039–5042. doi:10.1210/jc.2003-030093 PMID:14557492

Collins, J. E., Heward, J. M., Howson, J. M., Foxall, H., Carr-Smith, J., Franklyn, J. A., & Gough, S. C. (2004). Common allelic variants of exons 10, 12, and 33 of the thyroglobulin gene are not associated with autoimmune thyroid disease in the United Kingdom. *The Journal of Clinical Endocrinology and Metabolism*, *89*(12), 6336–6339. doi:10.1210/jc.2004-1336 PMID:15579800

Criswell, L. A., Pfeiffer, K. A., Lum, R. F., Gonzales, B., Novitzke, J., Kern, M., ... Gregersen, P. K. (2005). Analysis of families in the multiple autoimmune disease genetics consortium (MADGC) collection: The PTPN22 620W allele associates with multiple autoimmune phenotypes. *American Journal of Human Genetics*, *76*(4), 561–571. doi:10.1086/429096 PMID:15719322

Criswell, L. A., Pfeiffer, K. A., Lum, R. F., Gonzales, B., Novitzke, J., Kern, M., ... Gregersen, P. K. (2005). Analysis of families in the multiple autoimmune disease genetics consortium (MADGC) collection: The PTPN22 620W allele associates with multiple autoimmune phenotypes. *American Journal of Human Genetics*, *76*(4), 561–571. doi:10.1086/429096 PMID:15719322

Dahlgren, M., Khosroshahi, A., Nielsen, G. P., Deshpande, V., & Stone, J. H. (2010). Riedel's thyroiditis and multifocal fibrosclerosis are part of the IgG4-related systemic disease spectrum. *Arthritis Care & Research (Hoboken)*, *62*(9), 1312–1318. doi:10.1002/acr.20215 PMID:20506114

de Freitas, C. U., Grimaldi-Campos, R. A., Rodrigues-Silva, M. A., Panachão, M. R., de Moraes, J. C., Waissmann, W., ... Santos, R. T. (2010). Can living in the surroundings of a petrochemical complex be a risk factor for *autoimmune thyroid disease? Environmental Research*, *110*(1), 112–117. doi:10.1016/j.envres.2009.10.009 PMID:19913221

Desailloud, R., & Hober, D. (2009). Viruses and thyroiditis: An update. *Virology Journal*, *6*(1), 5–11. doi:10.1186/1743-422X-6-5 PMID:19138419

Dong, Z., Takakuwa, T., Takayama, H., Luo, W. J., Takano, T., Amino, N., ... Aozasa, K. (2002). Fas and Fas ligand gene mutations in Hashimoto's thyroiditis. *Laboratory Investigation*, *82*(12), 1611–1616. doi:10.1097/01.LAB.0000041700.09232.9C PMID:12480911

Donner, H., Braun, J., Seidl, C., Rau, H., Finke, R., Ventz, M., ... Badenhoop, K. (1997). Codon 17 polymorphism of the cytotoxic T lymphocyte antigen 4 gene in Hashimoto's thyroiditis and Addison's disease. *The Journal of Clinical Endocrinology and Metabolism*, *82*, 4130–4132. PMID:9398726

Duchatelet, S., Caillat-Zucman, S., Dubois-Laforgue, D., Blanc, H., Timsit, J., & Julier, C. (2008). FCRL3–169CT functional polymorphism in type 1 diabetes and autoimmunity traits. *Biomedicine and Pharmacotherapy*, *62*(3), 153–157. doi:10.1016/j.biopha.2007.09.003 PMID:17961971

Dultz, G., Matheis, N., Dittmar, M., Röhrig, B., Bender, K., & Kahaly, G. J. (2009). The protein tyrosine phosphatase non-receptor type 22 C1858T polymorphism is a joint susceptibility locus for immunthyroiditis and autoimmune diabetes. *Thyroid*, *19*(2), 14–148. doi:10.1089/thy.2008.0301 PMID:19090780

Duntas, L. H. (2010). Environmental factors and autoimmune thyroiditis. *Nature Clinical Practice. Endocrinology & Metabolism*, *4*(8), 454–460. doi:10.1038/ncpendmet0896 PMID:18607401

Elfström, P., Montgomery, S. M., Kämpe, O., Ekbom, A., & Ludvigsson, J. F. (2008). Risk of Thyroid disease in individuals with Celiac disease. *The Journal of Clinical Endocrinology and Metabolism*, *93*(10), 3915–3921. doi:10.1210/jc.2008-0798 PMID:18611971

Figueroa-Vega, N., Alfonso-Pérez, M., Benedicto, I., Sánchez-Madrid, F., González-Amaro, R., & Marazuela, M. (2010). Increased circulating pro-inflammatory cytokines and Th17 lymphocytes in Hashimoto's thyroiditis. *The Journal of Clinical Endocrinology and Metabolism*, *95*(2), 953–962. doi:10.1210/jc.2009-1719 PMID:20016049

Fountoulakis, S., Philippou, G., & Tsatsoulis, A. (2007). The role of iodine in the evolution of thyroid disease in Greece: From endemic goiter to thyroid autoimmunity. *Hormones (Athens, Greece)*, *6*, 25–35. PMID:17324915

Fountoulakis, S., Vartholomatos, G., Kolaitis, N., Frillingos, S., Philippou, G., & Tsatsoulis, A. (2008). Differential expression of Fas system apoptotic molecules in peripheral lymphocytes from patients with Graves' disease and Hashimoto's thyroiditis. *European Journal of Endocrinology*, *158*(6), 853–859. doi:10.1530/EJE-08-0092 PMID:18505906

Fountoulakis, S., Vartholomatos, G., Kolaitis, N., Frillingos, S., Philippou, G., & Tsatsoulis, A. (2008). HLA-DR expressing peripheral T regulatory cells in newly diagnosed patients with different forms of autoimmune thyroid disease. *Thyroid*, *18*(11), 1195–1200. doi:10.1089/thy.2008.0089 PMID:18925837

Fujimoto, T., Doi, K., Koyanagi, M., Tsunoda, T., Takashima, Y., Yoshida, Y., ... Shirasawa, S. (2009)..... Shirasawa, S. (2009). ZFAT is an antiapoptotic molecule and critical for cell survival in MOLT-4 cells. *FEBS Letters*, *583*(3), 568–572. doi:10.1016/j.febslet.2008.12.063 PMID:19162026

Gartner, R., Schopohl, D., Schaefer, S., Dugrillon, A., Erdmann, A., Toda, S., & Bechtner, G. (1997). Regulation of transforming growth factor beta-1 messenger ribonucleic acid expression in porcine thyroid follicles *in vitro* by growth factors, iodine, or delta-iodolactone. *Thyroid*, *7*(4), 633–640. doi:10.1089/thy.1997.7.633 PMID:9292955

Gibson, A. W., Li, F. J., Wu, J., Edberg, J. C., Su, K., Cafardi, J., ... Davis, R. S. (2009). The FCRL3–169CT promoter single-nucleotide polymorphism, which is associated with systemic lupus erythematosus in a Japanese population, predicts expression of receptor protein on CD19+B cells. *Arthritis & Rheumatology (Hoboken, N.J.), 60*(11), 3510–3512. doi:10.1002/art.24915 PMID:19877046

Giordano, C., Stassi, G., De Maria, R., Todaro, M., Richiusa, P., Papoff, G., ... Galluzzo, A. (1997, February 14). Potential involvement of Fas and its ligand in the pathogenesis of Hashimoto's thyroidiitis. *Science, 275*(5302), 960–965. doi:10.1126cience.275.5302.960

Giordano, C., Stassi, G., De Maria, R., Todaro, M., Richiusa, P., Papoff, G., ... Galluzzo, A. (1997). Potential involvement of Fas and its ligand in the pathogenesis of Hashimoto's thyroiditis. *Science, 275*(5302), 960–963. doi:10.1126cience.275.5302.960 PMID:9020075

Gokowski, F., Buziak-Bereza, M., Trofimiuk, M., Badys-Waligórska, A., Szybiski, Z., & Huszno, B. (2007). Increased prevalence of hyperthyroidism as an early and transient side-effect of implementing iodine prophylaxis. *Public Health Nutrition, 10*(8), 799–802. doi:10.1017/S1368980007585939 PMID:17381939

Green, L. M., Lazarus, J. P., LaBue, M., & Shah, M. M. (1995). Reduced cell-cell communication in a spontaneous murine model of autoimmune thyroid disease. *Endocrinology, 136*(8), 3611–3618. doi:10.1210/endo.136.8.7628400 PMID:7628400

Guimaraes, V. C., Quintans, J., Fisfalen, M. E., Straus, F. H., Fields, P. E., & Medeiros-Neto DeGroot, L. J. (1996). Immunosupression of thyroiditis. *Endocrinology, 137*(6), 2199–2207. doi:10.1210/endo.137.6.8641166 PMID:8641166

Hamano, H., Kawa, S., Horiuchi, A., Unno, H., Furuya, N., Akamatsu, T., ... Kiyosawa, K. (2001). High serum IgG4 concentrations in patients with sclerosing pancreatitis. *The New England Journal of Medicine, 344*(10), 737–328. doi:10.1056/NEJM200103083441005 PMID:11236777

Hawkins, B. R., Lam, K. L., Ma, J. C., Wang, C., & Yeung, R. T. (1987). Strong association between HLA-DRw9 and Hashimoto's thyroiditis in Southern Chinese. *Acta Endocrinologica*, *114*(4), 543–546. doi:10.1530/acta.0.1140543 PMID:3472422

Heydarian, P., Ordookhanim, A., & Azizim, F. (2007). Goiter rate, serum thyrotropin, thyroid autoantibodies and urinary iodine concentration in Tehranian adults before and after national salt iodization. *Journal of Endocrinological Investigation*, *30*(5), 404–410. doi:10.1007/BF03346318 PMID:17598973

Hidaka, Y., Amino, N., Iwatani, Y., Kaneda, T., Nasu, M., Mitsuda, N., ... Miyai, K. (1992). Increase in peripheral natural killer cell activity in patients with autoimmune thyroid disease. *Autoimmunity*, *11*(4), 239–243. doi:10.3109/08916939209035161 PMID:1581468

Hollowell, J. G., Staehling, N. W., Flanders, W. D., Hannon, W. H., Gunter, E. W., Spencer, C. A., & Braverman, L. E. (2002). Serum TSH, T(4), and thyroid antibodies in the United States population (1988 to 1994): National Health and Nutrition Examination Survey (NHANES III). *The Journal of Clinical Endocrinology and Metabolism*, *87*(2), 489–499. doi:10.1210/jcem.87.2.8182 PMID:11836274

Honda, K., Tamai, H., Morita, T., Kuma, K., Nishimura, Y., & Sasazuki, T. (1989). Hashimoto's thyroiditis and HLA in Japanese. *The Journal of Clinical Endocrinology and Metabolism*, *69*(6), 1268–1273. doi:10.1210/jcem-69-6-1268 PMID:2584361

Hunt, P. J., Marshall, S. E., Weetman, A. P., Bunce, M., Bell, J. I., Wass, J. A., & Welsh, K. I. (2001). Histocompatibility leucocyte antigens and closely linked immunomodulatory genes in autoimmune thyroid disease. *Horumon To Rinsho*, *55*(4), 491–499. doi:10.1046/j.1365-2265.2001.01356.x PMID:11678832

Ikari, K., Momohara, S., Nakamura, T., Hara, M., Yamanaka, H., Tomatsu, T., & Kamatani, N. (2006). Supportive evidence for a genetic association of the FCRL3 promoter polymorphism with rheumatoid arthritis. *Annals of the Rheumatic Diseases*, *65*(5), 671–673. doi:10.1136/ard.2005.043489 PMID:16176992

Ikegami, H., Awata, T., Kawasaki, E., Kobayashi, T., Maruyama, T., Nakanishi, K., ... Ogihara, T. (2006). The association of CTLA4 polymorphism with type 1 diabetes is concentrated in patients complicated with autoimmune thyroid disease: A multicenter collaborative study in Japan. *The Journal of Clinical Endocrinology and Metabolism*, *91*(3), 1087–1092. doi:10.1210/jc.2005-1407 PMID:16352685

Inoue, N., Watanabe, M., Morita, M., Tomizawa, R., Akamizu, T., Tatsumi, K., ... Iwatani, Y. (2010). Association of functional polymorphisms related to the transcriptional level of FOXP3 with prognosis of autoimmune thyroid diseases. *Clinical and Experimental Immunology*, *162*(3), 402–406. doi:10.1111/j.1365-2249.2010.04229.x PMID:20942809

Inoue, N., Watanabe, M., Nanba, T., Wada, M., Akamizu, T., & Iwatani, Y. (2009). Involvement of functional polymorphisms in the TNFA gene in the pathogenesis of autoimmune thyroid diseases and production of anti-thyrotropin receptor antibody. *Clinical and Experimental Immunology*, *156*(2), 199–204. doi:10.1111/j.1365-2249.2009.03884.x PMID:19250279

Ito, C., Watanabe, M., Okuda, N., Watanabe, C., & Iwatani, Y. (2006). Association between the severity of Hashimoto's disease and the functional +874A/T polymorphism in the interferon-gamma gene. *Endocrine Journal*, *53*(4), 473–478. doi:10.1507/endocrj.K06-015 PMID:16820703

Itoh, M., Takahashi, T., Sakaguchi, N., Kuniyasu, Y., Shimizu, J., Otsuka, F., & Sakaguchi, S. (1999). Thymus and Autoimmunity: Production of CD25+CD4+ naturally anergic and suppressive T Cells as a key function of the thymus in maintaining immunologic self-tolerance. *Journal of Immunology (Baltimore, Md.: 1950)*, *162*, 5317–5326. PMID:10228007

Jacobson, E. M., Huber, A., & Tomer, Y. (2008). The HLA gene complex in thyroid autoimmunity: From epidemiology to etiology. *Journal of Autoimmunity*, *30*(1-2), 58–62. doi:10.1016/j.jaut.2007.11.010 PMID:18178059

Jacobson, E. M., & Tomer, Y. (2007). The CD40, CTLA-4, thyroglobulin, TSH receptor, and PTPN22 gene quintet and its contribution to thyroid autoimmunity: Back to the future. *Journal of Autoimmunity*, *28*(2-3), 85–98. doi:10.1016/j.jaut.2007.02.006 PMID:17369021

Jiang, X., Feng, X., Li, G., Zhao, Q., & Yin, H. (2010). Differential expression of connexin 43 in human autoimmune thyroid disease. *Acta Histochemica, 112*(3), 278–283. doi:10.1016/j.acthis.2009.02.001 PMID:19321193

Jublanc, C., Beaudeux, J. L., Aubart, F., Raphael, M., Chadarevian, R., Chapman, M. J., ... Brucker.t, E. (2010). Serum l.evels of adhesion molecules ICAM-1 and VCAM-1 and tissue inhibitor of metallo-proteinases, TIMP-1, are elevated in patients with autoimmune thyroid disorders: Relevance to vascular inflammation N*utriti.on. Metabolism and Cardiovascular Disease, 10*, 817–822.

Kaczmarek, E., Lacka, K., Jarmolowska-Jurczyszyn, D., Sidor, A., & Majewski, P. (2011). Changes of B and T lymphocytes and selected apopotosis markers in Hashimoto's thyroiditis. *Journal of Clinical Pathology, 64*(7), 626–630. doi:10.1136/jcp.2010.086553 PMID:21242329

Kahaly, G. J., Dienes, H. P., Beyer, J., & Hommel, G. (1998). Iodide induces thyroid autoimmunity in patients with endemic goitre: A randomised, double-blind, placebo-controlled trial. *European Journal of Endocrinology, 139*(3), 290–297. doi:10.1530/eje.0.1390290 PMID:9758438

Kahles, H., Ramos-Lopez, E., Lange, B., Zwermann, O., Reincke, M., & Badenhoop, K. (2005). Sex-specific association of PTPN22 1858T with type 1 diabetes but not with Hashimoto's thyroiditis or Addison's disease in the German population. *European Journal of Endocrinology, 153*(6), 895–899. doi:10.1530/eje.1.02035 PMID:16322396

Kakudo, K., Li, Y., Taniguchi, E., Mori, I., Ozaki, T., Nishihara, E., ... Miyauchi, A. (2012). IgG4-related disease of the thyroid glands [Review]. *Endocrine Journal, 59*(4), 273–281. doi:10.1507/endocrj.EJ11-0309 PMID:22133985

Karanikas, G., Shuetz, M., Wahl, K., Paul, M., Kontur, S., Pietschmann, P., ... Willheim, M. (2005). Relation of anti-TPO autoantibody titer and T lymphocyte cytokine production patterns in Hashimoto's thyroiditis. *Horumon To Rinsho, 63*, 191–196. PMID:16060913

Kasagi, K., Takahashi, N., Inoue, G., Honda, T., Kawachi, Y., & Izumi, Y. (2009). Thyroid function in Japanese adults as assessed by a general health checkup system in relation with thyroid-related antibodies and other clinical parameters. *Thyroid, 19*(9), 937–944. doi:10.1089/thy.2009.0205 PMID:19678737

Kavvoura, F. K., Akamizu, T., Awata, T., Ban, Y., Chistiakov, D. A., Frydecka, I., ... Ioannidis, J. P. (2007). Cytotoxic T-lymphocyte associated antigen 4 gene polymorphisms and autoimmune thyroid disease: A meta-analysis. *The Journal of Clinical Endocrinology and Metabolism, 92*(8), 3162–3170. doi:10.1210/jc.2007-0147 PMID:17504905

Kawakami, A., Eguchi, K., Matsouka, N., Tsuboi, M., Kawabe, Y., Ishikawa, N., ... Nagataki, S. (1996). Thyroid-stimulating hormons inhibits Fas antigen-mediated apoptosis of human thyrocytes *in vitro*. *Endocrinology, 137*(8), 3163–3169. doi:10.1210/endo.137.8.8754734 PMID:8754734

Kawakami, Y., Fisfalen, E., & DeGroot, L. J. (1992). Proliferative responses of peripheral blood mononuclear cells from patients with autoimmune thyroid disease to synthetic peptide epitopes of human thyroid peroxidase. *Autoimmunity, 13*(1), 17–26. doi:10.3109/08916939209014631 PMID:1384731

Kochi, Y., Myouzen, K., Yamada, R., Suzuki, A., Kurosaki, T., Nakamura, Y., & Yamamoto, K. (2009). FCRL3, an autoimmune susceptibility gene, has inhibitory potential on B-cell receptor-mediated signaling. *Journal of Immunology (Baltimore, Md.: 1950), 183*(9), 5502–5510. doi:10.4049/jimmunol.0901982 PMID:19843936

Komatsu, K., Hamano, H., Ochi, Y., Takayama, M., Muraki, T., Yoshizawa, K., ... Kawa, S. (2005). High prevalence of hypothyroidism in patients with autoimmune pancreatitis. *Digestive Diseases and Sciences, 50*(6), 1052–1057. doi:10.100710620-005-2703-9 PMID:15986853

Kong, Y. M., Morris, G. P., Brown, N. K., Yan, Y., Flynn, J. C., & David, C. S. (2009). Autoimmune thyroiditis: A model uniquely suited to probe regulatory T cell function. *Journal of Autoimmunity, 33*(3-4), 239–246. doi:10.1016/j.jaut.2009.09.004 PMID:19822405

Kordonouri, O., Hartmann, R., Badenhoop, K., Kahles, H., & Ilonen, J. (2010). PTPN22 1858T allele is associated with younger age at onset of type 1 diabetes and is not related to subsequent thyroid autoimmunity. *Human Immunology, 71*(7), 731–732. doi:10.1016/j.humimm.2010.04.002 PMID:20438787

Kosugi, S., Ban, T., Akamizu, T., & Kohn, L. D. (1992). Identification of separate determinants on the thyrotropin receptor reactive with Graves' thyroid-stimulating antibodies and with thyroid-stimulating blocking antibodies in idiopathic myxedema: These determinants have no homologous sequence on gonadotropin receptors. *Molecular Endocrinology (Baltimore, Md.)*, *6*, 168–180. PMID:1349156

Kotsa, K., Watson, P. F., & Weetman, A. P. (1997). A CTLA-4 gene polymorphism is associated with both Graves' disease and autoimmune hypothyroidism. *Horumon To Rinsho*, *46*(5), 551–554. doi:10.1046/j.1365-2265.1997.1710996.x PMID:9231050

Koyanagi, M., Nakabayashi, K., Fujimoto, T., Gu, N., Baba, I., Takashima, Y., ... Shirasawa, S. (2008). ZFAT expression in B and T lymphocytes and identification of ZFAT-regulated genes. *Genomics*, *91*(5), 451–457. doi:10.1016/j.ygeno.2008.01.009 PMID:18329245

Kyogoku, C., Langefeld, C. D., Ortmann, W. A., Lee, A., Selby, S., Carlton, V. E., ... Behrens, T. W. (2004). Genetic association of the R620W polymorphism of protein tyrosine phosphatase PTPN22 with human SLE. *American Journal of Human Genetics*, *75*(3), 504–507. doi:10.1086/423790 PMID:15273934

Langer, P., Tajtáková, M., Kocan, A., Petrík, J., Koska, J., Ksinantová, L., ... Klimes, I. (2007). Thyroid ultrasound volume, structure and function after long-term high exposure of large population to polychlorinated biphenyls, pesticides and dioxin. *Chemosphere*, *69*(1), 118–217. doi:10.1016/j.chemosphere.2007.04.039 PMID:17537484

Li, C., Yuan, J., Zhu, Y. F., Yang, X. J., Wang, Q., Xu, J., ... Zhang, J. A. (2016). Imbalance of Th17/Treg in Different Subtypes of Autoimmune Thyroid Diseases. *Cellular Physiology and Biochemistry*, *40*(1-2), 245–252. doi:10.1159/000452541 PMID:27855396

Li, Y., Bai, Y., Liu, Z., Ozaki, T., Taniguchi, E., Mori, I., ... Kakudo, K. (2009). Immunohistochemistry of IgG4 can help subclassify Hashimoto's autoimmune thyroiditis. *Pathology International*, *59*(9), 636–641. doi:10.1111/j.1440-1827.2009.02419.x PMID:19712131

Lin, W. Y., Wan, L., Tsai, C. H., Chen, R. H., Lee, C. C., & Tsai, F. J. (2006). Vitamin D receptor gene polymorphisms are associated with risk of Hashimoto's thyroiditis in Chinese patients in Taiwan. *Journal of Clinical Laboratory Analysis*, *20*(3), 109–112. doi:10.1002/jcla.20110 PMID:16721822

Lopez, E. R., Zwermann, O., Segni, M., Meyer, G., Reincke, M., Seissler, J., ... Badenhoop, K. (2004). A promoter polymorphism of the CYP27B1 gene is associated with Addison's disease, Hashimoto's thyroiditis, Graves' disease and type 1 diabetes mellitus in Germans. *European Journal of Endocrinology*, *151*, 193–197. doi:10.1530/eje.0.1510193 PMID:15296474

Maierhaba, M., Zhang, J. A., Yu, Z. Y., Wang, Y., Xiao, W. X., Quan, Y., & Dong, B. N. (2008). Association of the thyroglobulin gene polymorphism with autoimmune thyroid disease in Chinese population. *Endocrine*, *33*(3), 294–299. doi:10.100712020-008-9082-x PMID:19034705

Mao, C., Pan, H., Chen, Q., Wang, X., Ye, D., & Qiu, L. (2010). Association between Fc receptor-like 3 C169T polymorphism and risk of systemic lupus erythematosus: A meta-analysis. *Molecular Biology Reports*, *37*(1), 191–196. doi:10.100711033-009-9591-6 PMID:19565352

Martino, E., Bartalena, L., Bogazzi, F., & Braverman, L. E. (2001). The effects of amiodarone on the thyroid. *Endocrine Reviews*, *22*, 240–254. PMID:11294826

Matesanz, F., Fernandez, O., Milne, R. L., Fedetz, M., Leyva, L., Guerrero, M., ... Alcina, A. (2008). The high producer variant of the Fc-receptor like-3 (FCRL3) gene is involved in protection against multiple sclerosis. *Journal of Neuroimmunology*, *195*(1-2), 146–150. doi:10.1016/j.jneuroim.2008.01.004 PMID:18313765

McLachlan, S. M., Nagayama, Y., Pichurin, P. N., Mizutori, Y., Chen, C., Misharinl, A., ... Rapoportet, B. (2007). The link between Graves' disease and Hashimoto's thyroiditis: A role for regulatory T cells. *Endocrinology*, *148*(12), 5724–5733. doi:10.1210/en.2007-1024 PMID:17823263

Mitasíková, M., Lin, H., Soukup, T., Imanaga, I., & Tribulová, N. (2009). Diabetes and thyroid hormones affect connexin-43 and PKC-epsilon expression in rat heart atria. *Physiological Research*, *58*, 211–217. PMID:18380541

Mitsiades, N., Poulaki, V., Kotoula, V., Mastorakos, G., Tseleni-Balafouta, S., Koutras, D., & Tsokos, M. (1998). Fas/Fas ligand up-regulation and Bcl-2 down-regulation may be significant in the patogenesis of Hashimoto's thyroiditis. *The Journal of Clinical Endocrinology and Metabolism, 83*, 2199–2203. PMID:9626160

Mitsiades, N., Poulaki, V., Mitsiades, C. S., Koutras, D. A., & Chrousos, G. P. (2001). Apoptosis induced by FasL and TRAIL/Apo2L in the pathogenesis of thyroid diseases. *Trends in Endocrinology and Metabolism, 12*(9), 384–390. doi:10.1016/S1043-2760(01)00441-6 PMID:11595539

Mori, T., Akamizu, T., Kosugi, S., Sugawa, H., Inoue, D., Okuda, J., & Ueda, Y. (1994). Recent progress in TSH receptor studies with a new concept of "Autoimmune TSH receptor disease". *Endocrine Journal, 41*(1), 1–11. doi:10.1507/endocrj.41.1 PMID:7524929

Muixí, L., Carrascal, M., Alvarez, I., Daura, X., Martí, M., Armengol, M. P., ... Jaraquemada, D. (2008). Thyroglobulin peptides associate in vivo to HLA-DR in autoimmune thyroid glands. *Journal of Immunology (Baltimore, Md.: 1950), 81*(1), 795–807. doi:10.4049/jimmunol.181.1.795 PMID:18566446

Nagata, S., & Golstein, P. (1995). The Fas death factor. *Science, 267*(5203), 1449–1456. doi:10.1126cience.7533326 PMID:7533326

Nakano, A., Watanabe, M., Iida, T., Kuroda, S., Matsuzuka, F., Miyauchi, A., & Iwatani, Y. (2007). Apoptosis-induced decrease of intrathyroidal CD4(+) CD25(+) regulatory T cells in autoimmune thyroid diseases. *Thyroid, 17*(1), 25–31. doi:10.1089/thy.2006.0231 PMID:17274744

Nanba, T., Watanabe, M., Akamizu, T., & Iwatani, Y. (2008). The -590CC genotype in the IL4 gene as a strong predictive factor for the development of hypothyroidism in Hashimoto disease. *Clinical Chemistry, 54*(3), 621–623. doi:10.1373/clinchem.2007.099739 PMID:18310157

Nanba, T., Watanabe, M., Inoue, N., & Iwatani, Y. (2009). Increases of the Th1/Th2 cell ratio in severe Hashimoto's disease and in the proportion of Th17 cells in intractable Graves' disease. *Thyroid, 19*(5), 495–501. doi:10.1089/thy.2008.0423 PMID:19415997

Ng, H. P., & Kung, A. W. (2006). Induction of autoimmune thyroiditis and hypothyroidism by immunization of immunoactive T cell epitope of thyroid peroxidase. *Endocrinology, 147*(6), 3085–3092. doi:10.1210/en.2005-1130 PMID:16527849

Nielsen, C. H., Brix, T. H., Leslie, R. G., & Hegedüs, L. (2009). A role for autoantibodies in enhancement of proinflammatory cytokine responses to a self-antigen, thyroid perioxidise. *Clinical Immunology (Orlando, Fla.), 133*(2), 118–127. doi:10.1016/j.clim.2009.07.014 PMID:19726232

Nielsen, C. H., Hegedüs, L., Rieneck, K., Moeller, A. C., Leslie, R. Q., & Bendtzen, K. (2006). Production of interleukin (IL)-5 and IL-10 accompanies T helper cell type 1 (Th2) cytokine responses to a major thyroid self-antigen, thyroglobulin, in health and autoimmune thyroid disease. *Clinical and Experimental Immunology, 147*(2), 287–295. doi:10.1111/j.1365-2249.2006.03283.x PMID:17223970

Nithiyananthan, R., Heward, J. M., Allahabadia, A., Franklyn, J. A., & Gough, S. C. (2002). Polymorphism of the CTLA-4 gene is associated with autoimmune hypothyroidism in the United Kingdom. *Thyroid, 12*(1), 3–6. doi:10.1089/105072502753451896 PMID:11842815

Nystrom, E., Bengtsson, C., Lapidus, L., Petersen, K., & Lindstedt, G. (1993). Smoking--A risk factor for hypothyroidism. *Journal of Endocrinological Investigation, 16*(2), 129–131. doi:10.1007/BF03347665 PMID:8463548

Okamura, K., Sato, K., Yoshinari, M., Ikenoue, H., Kuroda, T., Nakagawa, M., ... Fujishima, M. (1990). Recovery of the thyroid function in patients with atrophic hypothyroidism and blocking type TSH binding inhibitor immunoglobulin. *Acta Endocrinologica, 122*(1), 107–114. doi:10.1530/acta.0.1220107 PMID:1968305

Pacini, F., Vorontsova, T., Molinaro, E., Kuchinskaya, E., Agate, L., Shavrova, E., ... Pinchera, A. (1998). Prevalence of thyroid autoantibodies in children and adolescents from Belarus exposed to the Chernobyl radioactive fallout. *Lancet, 352*(9130), 763–7666. doi:10.1016/S0140-6736(97)11397-6 PMID:9737280

Pan, G., Ni, J., Wei, Y. F., Yu, G., Gentz, R., & Dixit, V. M. (1997). An antagonist decoy receptor and a death domain-containing receptor for TRAIL. *Science, 277*(5327), 815–818. doi:10.1126cience.277.5327.815 PMID:9242610

Pan, G., O'Rourke, K., Chinnaiyan, A. M., Gentz, R., Ebner, R., Ni, J. K., & Dixit, V. M. (1997). The receptor for the cytotoxic ligand TRAIL. *Science*, *276*(5309), 111–113. doi:10.1126cience.276.5309.111 PMID:9082980

Park, Y. J., Chung, H. K., Park, D. J., Kim, W. B., Kim, S. W., Koh, J. J., & Cho, B. Y. (2000). Polymorphism in the promoter and exon 1 of the cytotoxic T lymphocyte antigen-4 gene associated with autoimmune thyroid disease in Koreans. *Thyroid*, *10*(6), 453–459. doi:10.1089/thy.2000.10.453 PMID:10907987

Petrone, A., Giorgi, G., Mesturino, C. A., Capizzi, M., Cascino, I., Nistico, L., ... Buzzetti, R. (2001)..... Buzzetti R. (2001). Association of DRB1*04-DQB1*0301 haplotype and lack of association of two polymorphic sites at CTLA-4 gene with Hashimoto's thyroiditis in an Italian population. *Thyroid*, *11*(2), 171–175. doi:10.1089/105072501300042901 PMID:11288988

Rose, N. R., Bonita, R., & Burek, C. L. (2002). Iodine: An environmental trigger of thyroiditis. *Autoimmunity Reviews*, *1*(1-2), 97–103. doi:10.1016/S1568-9972(01)00016-7 PMID:12849065

Sahin, M., Gursoy, A., & Erdogan, M. F. (2009). Cytotoxic T lymphocyte-associated molecule-4 polymorphism in Turkish patients with Hashimoto thyroiditis. *International Journal of Immunogenetics*, *36*(2), 103–106. doi:10.1111/j.1744-313X.2009.00831.x PMID:19284444

Sakaguchi, S., Yamaguchi, T., Nomura, T., & Ono, M. (2008). Regulatory T cells and immune tolerance. *Cell*, *133*(5), 775–787. doi:10.1016/j.cell.2008.05.009 PMID:18510923

Sakai, K., Shirasawa, S., Ishikawa, N., Ito, K., Tamai, H., Kuma, K., ... Sasazuki, T. (2001). Identification of susceptibility loci for autoimmune thyroid disease to 5q31-q33 and Hashimoto's thyroiditis to 8q23-q24 by multipoint affected sib-pair linkage analysis in Japanese. *Human Molecular Genetics*, *10*(13), 1379–1386. doi:10.1093/hmg/10.13.1379 PMID:11440990

Shevach, E. M. (2006). From vanilla to 28 flavours: Multiple varieties of T regulatory cells. *Immunity*, *25*(2), 195–201. doi:10.1016/j.immuni.2006.08.003 PMID:16920638

Shi, Y., Wang, H., Su, Z., Chen, J., Xue, Y., Wang, S., ... Xu, H. (2010). Differe.ntiation imbalance of Th1/Th17 in peripheral blood mononuclear cells might contribute to pathogenesis of Hashimoto's thyroiditis *Scandan.avian. Journal of Immunology (Baltimore, Md.: 1950)*, *72*, 250–255. PMID:20696023

Shirasawa, S., Harada, H., Furugaki, K., Akamizu, T., Ishikawa, N., Ito, K., ... Sasazuki, T. (2004). SNPs in the promoter of a B cell-specific antisense transcript, SAS-ZFAT, determine susceptibility to autoimmune thyroid disease. *Human Molecular Genetics*, *13*(19), 2221–2231. doi:10.1093/hmg/ddh245 PMID:15294872

Simmonds, M. J. (2013). GWAS in autoimmune thyroid disease: Redefining our understanding of pathogenesis. *Nature Reviews. Endocrinology*, *9*(5), 277–287. doi:10.1038/nrendo.2013.56 PMID:23529038

Smyth, D., Cooper, J. D., Collins, J. E., Heward, J. M., Franklyn, J. A., Howson, J. M., ... Todd, J. A. (2004). Replication of an association between the lymphoid tyrosine phosphatase locus (LYP/PTPN22) with type 1 diabetes, and evidence for its role as a general autoimmunity locus. *Diabetes*, *53*(11), 3020–3023. doi:10.2337/diabetes.53.11.3020 PMID:15504986

Stefani, M., Papi, S., Suver, M., Glavas-Obrovac, L., & Karner, I. (2008). Association of vitamin D receptor gene 3′-variants with Hashimoto's thyroiditis in the Croatian population. *International Journal of Immunogenetics*, *35*(2), 125–131. doi:10.1111/j.1744-313X.2008.00748.x PMID:18279374

Takakuwa, T., Dong, Z., Takayama, H., Matsuzuka, F., Nagata, S., & Aozasa, K. (2001). Frequent mutations of Fas gene. *Cancer Research*, *61*(4), 1382–1385. PMID:11245438

Takasu, N., Yamada, T., Takasu, M., Komiya, I., Nagasawa, Y., Asawa, T., ... Koizumi, Y. (1992). Disappe.arance of thyrotropin-blocking antibodies and spontaneous recovery from hypothyroidism in autoimmune thyroiditis. *The New England Journal of Medicine*, *326*(8), 513–518. doi:10.1056/NEJM199202203260803 PMID:1732791

Tamaki, H., Amino, N., Kimura, M., Hidaka, Y., Takeoka, K., & Miyai, K. (1990). Low prevalence of thyrotropin receptor antibody in primary hypothyroidism in Japan. *The Journal of Clinical Endocrinology and Metabolism*, *71*(5), 1382–1387. doi:10.1210/jcem-71-5-1382 PMID:1977757

Terauchi, M., Yanagawa, T., Ishikawa, N., Ito, K., Fukazawa, T., Maruyama, H., & Saruta, T. (2003). Interactions of HLA-DRB4 and CTLA-4 genes influence thyroid function in Hashimoto's thyroiditis in Japanese population. *Journal of Endocrinological Investigation*, *26*(12), 1208–1212. doi:10.1007/BF03349159 PMID:15055474

Thompson, C. B. (1995). Apoptosis in the pathogenesis and treatment of disease. *Science*, *267*(5203), 1456–1462. doi:10.1126cience.7878464 PMID:7878464

Thomson, C. D., Campbell, J. M., Miller, J., & Skeaff, S. A. (2011). Minimal impact of excess iodate intake on thyroid hormones and selenium status in older New Zealanders. *European Journal of Endocrinology*, *165*(5), 745–752. doi:10.1530/EJE-11-0575 PMID:21878580

Toda, S., Nishimura, T., Yamada, S., Koike, N., Yonemitsu, N., Watanabe, K., ... Sugihar.a, H. (1999). Immunoh.istochemical expression of growth factors in subacute thyroiditis and their effects on thyroid folliculogenesis and angiogenesis in collagen gel matrix culture. *The Journal of Pathology*, *188*, 415–422. doi:10.1002/(SICI)1096-9896(199908)188:4<415::AID-PATH380>3.0.CO;2-H PMID:10440753

Tomer, Y. (2010). Genetic susceptibility to autoimmune thyroid disease: Past, present, and future. *Thyroid*, *20*(7), 715–725. doi:10.1089/thy.2010.1644 PMID:20604685

Tomer, Y. (2010). Hepatitis C and interferon induced thyroiditis. *Journal of Autoimmunity*, *34*(3), 322–326. doi:10.1016/j.jaut.2009.11.008 PMID:20022216

Tomer, Y., Ban, Y., Concepcion, E., Barbesino, G., Villanueva, R., Greenberg, D. A., & Davies, T. F. (2003). Common and unique susceptibility loci in Graves and Hashimoto diseases: Results of whole-genome screening in a data set of 102 multiplex families. *American Journal of Human Genetics*, *73*(4), 736–747. doi:10.1086/378588 PMID:12973666

Tomer, Y., Greenberg, D. A., Barbesino, G., Concepcion, E., & Davies, T. F. (2001). CTLA-4 and not CD28 is a susceptibility gene for thyroid autoantibody production. *The Journal of Clinical Endocrinology and Metabolism*, *86*, 1687–1693. PMID:11297604

Tomer, Y., Greenberg, D. A., Concepcion, E., Ban, Y., & Davies, T. F. (2002). Thyroglobulin is a thyroid specific gene for the familial autoimmune thyroid diseases. *The Journal of Clinical Endocrinology and Metabolism*, *87*(1), 404–407. doi:10.1210/jcem.87.1.8291 PMID:11788684

Toubi, E., & Shoenfeld, Y. (2010). The role of vitamin D in regulating immune responses. *The Israel Medical Association Journal*, *12*, 174–175. PMID:20684184

Ueda, H., Howson, J. M., Esposito, L., Heward, J., Snook, H., Chamberlain, G., ... Gough, S. C. (2003). Association of the T-cell regulatory gene CTLA4 with susceptibility to autoimmune disease. *Nature*, *423*(6939), 506–511. doi:10.1038/nature01621 PMID:12724780

Velaga, M. R., Wilson, V., Jennings, C. E., Owen, C. J., Herington, S., Donaldson, P. T., ... Pearce, S. H. (2004). The codon 620 tryptophan allele of the lymphoid tyrosine phosphatase (LYP) gene is a major determinant of Graves' disease. *The Journal of Clinical Endocrinology and Metabolism*, *89*(11), 5862–5865. doi:10.1210/jc.2004-1108 PMID:15531553

Wan, X. L., Kimura, A., Dong, R. P., Honda, K., Tamai, H., & Sasazuki, T. (1989). HLA-A and -DRB4 genes in controlling the susceptibility to Hashimoto's thyroiditis. *Human Immunology*, *42*(2), 131–136. doi:10.1016/0198-8859(94)00089-9 PMID:7744616

Wang, S. H., Bretz, J. D., Phelps, E., Mezosi, E., Arscott, P. L., Utsugi, S., & Baker, J. R. Jr. (2002). A unique combination of inflammatory cytokines enhances apoptosis of thyroid follicular cells and transforms nondestructive to destructive thyroiditis in experimental autoimmune thyroiditis. *Journal of Immunology (Baltimore, Md.: 1950)*, *168*(5), 2470–2474. doi:10.4049/jimmunol.168.5.2470 PMID:11859140

Wang, S. H., Van-Antwerp, M., Kuick, R., Gauger, P. G., Doherty, G. M., Fan, Y. Y., & Baker, J. R. Jr. (2007). Microarray analysis of cytokine activation of apoptosis pathways in the thyroid. *Endocrinology*, *148*(10), 4844–4852. doi:10.1210/en.2007-0126 PMID:17640998

Wasserman, E. E., Nelson, K., Rose, N. R., Rhode, C., Pillion, J. P., Seaberg, E., ... Yolken, R. H. (2009). Infection and thyroid autoimmunity: A seroepidemiologic study of TPOa-Ab. *Autoimmunity*, *42*(5), 439–446. doi:10.1080/08916930902787716 PMID:19811261

Watanabe, M., Yamamoto, N., Marouka, H., Tamai, H., Matsuzuka, F., Miyauchi, A., & Iwatani, Y. (2002). Independent involvement of CD8+CD25+ cells and thyroid autoantibodies in disease severity of Hashimoto's disease. *Thyroid, 12*(9), 801–808. doi:10.1089/105072502760339370 PMID:12481946

Weetman, A. P. (2004). Cellular immune responses in autoimmune thyroid disease. *Horumon To Rinsho, 61*, 405–413. PMID:15473869

Xiao, C., & Rajewsky, K. (2009). MicroRNA control in the immune system: Basic principles. *Cell, 136*(1), 26–36. doi:10.1016/j.cell.2008.12.027 PMID:19135886

Xu, J., Yang, X., Guo, H., Hou, X., Liu, L., & Sun, X. (2006). Selenium supplement alleviated the toxic effects of excessive iodine in mice. *Biological Trace Element Research, 111*(1-3), 229–238. doi:10.1385/BTER:111:1:229 PMID:16943608

Yamada, H., Watanabe, M., Nanba, T., Akamizu, T., & Iwatani, Y. (2008). The +869T/C polymorphism in the transforming growth factor-beta1 gene is associated with the severity and intractability of autoimmune thyroid disease. *Clinical and Experimental Immunology, 151*(3), 379–382. doi:10.1111/j.1365-2249.2007.03575.x PMID:18190611

Yu, X., Li, L., Li, Q., Zang, X., & Liu, Z. (2011). TRAIL and DR5 Promote Thyroid Follicular Cell Apoptosis in Iodine Excess-Induced Experimental Autoimmune Thyroiditis in NOD Mice. *Biological Trace Element Research, 143*(2), 1064–1076. doi:10.100712011-010-8941-5 PMID:21225479

Zaletel, K., & Gaberscek, S. (2011). Hashimoto's thyroiditis: From genes to the disease. *Current Genomics, 12*(8), 576–588. doi:10.2174/138920211798120763 PMID:22654557

Zaletel, K., Krhin, B., Gaberscek, S., Bicek, A., Pajic, T., & Hojker, S. (2010). Association of CT60 cytotoxic T lymphocyte antigen-4 gene polymorphism with thyroid autoantibody production in patients with Hashimoto's and postpartum thyroiditis. *Clinical and Experimental Immunology, 161*, 41–47. PMID:20408864

Zaletel, K., Krhin, B., Gaberscek, S., & Hojker, S. (2006). Thyroid autoantibody production is influenced by exon 1 and promoter CTLA-4 polymorphisms in patients with Hashimoto's thyroiditis. *International Journal of Immunogenetics*, *33*(2), 87–91. doi:10.1111/j.1744-313X.2006.00574.x PMID:16611252

Zeitlin, A. A., Heward, J. M., Newby, P. R., Carr-Smith, J. D., Franklyn, J. A., Gough, S. C., & Simmonds, M. J. (2008). Analysis of HLA class II genes in Hashimoto's thyroiditis reveals differences compared to Graves' disease. *Genes and Immunity*, *9*(4), 358–363. doi:10.1038/gene.2008.26 PMID:18449200

Zhu, J., Zhang, Y., Zhang, W., Zhang, W., Fan, L., Wang, L., ... Huang, G. (2016). MicroRNA-142-5p contributes to Hashimoto's thyroiditis by targeting CLDN1. *Journal of Translational Medicine*, *14*(1), 166–168. doi:10.118612967-016-0917-6 PMID:27277258

Chapter 7 Diagnosis

ABSTRACT

Clinically, a diffuse, firm goiter with pyramidal lobe enlargement, and without signs of thyrotoxicosis, should suggest the diagnosis of Hashimoto's thyroiditis (HT). The association of goiter with hypothyroidism is almost diagnostic. The thyroid stimulating hormone (TSH) is the sensitive marker of hypothyroidism and diagnosis of subclinical hypothyroidism. Thyroid perioxidase antibodies (TPO-Ab) and, less frequently, thyroglobulin antibodies (Tg-Ab) are elevated in the serum of patients with HT. Ultrasound may display an enlarged gland with normal texture, focal, or diffuse glandular enlargement with coarse, heterogenous, and hypo-echoic pattern, or a suggestion of multiple ill-defined micro-nodules. Color Doppler shows extensive hyper-vascularity. Histologically, the thyroid gland shows diffuse lymphocytic and plasma cell infiltration with formation of lymphoid follicles. Atrophy of the thyroid parenchyma is usually evident. It also reveals scant colloid, and a few epithelial cells, which may show Hurthle cell change. This chapter explores the diagnosis of Hashimoto's disease.

DOI: 10.4018/978-1-5225-9655-4.ch007

INTRODUCTION

Diagnosis of Hashimoto's thyroiditis involves two considerations; (1) differential diagnosis of the thyroid lesion and (2) assessment of the metabolic status.

Clinical Evaluation

A diffuse, firm *goiter* with pyramidal lobe enlargement, and without signs of thyrotoxicosis, should suggest the diagnosis of Hashimoto's thyroiditis. Most often the gland is bosselated. It is usually symmetrical, although much variation in symmetry (as well as consistency) can occur. The trachea is rarely deviated or compressed. The association of goiter with *hypothyroidism* is almost diagnostic of Hashimoto's disease, but is also seen in certain syndromes due to defective hormone synthesis or hormone response.

Pain and tenderness are unusual but may be present. A rapid onset is also unusual, but the goiter may rarely grow from normal to several times the normal size in a few weeks. Most commonly the gland is 2-4 times the normal size. Satellite *lymph nodes* may be present, especially the Delphian node above the isthmus. Multinodular goiter (MNG) occurs in significant incidence in adult women; thus the association of MNG and Hashimoto's thyroiditis is not rare, and may provide the finding of a grossly nodular gland in a patient who is mildly hypothyroid and has positive antibody tests.

Symptoms (History-Taking)

Common, *early presenting symptoms of hypothyroidism*, such as fatigue, constipation, dry skin, and weight gain, are non-specific. Weight gain due to hypothyroidism is usually no greater than 10% of the baseline euthyroid weight and is mostly attributable to fluid accumulation in interstitial tissues.

Other symptoms of hypothyroidism include the following:

- Cold intolerance
- Hoarseness of voice and pressure symptoms in the neck from thyroid enlargement
- Laziness and loss of energy (chronic fatigue syndrome), and less frequently erectile dysfunction.

- Decreased sweating
- Mild nerve deafness
- Peripheral neuropathy
- Galactorrhea (may occur because of the increased prolactin levels).
- Depression, dementia, and other psychiatric disturbances. Hashimoto's when presenting as *mania* is known as *Prasad's syndrome* after ***Ashok Prasad***, the psychiatrist who first described it.
- Memory loss
- Joint pains and muscle cramps
- Hair loss from an autoimmune process directed against the hair follicles
- Menstrual irregularities (typically menorrhagia, infertility, and loss of libido). Increased prolactin secondary to increased thyrotropin-releasing hormone (TRH) leads to decreased luteinizing hormone (LH) and follicle-stimulating hormone (FSH) and to decreased response to gonadotropin-releasing hormone (GnRH), resulting in anovulatory cycles with menstrual irregularities
- Sleep apnea and daytime somnolence (obstructive sleep apnea in hypothyroidism is thought to be partly caused by hypofunction of upper airway muscles and weakness of the diaphragm).

Physical Examination

Physical findings are variable and depend on the extent of *hypothyroidism* and other factors such as *age* of the patient. Findings include the following:

- Puffy face and peri-orbital edema typical of hypothyroid facies
- Cold, dry skin, which may be rough and scaly. The skin may appear yellow but does not involve the sclera, which distinguishes it from the yellowing of jaundice due to hypercarotenemia
- Peripheral edema of hands and feet, typically non-pitting
- Thickened and brittle nails (may appear ridged)
- Hair loss involving the scalp, the lateral third of eyebrows, and possibly skin, genital, and facial hair
- Bradycardia
- Elevated blood pressure (typically diastolic hypertension); however, most often, blood pressure is normal or even low
- Diminished deep tendon reflexes and the classic prolonged relaxation phase, most notable and initially described at the Achilles tendon (although it may be present in other deep tendon reflexes as well)

- Macroglossia
- The thyroid gland is typically enlarged, firm, and rubbery, without any tenderness or bruit; it may be normal in size or not palpable at all.
- Hoarseness of voice
- Slow speech
- Impairment memory
- Peripheral neuropathy (either mono-neuropathy as exemplified by carpal tunnel syndrome, or poly-neuropathy due to involvement of several peripheral nerves, manifesting as paresthesia.
- Cerebellar ataxia.

Laboratory Tests

Thyroid function tests are commonly employed to assess the hormonal status of HT by assessing the levels of thyroid stimulating hormone (TSH), tri-iodothyronine (T3), tetra-iodothyronine (T4). Among these TSH is the sensitive marker of hypothyroidism and diagnosis of subclinical hypothyroidism. Frequent monitoring of TSH is needed to assess the response of the treatment and disease progression.

Thyroxin (T4) Level

Total thyroxine (TT4) and free thyroxine (FT4) concentrations range from low to high, but are most typically in the normal or low range (McConahey, Keating, Butt, & Owen, 1961). The radio-active iodine uptake (RAIU) (rarely required) is variable and ranges from below normal to elevated values, depending on such factors as TSH levels, the efficiency of use of iodide by the thyroid, and the nature of the components being released into the circulation. When the serum TSH and the free T4 levels are low in the outpatient setting, the case for central hypothyroidism is strengthened. However, in the acutely ill patient, non-thyroidal illness (euthyroid sick syndrome) is the more likely possibility. The TSH level cannot be reliably used in some clinical settings to distinguish central hypothyroidism from non-thyroidal illness. Physical findings suggestive of thyroid disease, as well as the presence of obvious or subtle clinical features of hypothyroidism, become pivotal in establishing the correct diagnosis.

Tri-iodothyronin ((T3) Level

A low *T3 level* and a high reverse T3 level may be of additional help in the diagnosis of non-thyroidal illness. Serum T3 levels are most often maintained within reference ranges (even in the very late stages of hypothyroidism), and T3 measurement has little value in the diagnosis of hypothyroidism. Furthermore, T3 levels may be low in up to 70% of hospitalized patients without hypothyroidism or any thyroid disease, as is the case with non-thyroidal illness.

Serum TSH Level

Serum TSH reflects the patient's metabolic status. However, some patients are clinically euthyroid, with normal FT4 and T3 levels, but have mildly elevated TSH. Whether this "subclinical hypothyroidism" represents partial or complete compensation is a matter of debate. In the outpatient setting, when there is no cause to suspect hypothalamic or pituitary disease and in the absence of non-thyroidal illness and of medications that suppress TSH production in the inpatient setting, a normal TSH level excludes primary hypothyroidism from any cause. Medications that suppress TSH production include steroids, dopamine, dobutamine, and octreotide.

Gamma-Globulin Level

Gamma-globulin levels may be elevated, although usually they are normal (Glynne & Thomson, 1972). This alteration evidently reflects the presence of high concentrations of circulating antibodies to thyroglobulin (Tg), for an antibody concentration as high as 5.2 mg/ml has been reported.

Thyroid Antibodies

Thyroid perioxidase antibodies (TPO-Ab), and less frequently, *thyroglobulin antibodies* (Tg-Ab) are found in the serum of patients with Hashimoto's thyroiditis. High levels are diagnostic of autoimmune thyroid disease. However, 10-15% of patients with Hashimoto thyroiditis may be antibody-negative. Anti-TPO-Abs are considered as the best serological marker to establish the diagnosis of Hashimoto thyroiditis. It is positive in about 95% of patients whereas anti-Tg-Abs are positive in 60- 80%. Young patients tend to have lower and occasionally negative levels. In this age group, even low titers signify the presence of thyroid autoimmunity (McConahey, Keating, Butt, & Owen, 1961).

Histology / Cytology

Hashimoto thyroiditis is a histological diagnosis. Fine-needle aspiration (FNA) can be a useful diagnostic procedure but is *infrequently* required, except in patients that seem to have a discreet *nodule* in the gland. Typically, the thyroid gland shows diffuse lymphocytic and plasma cell infiltration with formation of lymphoid follicles from follicular hyperplasia and damage to the follicular basement membrane. Atrophy of the thyroid parenchyma is usually evident. It also reveals *scant* colloid, and a few epithelial cells which may show *Hurthle cell change*. In this context, Hurthle cells do *not* represent a discrete adenoma. However, if only abundant Hurthle cells dominate the specimen, and there are few or no lymphocytes or macrophages, the **biopsy** must be interpreted as a possible Hurthle cell tumor. Correlation of FNA findings with the presence of thyroid auto-antibodies, namely anti-TPO and anti-Tg, is helpful in confirming the diagnosis of Hashimoto's thyroiditis. Biopsy results are less frequently diagnostic in children (Monteleone, Davis, Tung, Ramos, & Peden, 1973).

Isotope Scanning

Thyroid isotope scan is *not* usually necessary, but can be helpful. The image is characteristically that of a diffuse or mottled uptake in an enlarged gland, in striking contrast to the focal "cold" and "hot" areas of multinodular goiter. Focal loss of isotope accumulation may occur in severely diseased portions of the thyroid. A cold thyroid nodule would indicate a higher risk for malignancy and therefore a need for fine-needle aspiration (FNA).

Ultrasound Imaging

Ultrasound (US) may display an enlarged gland with *normal* texture, focal or diffuse *glandular enlargement* with coarse, heterogenous and hypo-echoic pattern, or a suggestion of multiple ill-defined *nodules* (Figure 1) (Kawakami, Fisfalen, & DeGroot, 1992). The presence of discrete hypo-echoic micro-nodules (1-6 mm) is strongly suggestive of chronic thyroiditis. Fine echogenic fibrous septa may produce pseudo-lobulated appearance. *Color Doppler* shows extensive hyper-vascularity.

Although features of Hashimoto thyroiditis are usually identifiable on US, it is usually not necessary for diagnosing the condition. However, US is useful for assessing thyroid size, echotexture, and, most importantly, whether *thyroid nodules a*re present. Ultrasonographic study aids in confirming the presence of a thyroid nodule, in defining a nodule as solid or cystic, and in defining features suggestive of malignancy, such as irregular margins, a poorly defined halo, micro-calcification, and increased vascularity on Doppler examination.

Ultrasonography is also useful in facilitating FNA of nodules in general and, in particular, small or poorly-defined nodules when indicated and in patients with distorted neck anatomy. A definite diagnosis of benign *versus* malignant thyroid lesion can be confirmed only by cytological or histological examination of thyroid tissue.

Evaluating Variations in Presentation of Hashimoto's Thyroiditis

Small *atrophic gland* may be present at end stage of disease. *Nodular* form may be present in background of diffuse thyroiditis seen on ultrasound. *Benign*

Figure 1. Ultrasound imaging of the thyroid gland (right lobe longitudinal) in a person with Hashimoto thyroiditis

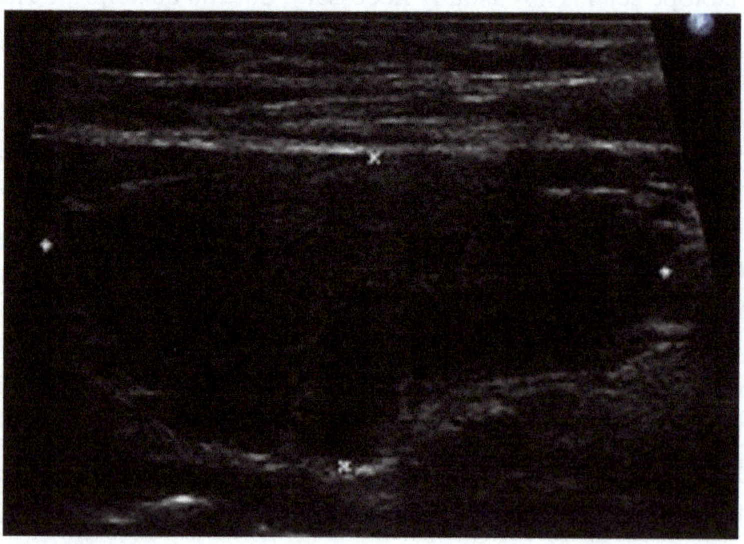

and malignant nodules may coexist in the background of diffuse thyroiditis. For differentiation between both, FNAC is needed.

Evaluating Complications of Hypothyroidism

The following tests are *not* necessary for the diagnosis of primary hypothyroidism but may be performed to evaluate complications of hypothyroidism in some patients, when clearly indicated.

Complete Blood Count

Up to 30-40% of patients with hypothyroidism have *anemia*, usually from decreased erythropoiesis. In 15% of patients, it is a microcytic, hypochromic iron deficiency anemia. Although this can be a normocytic normochromic anemia, the most common morphological abnormality is a macrocytic anemia that may be partially due to insufficient vitamin B_{12} and folate intake.

Total and Fractionated Lipid Profile

Total cholesterol, Low-density lipid (LDL), and triglyceride levels may be *elevated* in hypothyroidism and may be responsive to levothyroxine (L-T4) replacement.

Basic Metabolic Panel

Glomerular filtration rate, renal plasma flow, and renal free water clearance are all *decreased* in hypothyroidism and may result in hyponatremia.

Creatine Kinase

Creatine kinase levels, predominantly the MM isoenzyme from skeletal muscle and the aldolase enzyme, are frequently *elevated* in severe hypothyroidism.

Prolactin

Prolactin may be *elevated* in primary hypothyroidism, probably due to overlap secretion due to stimulation of the lactotroph by the elevated TRH level. The decreased clearance of prolactin in hypothyroidism may also play a contributory role. The elevated prolactin level leads to decreased gonadotropin secretion and decreased responsiveness to GnRH. The result of this is anovulatory cycles with menstrual abnormalities, galactorrhea, and infertility in some patients.

Additional Studies

Other studies that are usually *not* routinely necessary for diagnosis or evaluation of hypothyroid patients, but may be performed for evaluation of complications of primary hypothyroidism (when indicated) include:

- *Chest X-ray*: It may show small pleural effusions
- *Electrocardiogram (ECG):* It may show low-voltage QRS tracing, nonspecific ST-wave changes, and premature ventricular contractions; prolongation of the QT interval, and ventricular tachycardia may be noted
- *Echocardiogram*: It may show some pericardial effusion in severe cases of hypothyroidism.

Table 1. Characteristic diagnostic features of Hashimoto's thyroiditis

Parameters	Characteristic Features
Clinical - Gender - Age - Physical findings	Female: male ratio ranges from 3:1 to 15:1 Most common in the 3rd-4th decades) or 4th-6th decade (USA - Goiter: Usually diffuse, less commonly nodular) - Pain and tenderness may be present - Satellite LNs may be present
Biochemical - Thyroid function (TSH,T3,T4) - Thyroid antibodies	Early: hyperthyroid Later: hypothyroid: Subclinical or overt. Anti-TPO and anti-Tg antibodies: Elevated in > 90% of cases
Imaging (Ultrasound)	Enlarged gland with *normal* texture, focal or diffuse *glandular enlargement* with coarse, heterogenous and hypo-echoic pattern, or multiple ill-defined hypo-echoic micro-nodules.
Histological / Cytological	- Diffuse lymphocytic and plasma cell infiltration with formation of lymphoid follicles. - Lymphoid: epithelial ratio ranges from 2:1 to 10:1. - Scant colloid and a few epithelial cells which may show Hurthle cell change. - Paradoxical presence of colloid is not unusual due to Iodine supplementation and autoimmunity. - Associated lesions may occur: colloid goiter, cellular adenoma, follicular neoplasm, Hurthle cell neoplasm, PTC, non-Hodgkins lymphoma and follicular carcinoma; most commonly (PTC) and primary thyroid lymphoma.

LNs: lymph nodes, TSH: thyroid stimulating hormone, T4: thyroxine, T3: triiodothyronine, TPO: thyroid perioxidase, Tg: thyroglobulin, PTC: papillary thyroid carcinoma

Summary of Characteristic Features of Hashimoto's Thyroiditis

The main characteris clinical, biochemical, imaging and histological feature of Hashimoto's thyroiditis are summarized in Table 1 below (Singh, 2009; Bhatia, 2007; Larson, 2007; Thomas, 2014; Jayaram, 2007; Marconi, 1991; Marwaha, 1998;, Kumar, 2002; Poropatich, 1994).

REFERENCES

Bhatia, A., Rajwanshi, A., Dash, R. J., Mittal, B. R., & Saxena, A. K. (2007). Lymphocytic thyroiditis - is cytological grading significant? A correlation of grades with clinical, biochemical, ultrasonographic and radionuclide parameters. *CytoJournal*, *4*(1), 10–15. doi:10.1186/1742-6413-4-10 PMID:17470291

Glynne, A., & Thomson, J. A. (1972). Serum immunoglobulin levels in thyroid disease. *Clinical and Experimental Immunology*, *12*, 71–77. PMID:4628405

Jayaram, G., Iyengar, K. R., Sthaneshwar, P., & Hayati, J. N. (2007). Hashimoto's thyroiditis - A Malaysian perspective. *Journal of Cytology / Indian Academy of Cytologists*, *24*(3), 119–124. doi:10.4103/0970-9371.41898

Kawakami, Y., Fisfalen, M. E., & DeGroot, L. J. (1992). Proliferative responses of peripheral blood mononuclear cells from patients with autoimmune thyroid disease to synthetic peptide epitopes of human thyroid peroxidase. *Autoimmunit*, *13*(1), 17–26. doi:10.3109/08916939209014631 PMID:1384731

Kumar, N., Ray, C., & Jain, S. (2002). Aspiration cytology of Hashimoto's thyroiditis in an endemic area. *Cytopathology*, *13*(1), 31–39. doi:10.1046/j.1365-2303.2002.00366.x PMID:11985566

Larson, S. D., Jackson, L. N., Riall, T. S., Uchida, T., Thomas, R. P., Qiu, S., & Evers, B. M. (2007). Increased incidence of well-differentiated thyroid cancer associated with Hashimoto's thyroiditis and the role of the PI3k/Akt pathway. *Journal of the American College of Surgeons*, *204*(5), 764–773. doi:10.1016/j.jamcollsurg.2006.12.037 PMID:17481480

Marcocci, C., Vitti, P., Cetani, F., Catalano, F., Concetti, R., & Pinchera, A. (1991). Thyroid ultrasonography helps to identify patients with diffuse lymphocytic thyroiditis who are prone to develop hypothyroidism. *The Journal of Clinical Endocrinology and Metabolism*, *72*(1), 209–213. doi:10.1210/jcem-72-1-209 PMID:1986019

Marwaha, R. K., Sankar, R., Magdum, M., Nijahvan, V. S., Khanna, C. M., Jaggi, C. B., ... Jain, S. K. (1998). Clinical, biochemical and cytomorphological observations in juvenile chronic lymphocytic thyroiditis. *Indian Pediatrics*, *35*, 967–973. PMID:10216719

McConahey, W. M., Keating, F. R. Jr, Butt, H. R., & Owen, C. A. Jr. (1961). Comparison of certain laboratory tests in the diagnosis of Hashimoto's thyroiditis. *The Journal of Clinical Endocrinology and Metabolism*, *21*(8), 879–883. doi:10.1210/jcem-21-8-879 PMID:13773811

Monteleone, J. A., Davis, R. K., Tung, K. K., Ramos, C. V., & Peden, V. H. (1973). Differentiation of chronic lymphocytic thyroiditis and simple goiter in pediatrics. *The Journal of Pediatrics*, *83*(3), 381–385. doi:10.1016/S0022-3476(73)80259-8 PMID:4125140

Poropatich, C., Marcus, D., & Oertel, Y. C. (1994). Hashimoto's thyroiditis: Fine-needle aspirations of 50 asymptomatic cases. *Diagnostic Cytopathology*, *11*(2), 141–145. doi:10.1002/dc.2840110207 PMID:7813361

Singh, N., Kumar, S., Negi, V. S., & Siddaraju, N. (2009). Cytomorphologic study of Hashimoto's thyroiditis and its serologic correlation: A study of 150 cases. *Acta Cytologica*, *53*(5), 507–516. doi:10.1159/000325377 PMID:19798877

Thomas, T., Sreedharan, S., Khadilkar, U. N., Deviprasad, D., Kamath, M. P., Bhojwani, K. M., & Alva, A. (2014). Clinical, biochemical and cytomorphologic study on Hashimoto's thyroiditis. *The Indian Journal of Medical Research*, *140*(6), 729–735. PMID:25758571

Chapter 8
Clinical Course

ABSTRACT

The various clinical presentations of Hashimoto's thyroiditis (HT) include euthyroidism and goiter, subclinical hypothyroidism and goiter, primary thyroid failure, hypothyroidism, adolescent goiter, painless thyroiditis or silent thyroiditis, post-partum painless thyrotoxicosis, and alternating hypo- and hyper-thyroidism. Generally, the progress from euthyroidism to hypothyroidism is considered "irreversible" due to thyroid cell damage and loss of thyroidal iodine stores. Myxedema psychosis is a relatively uncommon consequence of hypothyroidism. Myxedema coma, a rare, life-threatening condition, occurs late in the progression of hypothyroidism when the body's compensatory responses to hypothyroidism are overwhelmed by a precipitating factor such as infection, medication, environmental exposure, or other metabolic-related stresses. Several unusual syndromes that are believed to be associated with HT include amyloidosis, interstitial pneumonitis, Vitiligo, hives, and alopecia. Hashimoto's encephalopathy and Hashimoto's ophthalmopathy are rare complications of HT. This chapter explores the clinical course of Hashimoto's disease.

DOI: 10.4018/978-1-5225-9655-4.ch008

INTRODUCTION

Hashimoto's thyroiditis begins as a gradual ***enlargement*** of the thyroid gland and gradual development of ***hypothyroidism***. It is often discovered by the patient, who finds a fullness of the neck or a new lump while self-examining because of a vague discomfort in the neck. Perhaps most often, it is found by the physician during the course of an examination for some other complaint.

There are many *symptoms* that are attributed to Hashimoto's thyroiditis or Hashimoto's disease. The most common symptoms include the following: fatigue, weight gain, pale or puffy face, feeling cold, joint and muscle pain, constipation, dry and thinning hair, heavy menstrual flow or irregular periods, depression, panic disorder, a slowed heart rate, and problems getting pregnant and maintaining pregnancy.

Hashimoto's disease is about seven times more common in women than in men. It can occur in teens and young women, but more commonly shows up in middle age, particularly for men. People who develop Hashimoto's disease often have family members who have thyroid or *other autoimmune diseases*, and sometimes have other autoimmune diseases themselves. Hashimoto's disease is also characterized by invasion of the thyroid tissue by leukocytes, mainly T-lymphocytes. A rare but serious complication is thyroid *lymphoma*, generally the B-cell type, non-Hodgkin lymphoma.

The various clinical presentations of Hashimoto's thyroiditis are summarized in Table 1.

Goiter (Neck Swelling)

In some cases the thyroid gland may become firm, large, and lobulated; rarely causing *pressure symptoms* such as dyspnea or dysphagia, or *mild pain* and *tenderness*. The goiter of Hashimoto's thyroiditis may remain unchanged for decades (Tunbridge et al., 1977), but usually it gradually increases in size.

Table 1. Presentations of Hashimoto's thyroiditis

1. Euthyroidism and goiter
2. Subclinical hypothyroidism and goiter
3. Primary thyroid failure
4. Hypothyroidism
5. Adolescent goiter
6. Painless thyroiditis or silent thyroiditis
7. Post-partum painless thyrotoxicosis
8. Alternating hypo- and hyper-thyroidism

Enlargement of the thyroid gland in Hashimoto's disease (thyroiditis) is due to lymphocytic infiltration and fibrosis rather than tissue hypertrophy.

Occasionally, the patients presents with symptoms of *mild thyrotoxicosis*, especially during the early phase of the disease (known as ***Hashi-toxicosis***). Symptoms and signs of *mild hypothyroidism* may be present in 20% of patients when first seen (Gordin, Saarinen, Pelkonen, & Lamberg, 1974), or commonly develop over a period of several years. Progression from ***subclinical hypothyroidism*** (normal FT4 but elevated TSH) to ***overt hypothyroidism*** (low FT4 but elevated TSH) occurs in approximately 3-5% of patients each year. Eventually, thyroid atrophy and ***myxedema*** may develop (Buchanan and Harden, 1965). This assertion is based on the clinical observation that patients with Hashimoto's thyroiditis often develop myxedema, and the knowledge that patients with myxedema due to atrophy of the thyroid have a high incidence of Tg-Ab in their serum. The disease frequently produces goitrous myxedema in young women.

Pain / Tenderness

Occasionally, patients with Hashimoto's thyroiditis have persistent pain, which is unresponsive to non-steroidal anti-inflammatory drugs (NSAIDs), replacement with L-thyroxine, and recurs after therapy with steroids. Kon and DeGroot (2003) reported seven patients who finally underwent subtotal or near-total thyroidectomy, some of whom received subsequent radioactive iodide (RAI) thyroid ablation, with final relief of symptoms.

Hypothyroidism

Generally, the progress from euthyroidism to hypothyroidism has been considered an ***irreversible*** process due to thyroid cell damage and loss of thyroidal iodine stores. However, it is currently evident that up to 25% of patients who are hypothyroid may *spontaneously return to normal function* over the course of several years. This sequence may reflect the initial effect of high titers of thyroid stimulation blocking antibodies, which fall with time and allow thyroid function to return (Takasu et al., 1992).

At 5 years of follow-up of the natural course of euthyroid Hashimoto's thyroiditis in Italian children, more than 50% of the patients remained or became euthyroid (Radetti et al., 2006). The presence of goiter and elevated Tg-Ab at presentation, together with progressive increase in both TPO-Ab and

TSH, may be predictive factors for the future development of hypothyroidism (Caturegli, Remigis, & Rose, 2014).

Myxedema Psychosis

Myxedema psychosis, more colloquially known as *"myxedema madness"*, is a relatively uncommon consequence of hypothyroidism, such as in Hashimoto's thyroiditis or in patients who have had their thyroids removed surgically, and are not taking thyroxine replacement therapy. A chronically under-active thyroid can lead to slowly progressive dementia, delirium, and in extreme cases to hallucinations, coma, or psychosis, particularly in the elderly (Mavroson, Patel, & Akker, 2017). It was first recognized by Dr. *Richard Ashe*r of London in 1949. Treatment is via the standard treatment for hypothyroidism with levothyroxine replacement, or in especially acute cases, liothyronine (sodium salt of T_3). Hormone replacement in these patients usually reverses the psychotic symptoms, but may not help with cognitive deficits caused by changes in metabolic activity in the central nervous system (CNS). The "myxedema" part of the name simply refers to the non-pitting edema common to hypothyroidism.

Myxedema Coma

Myxedema coma, a rare, life-threatening condition, occurs late in the progression of hypothyroidism. It occurs when the body's compensatory responses to hypothyroidism are overwhelmed by a precipitating factor such as infection, medication, environmental exposure, or other metabolic-related stresses. A common misconception is that a patient must be comatose to be diagnosed with myxedema coma. However, myxedema coma is a misnomer because most patients exhibit neither the non-pitting edema known as myxedema nor coma (Jordan, 1995; Nicoloff, 1993). Instead, the cardinal manifestation of myxedema coma is a deterioration of the patient's mental status.

Epidemiology

Myxedema coma occurs rarely, appearing in 0.1% of all cases of hypothyroidism. When only comatose patients are considered, myxedema coma is exceedingly rare: one study reports 200 cases between 1953 and 1996 (Werner, Ingbar,

Braverman, & Utiger, 2000). A study by Ono et al estimated the annual incidence of myxedema coma in Japan to be 1.08 per million people (ono et al., 1992).

Hypothyroidism is four times more common in women than in men; 80% of cases of myxedema coma occur in females (Davis, 1984; Bailes, 1999). Myxedema coma occurs almost exclusively in persons 60 years and older (Davis and Davis, 1984). Thus, the condition is seen typically in elderly women.

Etiology

Within the United States and developed nations, the major causes of hypothyroidism are autoimmune destruction of the thyroid gland (eg, Hashimoto thyroiditis) and iatrogenic secondary to the treatment of Graves' disease (surgical or radioactive iodine ablation of the thyroid gland). Primary hypothyroidism (dysfunction of the thyroid gland) accounts for up to 90-95% of cases. Secondary hypothyroidism (dysfunction of the pituitary or hypothalamus) accounts for most of the remainder of cases.

Primary causes include autoimmune, idiopathic, post-operative, and congenital etiologies; radiation; radioiodine therapy; iodine deficiency; metabolic disorders; and medications (eg, lithium, amiodarone, phenytoin, carbamazepine, iodides). Furthermore, those with underlying autoimmune thyroiditis are susceptible to disease progression while taking these medications. Antineoplastic agents are also recognized to cause thyroid dysfunction in 20-50% of patients (Hamnvik, Larsen, & Marqusee, 2011). *Secondary* causes include pituitary and hypothalamic disorders such as trauma, neoplasm, irradiation, and infiltrative diseases including sarcoidosis or amyloidosis.

Pathophysiology

Hypothyroidism can be caused by permanent loss or atrophy of functional thyroid tissue (primary hypothyroidism); insufficient stimulation of a normal thyroid gland as a result of hypothalamic or pituitary disease (secondary hypothyroidism, often accompanied by compensatory thyroid gland enlargement); or a defect in the TSH molecule (control hypothyroidism).

Precipitating Event

Decompensation into myxedema coma occurs when the hypothyroid patient's homeostatic mechanisms are disrupted. Multiple factors can precipitate myxedema coma (Table 2). (Mazonson, 1984; Waldman, 1989; Tsitouras, 1995; Ulsen, 1995; Smallride, 1992). Some of the more common precipitating factors include infections, particularly pneumonia and urosepsis, and certain medications. Another potential risk factor is failure to reinstate thyroid replacement therapy during hospitalization.

History –Taking

Patients with myxedema coma usually have longstanding hypothyroidism, although it may not have been previously diagnosed. They often demonstrate classic symptoms of hypothyroidism: fatigue; constipation; weight gain; cold intolerance; a deep voice; coarse hair; and dry, pale, cool skin. However, elderly patients with hypothyroidism often have atypical presentations, such as decreased mobility (Mintzer, 1991), and some patients with compensated hypothyroidism are asymptomatic (Robuschi, Safran, Braverman, Gnudi, & Roti, 1987).

Physical Findings

As shown in Table 3 (Ono, 2017; Bardin, 1997; Orr, 1981; Parving, 1982; Martinez, 1982), physical findings in myxedema coma may include the classic myxedematous face, characterized by generalized puffiness, macroglossia,

Table 2. Factors known to precipitate myxedema coma

Carbon dioxide retention	
Gastrointestinal hemorrhage	
Hypoglycemia	
Hypothermia	
Stroke	
Injury	Burns, surgery, trauma
Infection	Pneumonia, influenza, urinary tract infection.
Medications	Amiodarone, Anesthetics, Narcotics, Barbiturates, Duiretics, β-blockers, Lithium, Phenothiazines, Phenytoin, Rifampin, Tranquilizers

ptosis, periorbital edema, and coarse, sparse hair. Non-pitting edema of the lower extremities is sometimes present. The findings from a thyroid examination are usually normal, but a goiter may be present in some patients. The presence of a scar on the neck might suggest post-surgical hypothyroidism and may be an important clue in the diagnosis of a comatosed patient. Neurological examination may reveal decreased reflex tendon relaxation and may reveal altered mentation.

Diagnostic Tests

Multiple diagnostic findings are reported in patients with myxedema coma. This disorder impacts thyroid hormone levels, electrolyte levels, creatine kinase (CPK) levels and other laboratory values (Table 4) (Doran, 1975; Derubertis, 1971; Skowsky, 1978; Lowe, 1962; Horton, 1976; Mazzaferri, 1999).

Imaging Studies

- *Chest radiography*: An enlarged cardiac silhouette in a chest radiograph may suggest pericardial effusion as shown in Figure 2. However, chest X-ray is reported to have a 30% false-negative rate in detecting hypothyroid pericardial effusions. Chest radiography can help detect pulmonary infections often associated with myxedema coma.
- *Acute abdominal series*: An ileus may be associated with hypothyroidism, and it may be present in myxedema coma.
- *Head CT scan (non-contrast):* In patients with altered mental status, the scan may be helpful in ruling out other etiologies such as intra-cerebral hemorrhage. The scan may be helpful in ruling out other etiologies of altered mental status, such as intracerebral hemorrhage.

Other Tests

- *Electrocardiogram:* Bradycardia, low voltage, prolonged PR interval, T-wave abnormalities, and electrical alternans (suggestive of effusion) may be present.
- *Core temperature:* Patients with myxedema coma have a temperature below 37°C (98.6°F) in 15% of cases. About 15% of those patients have a temperature below 29.5°C (85°F).

Table 3. Physical findings in myxedema coma

Mentation	There is a decline in mentation, which may be subtle, manifesting as apathy, neglect or a decrease in intellectual function; more obvious changes include confusion, psychosis and, rarely, coma.
Reflexes	Pseudomyotonic reflexes, prolonged relaxation phase, usually at least twice as long as the contraction phase
Hair	Alopecia; loss of axillary and pubic hair and outer 1/3 of eyebrows
Skin	Dry, cool, coarse, and thickened with a yellowish appearance
Subcutaneous tissue	Non-pitting edema; waxy, dry edema, secondary to accumulation of polysaccharide
Urinary system	Bladder dystonia and distension
Cardiovascular system	Elevated diastolic blood pressure (early), hypotension (late), bradycardia.
Gastrointestinal tract	Decreased motility, paralytic ileus, abdominal distention, fecal impaction, myxedema megacolon.
Respiratory system	- Hyperventilation / hypoventilation. - Hypoventilation results from decreased ventilatory response to hypoxia and hyper-capnia. - Respiratory dysfunction may lead to sleep apnea, and dynspnea may be exacerbated by myxedematous infiltration of the tongue and pharynx. - Diaphragmatic weakness induced by hypothyroidism is reversed by thyroid hormone replacement.
Hypothermia	Patient's temperature is usually < 35.5°C (95.9°F). Some patients present with a normal temperature.
Myxedematous face	Generalized swelling, macroglossia, ptosis, peri-orbital edema, course sparse hair (Figure 1)
Neck	Goiter, thyroidectomy scar may be present

Differential Diagnoses

Myxedema coma should be differentiated from depression and suicide, heart failure, hepatic encephalopathy, hypothermia, and septic shock

Management

Pre-Hospital Care

Acute life-threatening conditions should be stabilized in patients with hypothyroidism, and supportive therapy initiated.

Figure 1. Myxedematous face. Lips may be also swollen

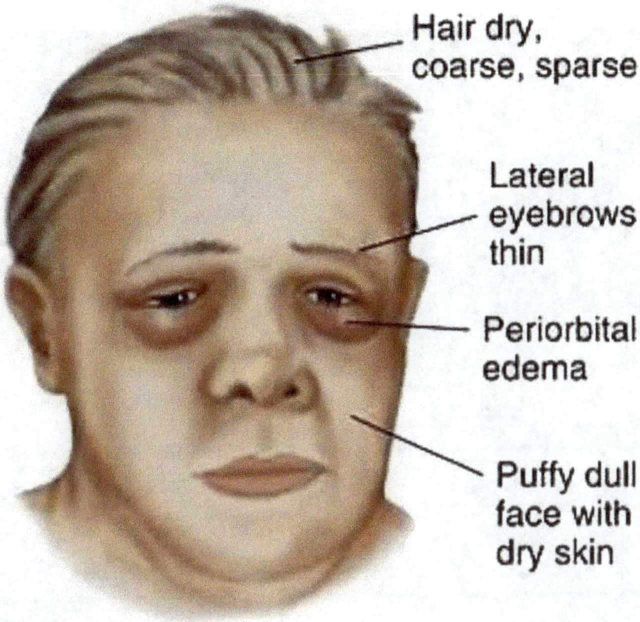

Table 4. Laboratory abnormalities in myxedema coma

Thyroid Hormones	Typically, patients with myxedema coma have primary hypothyroidism manifested by low serum levels of T_4 and T_3 and a high TSH level.
Elevated CPK and trans-aminases	Increased CPK (skeletl muscle source) and other transaminases result from altered membrane permeability.
Metabolic changes	- Hyperlipidemia. - Hypoglycemia, which result rom down-regulation of metabolism; and may also indicate the possibility of adrenal insufficiency.
Electrolyte changes	- Hyponatremia: It results from decreased free water clearance due to elevated levels of ADH and/or diminished blood flow to the kidneys. Serum creatinine is usually elevated. - The level of calcium is generally low, but may be elevated.
Arterial Blood Gases	Often reveal respiratory acidosis, hypoxia and hypercapnia.
Blood Picture	- Mild leucopenia - Normocytic anemia. Macrocytic anemia and pernicious anemia caused by associated immune dysfunction are sometimes present.
Lumbar puncture	Elevated protein levels.

CPK: creatinine phosphor-kinase; ADH: anti-diuretic hormone

Figure 2. Pericardial effusion. Note the "water-bottle" appearance of the cardiac silhouette.

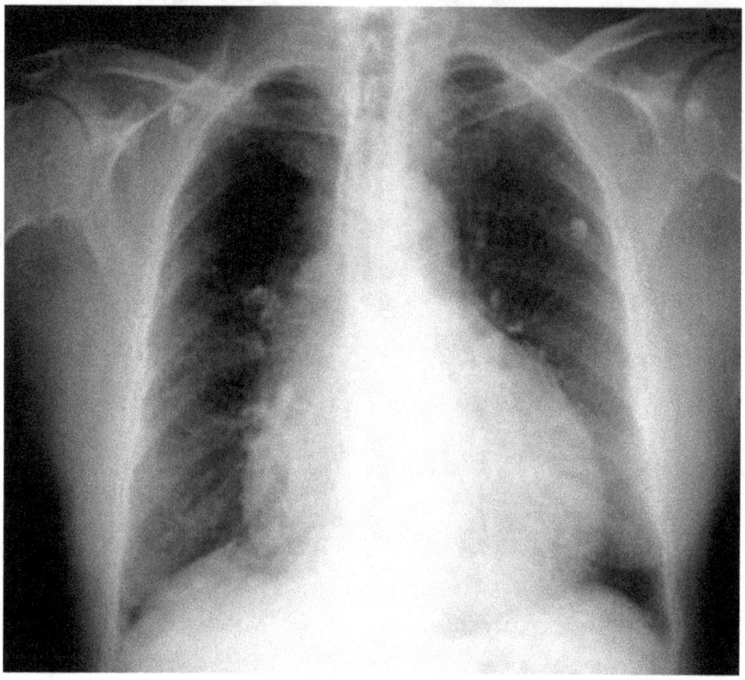

Emergency Department Care

Initial resuscitative measures should be implimented, including intravenous (IV) access, cardiac monitoring, and oxygen therapy, as indicated. Mechanical ventilation is indicated for patients with diminished respiratory drive or obtundation. Myxedema coma may lead to profound hemodynamic instability and airway compromise. A potentially difficult airway in patients with myxedema coma should be anticipated (Nicolof and Lopresti, 1993).

Inciting events such as infection should be investigated and treated immediately with appropriate antibiotics.

Hypotension may respond to crystalloid infusion. Occasionally, vasopressive agents are required. In refractory cases, hypotension may resolve with thyroid hormone replacement.

Treatment of hypothermia; most patients with myxedema coma respond to *passive* rewarming measures such as blankets and removal of cold or wet clothing; aggressive rewarming may lead to peripheral vasodilatation and hypotension. However, hemodynamically unstable patients with profound hypothermia require *active* rewarming measures.

Hyponatremia is treated initially with water restriction; however, if sodium levels are less than 120 mEq/L or any seizures occur, hypertonic saline is indicated.

Life-threatening causes of altered mental status are evaluated (eg, bedside glucose, pulse oximetry). If myxedema coma is suspected on clinical impression, *IV thyroid hormone treatment* should be started (prior to laboratory confirmation). The magnitude of hypothyroidism dictates the dose and route. Mild cases may be treated with gradual oral replacement, but patients with myxedema coma usually require large doses of IV replacement. General guidelines suggest administration of IV *levo-thyroxine* at a dose of 500-800 mcg. Alternatively, IV *liothyronine* can be given at a dose of 25 μg. The patient's heart should be monitored during hormone treatment, decreasing or discontinuing the dosage with any evidence of ischemia or dysrhythmia.

Physicians often recommend *glucocorticoid* replacement therapy because adrenal insufficiency may be concomitant (especially in patients with secondary hypothyroidism).

Medications such as sedatives, narcotics, and anesthetics should be vaoided. Metabolism of these agents may be slowed significantly, causing prolonged effects.

Further Inpatient Care

For further inpatient care, the patient should be admitted to the intensive care unit (ICU) and supportive ventilatory and hemodynamic management provided. Precipitating events such as infection are treated and rewarming continued as required. Diagnosis should be confirmed with laboratory testing and thyroid hormone replacement continued and converted to oral therapy when tolerated. Clinical improvement should be apparent within 24-36 hours of initiating thyroid hormone replacement.

Prognosis

The prognosis of hypothyroidism is good with early treatment. However, once the disease has progressed to myxedema coma, the mortality rate may exceed 20% in the treated population. Relapses occur if treatment is discontinued (Ono et al., 2017).

The mortality rate in myxedema coma has historically been as high as 80%. Some data suggest that aggressive management and early recognition have improved the mortality rate to 15-20%. However, a more recent observational study was unable to show significant differences in outcome based on replacement therapeutic methods, with a mortality rate remaining high at 40% (Beynon, Akhtar, & Kearney, 2008). Even with early detection and appropriate treatment, mortality ranges from 30 to 60 percent (Werner, Ingbar, Braverman, & Utiger, 2000).

Associated "Unusual" Syndromes

Within the past few years, several unusual syndromes believed to be associated with or part of the clinical spectrum of Hashimoto's thyroiditis have been described. Occasional patients develop ***amyloid*** *deposits* in the thyroid (Moriuchi et al., 1992). Shaw et al. (1991) described five patients with a relapsing steroid-responsive ***encephalopathy*** including episodes like stroke and seizures, high CSF protein, abnormal EEG, and normal CT scans. In the same year, Khardon et al. (1991) reported a steroid-responsive lymphocytic ***interstitial pneumonitis*** in four patients. It remains uncertain how these illnesses relate to lymphocytic thyroiditis, which has until now been largely identified as an organ-specific disease.

Hashimoto's thyroiditis and hypothyroidism are associated with Addison's disease, diabetes mellitus, hypogonadism, hypo-parathyroidism, and pernicious anemia. Such combinations are described as the ***polyglandular failure syndrome***. Two forms of polyglandular autoimmunity have been recognized (Eisenbart, Wilson, Ward, Buckley, & Lebovitz, 1979). In the ***Type I*** syndrome patients have hypoparathyroidism, muco-cutaneous candidiasis, Addison's disease, and occasionally hypothyroidism. ***Type II***, more frequent, often includes familial associations of diabetes mellitus, hypothyroidism, hypoadrenalism, and occasionally gonadal or pituitary failure. In these syndromes, antibodies reacting with the affected end organs are characteristically present. ***Vitiligo, hives, and alopecia*** are associated with thyroiditis. There is also a clear association with primary and secondary ***Sjogren's syndrome*** (Loviselli et al., 1988). Some patients appear to start with Hashimoto's thyroiditis, and progress with time to the picture of ***Riedel's thyroiditis*** including the frequently-associated ***retro-peritoneal fibrosis***. (Best, Munro, Burwell, & Volpe, 1991).

Musculoskeletal symptoms, including chest pain, fibrositis, and rheumatoid arthritis, occur in one-quarter of patients (Becker, Ferguson, & McConahey, 1963), and any of the musculoskeletal symptoms of hypothyroidism may likewise occur.

It has been suggested that thyroiditis predisposes to ***vascular** disease* and ***coronary*** occlusion. Abnormally elevated titers of thyroid auto-antibodies and the morphologic changes of thyroiditis are said to occur with an increased frequency among patients with coronary artery disease. Mild hypothyroidism associated with asymptomatic atrophic thyroiditis could predispose patients to heart disease (Bastenie et al., 1977). Others have failed to find increased Tg-Ab in patients with coronary artery disease or increased coronary disease in association with thyroiditis (Heinonen et al., 1972).

In *children*, retarded growth, retarded bone age, decreased hydroxyproline excretion, and elevated cholesterol levels may be seen.

The autoimmune phenomena that may occur or be found in association with Hashimoto thyroiditis are summarized in Table 5.

Neoplastic Transformation

Although chronic inflammation, leading to neoplastic transformation, is a well-established clinical phenomenon, the link between Hashimoto's thyroiditis and thyroid cancer remains controversial (Jankovic, 2013; Lee, 2013). Larson et al. (2007) reported that patients with Hashimoto's thyroiditis were three times more likely to have thyroid cancer, suggesting a strong link between chronic inflammation and cancer development. PI3K/Akt expression was increased in both Hashimoto's thyroiditis and well-differentiated thyroid

Table 5. Autoimmune phenomena associated with Hashimoto's thyroiditis

- Addison disease
- Alopecia (areata, totalis, and universalis)
- Autoimmune gastritis (pernicious anemia)
- Chronic active hepatitis (CAH)
- Idiopathic hypo-parathyroidism
- Poly-myalgia rheumatica and giant cell arteritis
- Primary biliary cirrhosis (PBC)
- Primary ovarian or testicular failure
- Rheumatoid arthritis
- Sjögren syndrome
- Systemic lupus erythematosus (SLE)
- Systemic sclerosis (scleroderma)
- Type-1 diabetes mellitus (DM)
- Vitiligo

cancer (WDTC), suggesting a possible molecular mechanism for thyroid carcinogenesis. Several authors reported that thyroid cancer may be associated with less aggressive disease and better outcome in patients with coexisting Hashimoto's thyroiditis (Dvorkin, 2013; Marotta, 2013).

Remission of Hashimoto's Thyroiditis - Pregnancy

Remission of Hashimoto's thyroiditis, with loss of goiter, hypothyroidism, and serum thyroid auto-antibodies, has been reported during pregnancy, with relapse after delivery (Amino et al., 1976). Antibody levels usually fall during pregnancy (Amino et al., 1978). These phenomena may reflect the immunosuppressive effects of pregnancy. After delivery thyroid auto-antibody levels rise, and after 2-6 months there may be sudden development of goiter and hypothyroidism (Amino et al., 1977). Endocrine Society Clinical Practice Guidelines were developed for the management of thyroid dysfunction during pregnancy and post-partum (Abalovich et al., 2007). In such cases, management requires special considerations because pregnancy induces major changes in thyroid function, and maternal thyroid disease can have adverse effects on the pregnancy and the fetus. Avoiding maternal (and fetal) hypothyroidism is of major importance because of potential damage to fetal neural development, an increased incidence of miscarriage, and preterm delivery.

Women who have low thyroid function that has not been stabilized are at greater risk of having an infant with: low birth weight, neonatal respiratory distress, hydrocephalus, hypospadias, miscarriage, and preterm delivery. Successful pregnancy outcomes are improved when Hashimoto's is treated. Recommendations are to only treat pregnant women who are TPOAb-positive throughout the entirety of their pregnancies and to screen all pregnant women for thyroid levels. Close cooperation between the endocrinologist and obstetrician benefits the woman and the infant. The Endocrine Society recommends screening in pregnant women who are considered high-risk for thyroid autoimmune disease.

Maternal *hyperthyroidism* and its treatment may be accompanied by coincident problems in fetal thyroid function. Autoimmune thyroid disease is associated with both increased rates of *miscarriage* and *post-partum thyroiditis* (PPT). Fine-needle aspiration cytology (FNAC) should be performed for dominant thyroid nodules discovered in pregnancy. Radioactive isotopes must be *avoided* during pregnancy and lactation. Universal screening of pregnant women for thyroid disease is *not* yet supported by adequate studies, but case finding targeted to specific groups of patients who are at increased risk is strongly supported. One study recommended screening all pregnant women for autoimmune thyroid disease in the first trimester in terms of cost-effectiveness (Dosiou, Sanders, Araki, & Crapo, 2008).

Maternal antibodies are known to cross the placenta, and as in Graves' disease, may affect the fetus and neonate. The TPO-Ab and Tg-Ab typically appear to have no adverse effect. Some evidence suggests cytotoxic antibodies, which are thought to be different from TPO-Ab or Tg-Ab, could cause fetal hypothyroidism (Amino, Tada, & Hidaka, 1999). However, TSH-Ab can rarely produce neonatal hypothyroidism, which is self-limiting over 4-6 weeks as the maternal IgG is metabolized. Women with positive TPO antibody before assisted reproduction have a significantly increased risk for miscarriage (Poppe et al., 2003).

Testing of thyroid peroxide (TPO) antibodies is recommended for women who have ever been pregnant regardless of pregnancy outcome. Previous pregnancy plays a major role in development of autoimmune overt hypothyroidism in pre-menopausal women, and the number of previous pregnancies should be taken into account when evaluating the risk of hypothyroidism in young women.

Painless (Silent) and Post-Partum Thyroiditis (PPT)

Silent (painless) thyroiditis is a syndrome that has a clinical course of thyroid dysfunction similar to subacute thyroiditis but with no anterior neck pain and no thyroid tenderness. Initially, patients have a thyrotoxic phase, later passing through euthyroidism to hypothyroidism and, finally, return to euthyroidism.

Post-partum thyroiditis (PPT) occurs within 6 months after delivery and runs an identical clinical course (Amino, Tada, & Hidaka, 1999). It is now considered to be identical to silent thyroiditis, and this term is used for patients who developed silent thyroiditis in the post-partum period. (Parving et al., 1982).

After delivery, *other forms of autoimmune thyroid dysfunction* also occur, including Graves' disease, transient hypothyroidism without preceding destructive thyrotoxicosis, and persistent hypothyroidism. In recent years, the term painless thyroiditis also has been used frequently, and the same disorder has been described using different names, such as thyrotoxicosis with painless thyroiditis (Woolf and Daly, 1976), occult subacute thyroiditis (Hamburger, 1976), hyper-thyroiditis (Woolf, 1980), lymphocytic thyroiditis with spontaneously resolving hyperthyroidism (Nikolai, Brosseau, Kettrick, Roberts, & Beltaos, 1980), painless thyroiditis and transient hyperthyroidism without goiter (Dorfman et al., 1977), and transient hyperthyroidism with lymphocytic thyroiditis (Gorman, Duick, Woolner, & Wahner, 1978). The thyrotoxicosis is induced by leakage of intra-thyroidal hormones into the circulation caused by damage to thyroid epithelial cells from inflammation. Thus, the thyroid radioactive iodine uptake (RAIU) is low (Gluck, Nusynowitz, & Plymate, 1975). Therefore, the early phase of thyrotoxicosis in silent thyroiditis, PPT, and subacute thyroiditis can be grouped together as destruction-induced thyrotoxicosis or simply as destructive thyrotoxicosis (Amino et al, 1978). When the measurement of RAIU is difficult, the measurement of anti-TSH receptor antibody and/or thyroid blood flow by ultrasonography (US) may be useful to differentiate between destruction-induced thyrotoxicosis and Graves' thyrotoxicosis. The quantitative measurement by power Doppler US was more effective than that of anti-TSH receptor antibody for differential diagnosis of these two types of thyrotoxicosis and may omit the radioactive iodine uptake test (ota et al., 2007).

During the clinical course of subclinical or very mild autoimmune thyroiditis, *aggravating factors* cause exacerbation of the destructive process. All women with subclinical autoimmune thyroiditis (Yoshida et al., 1978) and antithyroid microsomal antibodies of more than 1:5120 before pregnancy develop post-partum thyroiditis (Amino, Tada, & Hisaka, 1999). A significant percentage of patients with silent thyroiditis have personal or family history of autoimmune thyroid disease. Most patients have a complete remission, but some develop persistent hypothyroidism (Amino, Tada, & Hidaka, 1996). Some patients have had alternating episodes of typical "high-uptake" thyrotoxicosis and episodes of "transient" low-uptake thyrotoxicosis (Taylor and Sheelero, 1982).

Recurrence of disease is common in silent thyroiditis but very rare in subacute thyroiditis. Considering all these data, it is conceivable that silent thyroiditis is caused by an exacerbation of autoimmune thyroiditis induced by aggravating factors. Thyroiditis frequently recurs, and seasonal *allergic rhinitis* is reported to be an initiation factor (Yamamoto, Shibuya, Chen, & Ogata, 1988). Physically vigorous *massage on the neck* also was reported to be a contributing factor for silent thyroiditis (Tachi, Amino, & Miyai, 1990). The prevalence of silent thyroiditis, including post-partum disease, is approximately 5% of all types of thyrotoxicosis. Spontaneous silent thyroiditis is three times more frequent than PPT.

An immune rebound mechanism has been established for the induction of PPT. Post-partum thyroid destruction is associated with an increase in NK-cell counts and activity. Cessation of steroid therapy has initiated silent thyroiditis in a patient with autoimmune thyroiditis and *rheumatoid arthritis* (Maruyama, Kato, Mizuno, Kataoka, & Matusi, 1982), presumably because this also allows immune rebound. In patients with *Cushing's syndrome* who have associated subclinical autoimmune thyroiditis, silent thyroiditis has occurred after unilateral adrenalectomy (Takasu, Komiya, Nagasawa, Asawa, & Yamada, 1990).

Typically, painless thyroiditis or destructive thyrotoxicosis occurs at 2-4 months post-partum. The prevalence of PPT ranges from 3 to 8% of all pregnancies. Possible prevention of PPT, in a randomized prospective controlled study, 77 TPO+ pregnant women received 200 ug seleno-methionine daily starting at the 12th week of pregnancy, and 74 TPO+ women received a placebo. The treated group had significantly lower TPO antibody levels at the end of pregnancy and during the post-partum while on treatment. The incidence of PPT was reduced from 48.6 to 28.6% in the treated group, and the incidence of permanent hypothyroidism was equivalently reduced. Thyroid hormone levels did not differ (Negro et al., 2007).

Hashimoto's Encephalopathy

Hashimoto's encephalopathy or encephalitis is a *very rare* complication of Hashimoto's thyroiditis. Neurological complications are sometimes associated with thyroid dysfunction but patients with this encephalopathy are usually euthyroid. It a is treatable, steroid-responsive, progressive or relapsing encephalopathy associated with elevation of thyroid specific auto-antibodies (Peschen-rosin, Schabet, & Dichgans, 1999). Details will be discussed further in chapter 9.

Hashimoto's Ophthalmopathy

Thyroid-associated orbitopathy (TAO) usually occurs in Gravess' disease with hyperthyroidism, and sometimes in euthyroid and hypothyroid patients. Since most euthyroid and hypothyroid patients with orbitopathy are thyrotropin receptor antibody (TRAb)-positive, they are diagnosed as having euthyroid Graves' disease or hypothyroid Graves' disease. When euthyroid and hypothyroid patients with orbitopathy are TRAb-negative but associated with

Hashimoto's thyroiditis, "Hashimoto's ophthalmopathy" may be considered (Gateno, 2011; Yoshihara, 2011). Because patients with Hashimoto's thyroiditis test negative for TRAb, other auto-antibodies against an eye muscle antigen, such as calsequestrin, flavoprotein, or G2s were postulated (skillern et al., 1956). Details will be discussed further in chapter 10.

Summary of Hashimoto's Thyroiditis Presentations

Hashimoto's thyroiditis presents at the age group of 40-60 years with female predominance as painless enlargement of thyroid gland. Cases of painful goiter in Hashimoto's thyroiditis have been reported. Clinically, the patient can be euthyroid, hyperthyroid or hypothyroid based on the degree of thyroid destruction. Patients with Hashimoto's thyroiditis present initially with features of hyperthyroidism due to release of preformed thyroxine from the destroyed thyroid follicles. The disease then progresses to subclinical and overt hypothyroidism and ultimately thyroid failure.

There can be *local compressive* effect of the goiter such as dysphagia (esophagus), dysphonia (recurrent laryngeal nerve), and dyspnea (trachea). In the fibrous form, the thyroid gland appears lobulated with features of hypothyroidism. In the ***fibrous atrophy variant***, the gland may not be palpable and the patient presents with *idiopathic myxedema*. The ***IgG4-variant*** presents at the 5th decade with female to male ratio of 3:1 and has a rapid and aggressive course. The ***juvenile variant*** presents before the 18 years of age, and is usually asymptomatic. The ***Hashi-toxicosis variant*** has clinical features similar to Graves' hyperthyroidism initially, but finally hypothyroidism evolves. ***Painless (silent variant)*** occurs within 12 months after delivery (also known as ***post-partum thyroiditis***). Spontaneous recovery is possible after a period of time (Caturegli, De Remigis, Rose, 2014).

REFERENCES

Abalovich, M., Amino, N., Barbour, L. A., Cobin, R. H., De Groot, L. J., Glinoer, D., ... Stagnaro-Green, A. (2007). A. Management of thyroid dysfunction during pregnancy and postpartum: An Endocrine Society Clinical Practice Guideline. *The Journal of Clinical Endocrinology and Metabolism*, *92*(8Suppl), S1–S47. doi:10.1210/jc.2007-0141 PMID:17948378

Amino, N., Kuro, R., Tanizawa, O., Tanaka, F., Hayashi, C., Kotani, K., ... Kumahara, Y. (1978). Changes. of serum antithyroid antibodies during and after pregnancy in autoimmune thyroid diseases. *Clinical and Experimental Immunology*, *31*, 30–35. PMID:639347

Amino, N., Miyai, K., Kuro, R., Tanizawa, O., Azukizawa, M., Takai, S., ... Kumahara, Y. (1977). Transient postpartum hypothyroidism. Fourteen cases with autoimmune thyroiditis. *Annals of Internal Medicine*, *87*(2), 155–159. doi:10.7326/0003-4819-87-2-155 PMID:889196

Amino, N., Miyai, K., Onishi T., Hashimoto, T., Arai, K., Ishibashi, K., & Kumahara, Y. (1976). Transient hypothyroidism after delivery in autoimmune thyroiditis. *Journal of Clinical Endocrinology and Metabolism, 42*, 296-301.

Amino, N., Tada, H., & Hidaka, Y. (1996). Autoimmune thyroid disease and pregnancy. *Journal of Endocrinological Investigation*, *19*(1), 59–64. doi:10.1007/BF03347860 PMID:8851694

Amino, N., Tada, H., & Hidaka, Y. (1999). Postpartum autoimmune thyroid syndrome: A model of aggravation of autoimmune disease. *Thyroid*, *9*(7), 705–713. doi:10.1089/thy.1999.9.705 PMID:10447018

Amino, N., Yabu, Y., Miyai, K., Fujie, T., Azukizawa, M., Onishi, T., & Kumahara, Y. (1978). Differentiation of thyrotoxicosis induced by thyroid destruction from Graves' disease. *Lancet*, *2*(8085), 344–346. doi:10.1016/S0140-6736(78)92943-4 PMID:79711

Bailes, B. K. (1999). Hypothyroidism in elderly patients. *The Association of Pre-operative Registered Nurses*, *69*(5), 1026–1030. doi:10.1016/S0001-2092(06)62302-8 PMID:10332556

Bardin, C. W. (Ed.). (1997). *Current therapy in endocrinology and metabolism* (6th ed.). St. Louis, MO: Mosby.

Bastenie, P. A., Vanhaelst, L., Golstein, J., Smets, P., Keys, M. J., Karvonen, M. J., & Punsar, S. (1977). Asymptomatic autoimmune thyroiditis and coronary heart-disease. *Lancet, 1*, 155–159. doi:10.1016/S0140-6736(77)90177-5 PMID:69779

Becker, K. L., Ferguson, R. H., & McConahey, W. M. (1963). The connective-tissue diseases and symptoms associated with Hashimoto's thyroiditis. *The New England Journal of Medicine, 268*(6), 277–281. doi:10.1056/NEJM196302072680601 PMID:13970125

Best, T. B., Munro, R. E., Burwell, S., & Volpe, R. (1991). Riedel's thyroiditis associated with Hashimoto's thyroiditis, hypoparathyroidism, and retroperitoneal fibrosis. *Journal of Endocrinological Investigation, 14*(9), 767–772. doi:10.1007/BF03347912 PMID:1761813

Beynon, J., Akhtar, S., & Kearney, T. (2008). Predictors of outcome in myxoedema coma. *Critical Care (London, England), 12*(1), 111. doi:10.1186/cc6218 PMID:18254932

Buchanan, W. W., & Harden, R. M. (1965). Primary hypothyroidism and Hashimoto's thyroiditis. *Archives of Internal Medicine, 115*(4), 411–415. doi:10.1001/archinte.1965.03860160037006 PMID:14272368

Caturegli, P., De Remigis, A., & Rose, N. R. (2014). Hashimoto thyroiditis: Clinical and diagnostic criteria. *Autoimmunity Reviews, 13*(4-5), 391–397. doi:10.1016/j.autrev.2014.01.007 PMID:24434360

Caturegli, P., De Remigis, A., & Rose, N. R. (2014). Hashimoto thyroiditis: Clinical and diagnostic criteria. *Autoimmunity Reviews, 13*(4-5), 391–397. doi:10.1016/j.autrev.2014.01.007 PMID:24434360

Davis, P. J., & Davis, F. B. (1984). Hypothyroidism in the elderly. *Comprehensive Therapy, 10*, 17–23. PMID:6426851

Derubertis, F. R. Jr, Michelis, M. F., Bloom, M. E., Mintz, D. H., Field, J. B., & Davis, B. B. (1971). Impaired water excretion in myxedema. *The American Journal of Medicine, 51*(1), 41–53. doi:10.1016/0002-9343(71)90322-6 PMID:5570319

Doran, G. R., & Wilkinson, J. H. (1975). The origin of the elevated activities of creatine kinase and other enzymes in the sera of patients with myxoedema. *Clinica Chimica Acta, 62*(2), 203–211. doi:10.1016/0009-8981(75)90229-6 PMID:1149287

Dorfman, S. G., Copperman, M. T., Nelson, R. L., Depuy, H., Peake, R. L., & Young, R. L. (1977). Painless thyroiditis and transient hyperthyroidism without goiter. *Annals of Internal Medicine*, *86*(1), 24–28. doi:10.7326/0003-4819-86-1-24 PMID:576376

Dosiou, C., Sanders, G. D., Araki, S. S., & Crapo, L. M. (2008). Screening pregnant women for autoimmune thyroid disease: A cost-effectiveness analysis. *European Journal of Endocrinology*, *158*(6), 841–851. doi:10.1530/EJE-07-0882 PMID:18505905

Dvorkin, S., Robenshtok, E., Hirsch, D., Strenov, Y., Shimon, I., & Benbassat, C. A. (2013). Differentiated thyroid cancer is associated with less aggressive disease and better outcome in patients with coexisting Hashimotos thyroiditis. *The Journal of Clinical Endocrinology and Metabolism*, *98*(6), 2409–2414. doi:10.1210/jc.2013-1309 PMID:23609834

Eisenbart, G. S., Wilson, P. W., Ward, F., Buckley, C., & Lebovitz, H. (1979). The polyglandular failure syndrome. Disease inheritance, HLA type, and immune function. *Annals of Internal Medicine*, *1*(4), 528–533. doi:10.7326/0003-4819-91-4-528 PMID:314765

Gluck, F. B., Nusynowitz, M. L., & Plymate, S. (1975). Chronic lymphocytic thyroiditis, thyrotoxicosis, and low radioactive iodine uptake: Reports of four cases. *The New England Journal of Medicine*, *292*(13), 624–628. doi:10.1056/NEJM197509252931302 PMID:1089876

Gordin, A., Saarinen, P., Pelkonen, A., & Lamberg, B. A. (1974). Serum thyroglobulin and the response to thyrotropin releasing hormone in symptomless autoimmune thyroiditis and in borderline and overt hypothyroidism. *Acta Endocrinologica*, *75*(2), 274–279. doi:10.1530/acta.0.0750274 PMID:4133483

Gorman, C. A., Duick, D. S., Woolner, L. B., & Wahner, H. W. (1978). Transient hyperthyroidism in patients with lymphocytic thyroiditis. *Mayo Clinic Proceedings*, *53*, 359–365. PMID:580628

Hamburger, J. I. (1976). Occult subacute thyroiditis: Diagnostic challenge. *Michigan Medicine*, *70*, 1125–1129. PMID:5118969

Hamnvik, O. P., Larsen, P. R., & Marqusee, E. (2011). Thyroid dysfunction from antineoplastic agents. *Journal of the National Cancer Institute*, *103*(21), 1572–1587. doi:10.1093/jnci/djr373 PMID:22010182

Heinonen, O. P., Aho, K., Pyorala, K., Gordin, A., Punsar, S., & Puro, K. (1972). Symptomless autoimmune thyroiditis in coronary heart disease. *Lancet*, *1*(7754), 785–789. doi:10.1016/S0140-6736(72)90534-X PMID:4111258

Horton, L., Coburn, R. J., England, J. M., & Himsworth, R. L. (1976). The haematology of hypothyroidism. *The Quarterly Journal of Medicine*, *45*, 101–123. PMID:1257398

Jankovic, B., Le, K. T., & Hershman, J. M. (2013). Clinical Review: Hashimoto's thyroiditis and papillary thyroid carcinoma: is there a correlation? *The Journal of Clinical Endocrinology and Metabolism*, *98*(2), 474–482. doi:10.1210/jc.2012-2978 PMID:23293329

Jordan, R. M. (1995). Myxedema coma: Pathophysiology, therapy, and factors affecting prognosis. *The Medical Clinics of North America*, *79*(1), 185–194. doi:10.1016/S0025-7125(16)30091-8 PMID:7808091

Khardori, R., Eagleton, L. E., Soler, N. G., & McConnachie, P. R. (1991). Lymphocytic interstitial pneumonitis in autoimmune thyroid disease. *The American Journal of Medicine*, *90*(1), 649–652. doi:10.1016/0002-9343(91)90645-E PMID:2029024

Kon, Y. C., & Degroot, L. J. (2003). Painful Hashimoto's thyroiditis as an indication for thyroidectomy: Clinical characteristics and outcome in seven patients. *The Journal of Clinical Endocrinology and Metabolism*, *88*(6), 2667–2672. doi:10.1210/jc.2002-021498 PMID:12788871

Larson, S. D., Jackson, L. N., Riall, T. S., Uchida, T., Thomas, R. P., Qiu, S., & Evers, B. M. (2007). Increased incidence of well-differentiated thyroid cancer associated with Hashimoto thyroiditis and the role of the PI3k/Akt pathway. *Journal of the American College of Surgeons*, *204*(5), 764–673. doi:10.1016/j.jamcollsurg.2006.12.037 PMID:17481480

Lee, J. H., Kim, Y., Choi, J. W., & Kim, Y. S. (2013). The association between papillary thyroid carcinoma and histologically proven Hashimoto's thyroiditis: A meta-analysis. *European Journal of Endocrinology*, *168*(3), 343–349. doi:10.1530/EJE-12-0903 PMID:23211578

Loviselli, A., Mathieu, A., Pala, R., Mariotti, S., Cau, S., Marongiu, C., ... Martino, E. (1988). Development of thyroid disease in patients with primary and secondary Sjogren's syndrome. *Journal of Endocrinological Investigation*, *11*(9), 653–657. doi:10.1007/BF03350206 PMID:3221041

Lowe, C. E., Bird, E. D., & Thomas, W. C. Jr. (1962). Hypercalcemia in myxedema. *The Journal of Clinical Endocrinology and Metabolism*, *22*(3), 261–267. doi:10.1210/jcem-22-3-261 PMID:14466928

Marotta, V., Guerra, A., Zatelli, M. C., Uberti, E. D., Di Stasi, V., Faggiano, A., ... Vitale, M. (2013). BRAF mutation positive papillary thyroid carcinoma is less advanced when Hashimoto's thyroiditis lymphocytic infiltration is present. *Clinical Endocrinology*, *79*(5), 733–738. PMID:23469895

Martinez, F. J., Bermudez-Gomez, M., & Celli, B. R. (1989). Hypothyroidism. A reversible cause of diaphragmatic dysfunction. *Chest*, *96*(5), 1059–1063. doi:10.1378/chest.96.5.1059 PMID:2805837

Maruyama, H., Kato, M., Mizuno, O., Kataoka, K., & Matusi, S. (1982). Transient thyrotoxicosis occurred after cessation of steroid therapy in a patient with autoimmune thyroiditis and rheumatoid arthritis. *Endocrine Journal*, *29*(5), 583–588. doi:10.1507/endocrj1954.29.583 PMID:6897816

Mavroson, M. M., Patel, N., & Akker, E. (2017). Myxedema Psychosis in a Patient with Undiagnosed Hashimoto Thyroiditis. *The Journal of the American Osteopathic Association*, *117*(1), 50–57. doi:10.7556/jaoa.2017.007 PMID:28055088

Mazonson, P. D., Williams, M. L., Cantley, L. K., Dalldorf, F. G., Utiger, R. D., & Foster, J. R. (1984). Myxedema coma during long-term amiodarone therapy. *The American Journal of Medicine*, *77*(4), 751–754. doi:10.1016/0002-9343(84)90379-6 PMID:6486153

Mazzaferri, E. L., & Surks, M. I. (1999). Recognizing the faces of hypothyroidism. *Hospital Practice*, *34*(3), 109–110. doi:10.1080/21548331.1999.11443831 PMID:10089928

Mintzer, M. J. (1992). Hypothyroidism and hyperthyroidism in the elderly. *The Journal of the Florida Medical Association*, *79*, 231–235. PMID:1588294

Moriuchi, A., Yokoyama, S., Kashima, K., Andoh, T., Nakayama, I., & Noguchi, S. (1992). Localized primary amyloid tumor of the thyroid developing in the course of Hashimoto's thyroiditis. *Acta Pathologica Japonica*, *42*, 210–216. PMID:1570743

Negro, R., Greco, G., Mangieri, T., Pezzarossa, A., Dazzi, D., & Hassan, H. (2007). The influence of Selenium supplementation on postpartum thyroid status in pregnant women in thyroid perioxidase auto-antibodies. *The Journal of Clinical Endocrinology and Metabolism*, *92*(4), 1263–1268. doi:10.1210/jc.2006-1821 PMID:17284630

Nicoloff, J. T., & LoPresti, J. S. (1993). Myxedema coma. A form of decompensated hypothyroidism. *Endocrinology and Metabolism Clinics of North America*, *22*(2), 279–290. doi:10.1016/S0889-8529(18)30166-X PMID:8325287

Nikolai, T. F., Brosseau, J., Kettrick, M. A., Roberts, R., & Beltaos, E. (1980). Lymphocytic thyroiditis with spontaneously resolving hyperthyroidism (silent thyroiditis). *Archives of Internal Medicine*, *140*(4), 478–482. doi:10.1001/archinte.1980.00330160038023 PMID:6892676

Olsen, C. G. (1995). Myxedema coma in the elderly. *The Journal of the American Board of Family Practice*, *8*, 376–383. PMID:7484225

Ono, Y., Ono, S., Yasunaga, H., Matsui, H., Fushimi, K., & Tanaka, Y. (2017). Clinical characteristics and outcomes of myxedema coma: Analysis of a national inpatient database in Japan. *Journal of Epidemiology*, *27*(3), 117–122. doi:10.1016/j.je.2016.04.002 PMID:28142035

Ono, Y., Ono, S., Yasunaga, H., Matsui, H., Fushimi, K., & Tanaka, Y. (2017). Clinical characteristics and outcomes of myxedema coma: Analysis of a national inpatient database in Japan. *Journal of Epidemiology*, *27*(3), 117–122. doi:10.1016/j.je.2016.04.002 PMID:28142035

Orr, W. C., Males, J. L., & Imes, N. K. (1981). Myxedema and obstructive sleep apnea. *The American Journal of Medicine*, *70*(5), 1061–1066. doi:10.1016/0002-9343(81)90867-6 PMID:7234872

Ota, H., Amino, N., Morita, S., Kobayashi, K., Kubota, S., Fukata, S., ... Miyauchi, A. (2007). Quantitative measurement of thyroid blood flow for differentiation of painless thyroiditis from Graves' disease. *Horumon To Rinsho*, *67*(1), 41–45. doi:10.1111/j.1365-2265.2007.02832.x PMID:17437515

Parving, H. H., Helin, G., Garbarsch, C., Johansen, A. A., Jensen, B. A., Helin, P., ... Lyngsøe, J. (1982). Acid glycosaminoglycans in myxoedema. *Horumon To Rinsho*, *16*(2), 207–210. doi:10.1111/j.1365-2265.1982.tb03166.x PMID:6461440

Peschen-rosin, R., Schabet, M., & Dichgans, J. (1999). Manifestation of Hashimoto's encephalopathy years before onset of thyroid disease. *European Neurology*, *41*(2), 79–84. doi:10.1159/000008007 PMID:10023109

Poppe, K., Glinoer, D., Toumaye, H., Devroey, P., van Steirteghem, A., Kaufman, L., & Velkeniers, B. (2003). Assisted reproduction and thyroid autoimmunity: An unfortunate combination? *The Journal of Clinical Endocrinology and Metabolism*, *88*(9), 4129–4152. doi:10.1210/jc.2003-030268 PMID:12970279

Radetti, G., Gottardi, E., Bona, G., Corrias, A., Salardi, S., & Loche, S. (2006). Study Group for Thyroid Diseases of the Italian Society for Pediatric Endocrinology and Diabetes (SIEDP/ISPED).The natural history of euthyroid Hashimoto's thyroiditis in children. *The Journal of Pediatrics*, *149*(6), 827–832. doi:10.1016/j.jpeds.2006.08.045 PMID:17137901

Robuschi, G., Safran, M., Braverman, L. E., Gnudi, A., & Roti, E. (1987). Hypothyroidism in the elderly. *Endocrine Reviews*, *8*(2), 142–153. doi:10.1210/edrv-8-2-142 PMID:3301318

Shaw, P. J., Walls, T. J., Newman, P. K., Cleland, P. G., & Cartlidge, N. E. (1991). Hashimoto's encephalopathy: A steroid-responsive disorder associated with high antithyroid antibody titers -- report of five cases. *Neurology*, *41*(2, Part 1), 228–233. doi:10.1212/WNL.41.2_Part_1.228 PMID:1992366

Skillern, P. G., Crile, G. Jr, McCullaugh, E. P., Hazard, J. B., Lewis, L. A., & Brown, H. (1956). Struma lymphomatosa: Primary thyroid failure with compensatory thyroid enlargement. *The Journal of Clinical Endocrinology and Metabolism*, *16*(1), 35–39. doi:10.1210/jcem-16-1-35 PMID:13278381

Skowsky, W. R., & Kikuchi, T. A. (1978). The role of vasopressin in the impaired water excretion of myxedema. *The American Journal of Medicine*, *64*(4), 613–621. doi:10.1016/0002-9343(78)90581-8 PMID:645727

Smallridge, R. C. (1992). Metabolic and anatomic thyroid emergencies: A review. *Critical Care Medicine*, *20*(2), 276–291. doi:10.1097/00003246-199202000-00016 PMID:1737461

Tachi, J., Amino, N., & Miyai, K. (1990). Massage therapy on neck: A contributing factor for destructive thyrotoxicosis? *Thyroidology*, *2*, 25–27. PMID:1715747

Takasu, N., Komiya, I., Nagasawa, Y., Asawa, T., & Yamada, T. (1990). Exacerbation of autoimmune thyroid dysfunction after unilateral adrenalectomy in patients with Cushing's syndrome due to an adrenocortical adenoma. *The New England Journal of Medicine*, *322*(24), 1708–1712. doi:10.1056/NEJM199006143222404 PMID:2342537

Takasu, N., Yamada, T., Takasu, M., Komiya, I., Nagasawa, Y., Asawa, T., ... Koizumi, Y. (1992). Disappearance of thyrotropin-blocking antibodies and spontaneous recovery from hypothyroidism in autoimmune thyroiditis. *The New England Journal of Medicine*, *326*(8), 513–518. doi:10.1056/NEJM199202203260803 PMID:1732791

Tateno, F., Sakakibara, R., Kishi, M., & Ogawa, E. (2011). Hashimoto's ophthalmopathy. *The American Journal of the Medical Sciences*, *342*(1), 83–85. doi:10.1097/MAJ.0b013e318219bcf6 PMID:21701269

Taylor, H. C., & Sheeler, L. R. (1982). Recurrence and heterogeneity in painless thyrotoxic lymphocytic thyroiditis. Report of five cases. *Journal of the American Medical Association*, *248*(9), 1085–1088. doi:10.1001/jama.1982.03330090055029 PMID:6896731

Tsitouras, P. D. (1995). Myxedema coma. *Clinics in Geriatric Medicine*, *11*(2), 251–258. doi:10.1016/S0749-0690(18)30295-7 PMID:7606694

Tunbridge, W.G., Evered, D.C., Hall, R., Appleton, D., & Brewis, M., ... Smith, P.A. (1977). The spectrum of thyroid disease in a community. The Whickham Survey. *Horumon To Rinsho*, *7*, 481–485. PMID:598014

Waldman, S. A., & Park, D. (1989). Myxedema coma associated with lithium therapy. *The American Journal of Medicine*, *87*(3), 355–356. doi:10.1016/S0002-9343(89)80168-8 PMID:2773973

Werner, S. C., Ingbar, S. H., Braverman, L. E., & Utiger, R. D. (2000). *Werner & Ingbar's. The thyroid: a fundamental and clinical text* (8th ed.). Philadelphia, PA: Lipincott Williams &Wilkins.

Woolf, P. D. (1980). Transient painless thyroiditis with hyperthyroidism. A variant of lymphocytic thyroiditis. *Endocrine Reviews*, *1*(4), 411–416. doi:10.1210/edrv-1-4-411 PMID:7018893

Woolf, P. D., & Daly, R. (1976). Thyrotoxicosis with painless thyroiditis. *The American Journal of Medicine*, *60*(1), 73–79. doi:10.1016/0002-9343(76)90535-0 PMID:56130

Yamamoto, M., Shibuya, N., Chen, L. C., & Ogata, E. (1988). Seasonal recurrence of transient hypothyroidism in a patient with autoimmune thyroiditis. *Endocrine Journal*, *35*(1), 135–142. doi:10.1507/endocrj1954.35.135 PMID:3396511

Yoshida, H., Amino, N., Yagawa, K., Uemura, K., Satoh, M., Miyai, K., & Kumahara, Y. (1978). Association of serum antithyroid antibodies with lymphocytic infiltration of the thyroid gland: Studies of seventy autopsied cases. *The Journal of Clinical Endocrinology and Metabolism*, *46*(6), 859–863. doi:10.1210/jcem-46-6-859 PMID:263468

Yoshihara, A., Yoshimura, N. J., Nakachi, A., Ohye, H., Sato, S., Sekiya, K., ... Ito, K. (2011). Severe thyroid-associated orbitopathy in Hashimoto's thyroiditis. Report of two cases. *Endocrine Journal*, *58*(5), 343–348. doi:10.1507/endocrj.K11E-019 PMID:21427503

Chapter 9
Hashimoto's Encephalopathy

ABSTRACT

Hashimoto's encephalopathy is a relapsing encephalopathy occurring in association with Hashimoto's thyroiditis (HT) with high titers of anti-thyroid antibodies. The mechanism of pathogenesis is unknown. Auto-antibodies to α-enolase have been found to be associated with Hashimoto's encephalopathy. Recently, the crucial role of neuro-inflammation in the development of psychological disorders including depression and anxiety has received more attention. Because the majority of patients with Hashimoto's encephalopathy respond to steroids or immuno-suppressant treatment, this condition is now also referred to as "steroid-responsive encephalopathy." Initial treatment is usually with oral prednisone (50–150 mg/day) or high-dose IV methyl-Prednisolone (1 g/day) for 3-7 days. Thyroid hormone treatment is also included if required. This chapter explores Hashimoto's encephalopathy.

INTRODUCTION

Hashimoto's encephalopathy is an uncommon neurological condition associated with Hashimoto's thyroiditis and characterized by encephalopathy, thyroid autoimmunity, and good clinical response to steroids. It is sometimes referred to as a neuro-endocrine disorder, although the condition's relationship to the endocrine system is widely disputed (Graus et al., 2016).

Originally described in 1966, Hashimoto's encephalopathy remains a somewhat controversial disorder. It is most often characterized by a subacute onset of confusion with altered level of consciousness, seizures, and myoclonus.

DOI: 10.4018/978-1-5225-9655-4.ch009

In contrast to the cognitive dysfunction associated with hypothyroidism or hyperthyroidism, Hashimoto's encephalopathy is believed to be an immune-mediated disorder rather than representing the direct effect of an altered thyroid state on the central nervous system.

Up to the year 2005, there were almost 200 published case reports of Hashimoto's encephalopathy. From 1990 to 2000, 43 cases were published. Since that time, research has expanded and numerous cases are being reported by scientists around the world, suggesting that this rare condition is likely to have been significantly undiagnosed in the past. Over 100 scientific articles on Hashimoto's encephalopathy were published between 2000 and 2013 *(Brain, Jellinek, & Ball, 1966).*

Definition

Hashimoto's encephalopathy is a relapsing encephalopathy occurring in association with Hashimoto's thyroiditis, with high titers of anti-thyroid antibodies. Clinically, the condition may present one or more symptoms. Onset is often gradual and may go unnoticed by the patient and close associates to the patients. Symptoms sometimes resolve themselves within days to weeks, leaving a patient undiagnosed. For many other patients, the condition may result in ongoing problems with a variety of manifestations, often confusing clinicians due to the diffuse nature of symptoms.

Synonyms

Hashimoto's encephalopathy has also been known by the following alternative names:

- Steroid-responsive encephalopathy associated with autoimmune thyroiditis (SREAT).
- Non-vasculitic autoimmune meningo-encephalitis (NAIM)
- Encephalopathy associated with autoimmune thyroid disease (EAATD)

History

Brain et al. (1966) described the first case of Hashimoto's encephalopathy The patient was a 48-year-old man with hypothyroidism, multiple episodes of encephalopathy, and stroke-like symptoms as well as Hashimoto's thyroiditis confirmed by elevated anti-thyroid antibodies.

Epidemiology

The prevalence has been estimated to be 2.1/100,000 with a male to female ratio of 1:4. The mean age of onset is 44 with 20% of cases presenting before the age of 18 years *(Fujii et al., 2005).* Most reported cases occur during the patient's fifth decade of life.

Pathogenesis

The mechanism of pathogenesis is *unknown*. It does not appear to be directly related to hypothyroidism or hyperthyroidism, as the majority of reported patients are euthyroid at the time of presentation. A *toxic effect* of increased thyrotropin-releasing hormone on the central nervous system has been proposed, as some patients appear to improve with thyroid supplementation despite being euthyroid. However, these cases appear to be the exception rather than the rule. The bulk of evidence points to an *autoimmune* disorder similar to Hashimoto's thyroiditis as its name suggests (*autoimmune vasculitis*) or other inflammatory process, perhaps associated with immune complex deposition, and possibly disrupting the cerebral micro-vasculature.

Consistent with this hypothesis, auto-antibodies to α-enolase have been found to be associated with Hashimoto's encephalopathy (Payer, Petrovic, Lisy, & Langer, 2012). Since enolase is the penultimate step in glycolysis, if it were inhibited (for example by being bound by auto-antibodies) one would expect decreased energy production by each cell, leading to resulting *atrophy* of the affected organ.

This would occur most likely through each cell shrinking in size in response to the energy deficit (and/or in extreme situations from some cells dying via either apoptosis or necrosis, depending on location) (Ihejirika, 2014). This may occur as a result of there not being enough ATP to maintain cellular functions: notably failure of the Na/K ATPase, resulting in a loss of the gradient to drive the Na/Ca anti-porter, which normally keeps Ca^{++} out of cells so that it does not build to toxic levels that will rupture cell lysosomes leading to apoptosis. An additional feature of a low energy state is failure to maintain axonal transport via Dynein/Kinesin ATPases, which in many diseases results in neuronal injury to both the brain and/or periphery (Blanchin, 2007).

In fact, thyroid autoantibody from patients with Hashimoto's disease have been reported (in- vitro) to bind astrocytes (Moodley, Botha, Raidoo, & Naidoo, 2011). The presence of antigenic sites for thyroid autoantibodyon neural tissues also has been demonstrated (Berris, and Owen, 1965). Thus, these studies suggest that thyroid autoantibody may cross-react with auto-antigens expressed in the brain and modulate local immune responses. Please, discuss these findings in the sub-section.

Recently, the crucial role of neuro-inflammation in the development of psychological disorders including depression and anxiety has received more attention. Characteristic features of neuro-inflammation include the activation of microglia and astroglia and generation of pro-inflammatory cytokines (Cai et al., 2018). Using an animal model, Cai et al. (2018) reported that Hashimoto's thyroiditis (HT) mice showed intra-thyroidal monocyte infiltration and rising serum thyroid autoantibody levels accompanied by *normal* thyroid function, which defines euthyroid HT in humans. These mice displayed more anxiety- and depressive-like behaviors than controls despite a similar thyroid functional state between the two groups. In humans, several authors reported impairments of mental well-being in patients with HT that were shown to be independent of thyroid function (Hammar, 1975; Edvardsson, 2010; Pinelli, 1990; Hannan, 2016; Bektas, 2012).

Furthermore, HT mice showed microglia and astrocyte activation in the frontal cortex detected by immunohistochemistry (IHC), real-time polymerase chain reaction (RT-PCR), and transmission electron microscopy (TEM) with microglia showing phagocytic function and astrocytes tending to show features involved in active proteosynthesis. An increasing number of human studies have reported microglia activation in the CNS of patients with psychiatric disorders, such as depression, schizophrenia, and anxiety (Striano, 2006; Ferlazzo, 2006). Results from animal models have shown that neuro-inflammation is closely associated with abnormal emotional behavior, which could be improved after anti-inflammatory treatment (Canton, 2000; Al0Busaidi, 2017; Ashworth, 1965). Notably, studies on brain biopsy revealed activated microglia and reactive astrocytes in patients with Hashimoto's encephalopathy (Sinharay, 2002; Varrasi, 2017).

Cai et al. (2018) reported also that microglia and astrocyte activation in the frontal cortex (in HT mice) observations were also accompanied by enhanced gene expression of the pro-inflammatory cytokines interleukin 1L-1beta (*IL-1β*) and tumor necrosis-alpha (*TNF-α*) in the frontal cortex. Despite this inflammatory response, *no* signs of neuronal apoptosis were visible by the TUNEL staining (Terminal deoxynucleotidyl transferase-mediated dUTP-biotin nick end labeling staining) and transmission electron microscopy (TEM) in the frontal cortex of HT mice, which is in line with previous studies showing that increased brain inflammatory response was not functionally associated with neuronal apoptosis or neuronal damage (Ghihka-Schmid, 1996; Marshall, 2006; Yu, 2014; Salpetro, 2014). Additionally, Indoleamine-2,3-dioxygenase (IDO1) and serotonin transported (SERT), key serotonin-system-related genes activated by pro-inflammatory cytokines, were upregulated in HT mice, accompanied by reduced frontal cortex serotonin levels. In vivo studies have suggested that central inflammatory signaling activation significantly upregulates IDO1 and/or SERT, resulting in depressive-like behavior in animals (Berger, 2010; Shah, 2011; Hommat, 2007). Indeed, IDO-1 and SERT are crucial regulators of central 5-HT signaling, which plays vital roles in the development of psychiatric symptoms in humans and animals (Hilberath, Schmidt, & Wolf, 2014). These findings suggest that HT induces *neuro-inflammation* and alters related serotonin signaling in the euthyroid state, which may underlie the deleterious effects of HT itself on emotional function.

The *mechanisms* by which HT induces neuro-inflammation in the euthyroid state are still unknown. In an animal model, hypothyroidism was associated with an increased number of astrocyte cells in the brain (Graham et al., 2016). Moreover, different studies described the presence of antigenic sites for thyroid anto-antibodies (TA) on neural tissues (Pari, 2014; Ercoli, 2019), and most recently, anti-thyroglobulin (anti-Tg) has been shown to immunolocalize to vascular smooth muscle of all limbic regions, including frontal cortex (Sawka, Fatourechi, Boeve, & Mokri, 2002). In the study by Cai et al. (2018), they described the increased presence of TA in the frontal cortex of HT mice. It appears reasonable to then propose that TA may *cross-react* with auto-antigens expressed in the brain and modulate local immune responses.

Blanchin et al. (2008) explored the neurological targets of anti-thyroperoxidase (TPO) auto-antibodies in Hashimoto's encephalopathy. They reported that high levels of anti-TPO auto-antibodies were detected in Hashimoto's encephalopathy group's cerebrospinal fluids. In immuno-fluorescence assays on monkey brain cerebellum sections, both Hashimoto's encephalopathy patients' sera and anti-TPO monoclonal antibodies were able to bind cerebellar cells expressing glial fibrillary acid protein. Normal human astrocytes from primary cultures also reacted with anti-TPO monoclonal antibodies. Specific astrocyte binding of anti-TPO auto-antibodies suggests a role of these auto-antibodies in the pathogenesis of Hashimoto's encephalopathy.

Hashimoto's encephalopathy is not to be caused by thyroid dysfunction or antithyroid antibodies, but rather represents an *association of an uncommon autoimmune encephalopathy* with a common autoimmune thyroid disease (Sawka, Fatourechi, Boeve, & Mokri, 2002). Identification of antibodies to brain specific antigens may disclose the real pathogenesis of this condition. Recently, auto-antibodies against the amino NH_2-terminal of α-enolase (referred to as NAE) were reported to be highly specific in the serum of a limited number of Hashimoto's encephalopathy patients (11%, 2/17), but in none of controls (n=25) including those with other neurological or immunological conditions involving encephalopathy (Yoneda, 2007; Seo, 2003).

Steroid reversible cerebral hypo-metabolism was recently documented by PET-scan in this condition (Hosoi, Kono, Terada, Konishi, & Miyajima, 2013). There is a report that Hashimoto's encephalopathy is associated with elevated intra-thecal and serum IgG4 levels Ercoli, T., Defazio, G., & Muroni, A. (2019). Additional case studies, including histological investigations and measurements of IgG4, are needed to elucidate the pathological role of IgG4 in Hashimoto's encephalopathy.

Pathology

Very little is known about the pathology of Hashimoto's encephalopathy. Post-mortem studies of some individuals have shown lymphocytic vasculitis of venules and veins in the brain-stem and a diffuse gliosis involving gray matter more than white matter.

As mentioned above, auto-antibodies to alpha-enolase associated with Hashimoto's encephalopathy have been the most hypothesized mechanism of injury.

Recently, Ercoli et al. (2019) reviewed the literature (1965 to 2018) and identified 37 cases of cebellar disorders associated with Hashimoto encephalopathy.[(39)] Patients presented with signs of ataxia, mostly predictive of vermis involvement and frequent impairment of cerebellar hemispheres. Signs and symptoms consistent with a dysfunction of the flocculonodular lobe (vertigo, nystagmus) were only evident in a minority of patients. Additional neurological signs, such as dystonia (Tang, 2011; Termsarasab, 2018; Matsunaga, 2013), psychiatric symptoms (personality changes and depression) (Selim and Drachman, 2001), ocular disturbances (Alvarez, 2017; Lee, 2015; Avila, 2013; Castillo, 2006), and myoclonus, could also be found in Hashimoto's encephalopathy patients (Lee, 2015; Avila, 2013;

Castillo, 2006). When present, atrophy of vermis and often of both cerebellar hemispheres was the main pathological abnormality confirmed by imaging in Hashimoto encephalopathy (Tang et al., 2011).

Clinical Presentation

The onset of symptoms in Hashimoto's encephalopathy tends to be fairly gradual and to occur over 1–7 days.

Symptoms of Hashimoto's encephalopathy may include:

- Personality changes
- Aggression
- Delusional behavior
- Concentration and memory problems
- Coma
- Disorientation
- Headaches
- Jerks in the muscles (myoclonus – 65% of cases)
- Lack of coordination (ataxia – 65% of cases)
- Partial paralysis on the right side
- Psychosis
- Seizures (60% of cases)
- Sleep abnormalities (55% of cases)
- Speech problems (transient aphasia – 80% of cases)
- Status epilepticus (20% of cases)
- Tremors (80% of cases)

Diagnosis

General Laboratory Findings

- Increased liver enzyme levels (55% of cases)
- Increased thyroid-stimulating hormone (TSH) (55% of cases)
- Increased erythrocyte sedimentation rate (ESR) (25% of cases)

Cerebro-Spinal Fluid (CSF) Findings

- Raised protein (25% of cases)

- Negative for 14–3–3 protein
- May contain anti-thyroid antibodies.
- Thyroid Hormone Abnormalities (>80% of cases):
- Subclinical hypothyroidism (35% of cases)
- Overt hypothyroidism (20% of cases)
- Hyperthyroidism (5% of cases)
- Euthyroid on levothyroxine (10% of cases)
- Euthyroid not on levothyroxine (20% of cases)

Thyroid Antibodies

Both anti-thyroid peroxidase antibodies (anti-TPO, anti-thyroid microsomal antibodies, anti-M) and anti-thyroglobulin antibodies (anti-Tg) – in the disease are elevated but their levels do not correlate with the severity.

Radiological Findings

- *Magnetic resonance imaging* (MRI) abnormalities consistent with encephalopathy (26% of cases).
- *Single photon emission computed tomography* shows focal and global hypoperfusion (75% of cases)
- *Cerebral angiography* is normal

Electro-encephalogram (EEG) Studies

- While almost always abnormal (98% cases), are usually non-diagnostic.
- The most common findings are diffuse or generalized slowing or frontal intermittent rhythmic delta activity.
- Prominent tri-phasic waves, focal slowing, epileptiform abnormalities, photo-paroxysmal and photo-myogenic responses may be seen.

Differential Diagnosis

Hashimoto's encephalopathy should be differentiated from the following disorders:

- Alzheimer's disease
- Cerebro-vascular accidents (CVA) (stroke)

- Creutzfeldt–Jakob disease (CJD)
- Epilepsy
- Migraine (including basilar, hemiplegic, and retinal types)
- Other forms of autoimmune encephalitis, including forms of limbic encephalitis such as anti-NMDA receptor encephalitis
- Schizophrenia
- Spontaneous cerebrospinal fluid leak
- Viral encephalitis
- Transient ischemic attack

Treatment

Because the majority of patients with Hashimoto's encephalopathy respond to steroids or immuno-suppressant treatment, this condition is now also referred to as steroid-responsive encephalopathy. Initial treatment is usually with oral *prednisone* (50–150 mg/day) or high-dose IV methyl-prednisolone (1 g/day) for 3–7 days. *Thyroid hormone* treatment is also included if required.

Failure of some patients to respond to this first line treatment has produced a variety of alternative treatments that have been proposed and tried including *azathioprine, cyclophosphamide, chloroquine, methotrexate, periodic intravenous (IV) immunoglobulin and plasma exchange*. There have been no controlled trials so the optimal treatment is not known. *Seizures*, if present, are controlled with typical *anti-epileptic* agents.

Prognosis

Duration of treatment is usually between 2 and 25 years. Earlier reports suggested that 90% of cases stay in remission after discontinuation of treatment; however, this is at odds with more recent studies which suggest that relapse commonly occurs after initial high-dose steroid treatment *(Flanagan et al., 2010)*. Left untreated, this condition can result in coma and death.

REFERENCES

Al-Busaidi, M., Burad, J., Al-Belushi, A., & Gujjar, A. (2017). Super refractory status epilepticus in Hashimoto's encephalopathy. *Oman Medical Journal*, *32*(3), 247–250. doi:10.5001/omj.2017.46 PMID:28584608

Álvarez, B. G., Yusta, I. A., Carvalho, M. G., & Sánchez, I. (2017). Cerebellopathy secondary to anti-peroxidase antibody-mediated toxicity. A special case of Hashimoto encephalopathy. *Journal of Neuroimmunology*, *15*(312), 1–3. doi:10.1016/j.jneuroim.2017.08.007 PMID:28863961

Ashworth, B. (1965). Ataxia and hypothyroidism. *Bristol Medical- Chirurgical Journal*, *80*(1), 1–4. PMID:14286937

Avila, A., Serrado, A., Reig, L., Famades, A., & Maho, P. (2013). Early presentation of gait disturbance in a steroid-responsive encephalopathy associated with autoimmune thyroiditis. *European Journal of Neurology*, *10*(5), 601. doi:10.1046/j.1468-1331.2003.00667.x PMID:12940849

Bektas, Ö., Yılmaz, A., Kendirli, T., Sıklar, Z., & Deda, G. (2012). Hashimoto encephalopathy causing drug-resistant status epilepticus treated with plasmapheresis. *Pediatric Neurology*, *46*(2), 132–135. doi:10.1016/j.pediatrneurol.2011.11.009 PMID:22264710

Berger, I., Castiel, Y., & Dor, T. (2010). Paediatric Hashimoto encephalopathy, refractory epilepsy and immunoglobulin treatment unusual case report and review of the literature. *Acta Paediatrica (Oslo, Norway)*, *99*(12), 1903–1905. doi:10.1111/j.1651-2227.2010.01967.x PMID:20678162

Berris, B., & Owen, T. (1965). Unusual manifestations of myxedema. *Canadian Medical Association Journal*, *3*(93), 21–25. PMID:14308905

Blanchin, S., Coffin, C., Viader, F., Ruf, J., Carayon, P., Potier, F., ... Ballet, J. J. (2007). Anti-thyroperoxidase antibodies from patients with Hashimoto's encephalopathy bind to cerebellar astrocytes. *Journal of Neuroimmunology*, *192*(1-2), 13–20. doi:10.1016/j.jneuroim.2007.08.012 PMID:17963848

Brain, L., Jellinek, E. H., & Ball, K. (1966). Hashimoto's disease and encephalopathy. *Lancet*, *2*(7462), 512–514. doi:10.1016/S0140-6736(66)92876-5 PMID:4161638

Cai, Y., Wang, F., Chen, Z., Li, L., Wu, Z., Ge, J., ... Zhu, D. (2018). Hashimoto's thyroiditis induces neuroinflammation and emotional alterations in euthyroid mice. *Journal of Neuroinflammation*, *15*(1), 299. doi:10.118612974-018-1341-z PMID:30373627

Cantón, A., de Fàbregas, O., Tintoré, M., Mesa, J., Codina, A., & Simó, R. (2000). Encephalopathy associated to autoimmune thyroid disease: A more appropriate term for an underestimated condition? *Journal of the Neurological Sciences*, *176*(1), 65–69. doi:10.1016/S0022-510X(00)00302-6 PMID:10865094

Castillo, P., Woodruff, B., Caselli, R., Vernino, S., Lucchinetti, C., Swanson, J., ... Boeve, B. (2006). Steroid.-responsive encephalopathy associated with autoimmune thyroiditis. *Archives of Neurology*, *63*(2), 197–202. doi:10.1001/archneur.63.2.197 PMID:16476807

Edvardsson, B., & Persson, S. (2010). Subclinical hypothyroidism presenting with gait abnormality. *The Neurologist*, *16*(2), 115–116. doi:10.1097/NRL.0b013e3181be6fdb PMID:20220447

Ercoli, T., Defazio, G., & Muroni, A. (2019). Status epilepticus in Hashimoto's encephalopathy. *Seizure*, *70*, 1–5. doi:10.1016/j.seizure.2019.06.020 PMID:31228700

Ercoli, T., Defazio, G., & Muroni, A. (2019). Cerebellar syndrome associated with thyroid disorders. *Cerebellum (London, England)*, *18*(5), 932–940. doi:10.100712311-019-01059-9 PMID:31388971

Ferlazzo, E., Raffaele, M., Mazzù, I., & Pisani, F. (2006). Recurrent status epilepticus as the main feature of Hashimoto's encephalopathy. *Epilepsy & Behavior*, *8*(1), 328–330. doi:10.1016/j.yebeh.2005.11.005 PMID:16343998

Ferracci, F., Bertiato, G., & Moretto, G. (2004). Hashimoto's encephalopathy: Epidemiologic data and pathogenetic considerations. *Journal of the Neurological Sciences*, *217*(2), 165–168. doi:10.1016/j.jns.2003.09.007 PMID:14706219

Flanagan, E. P., McKeon, A., Lennon, V. A., Flanagan, E. P., McKeon, A., Lennon, V. A., ... Pittock, S. J. (2010). Autoimmune dementia: Clinical course and predictors of immunotherapy response. *Mayo Clinic Proceedings*, *85*(10), 881–887. doi:10.4065/mcp.2010.0326 PMID:20884824

Fujii, A., Yoneda, M., Ito, T., Yamamura, O., Satomi, S., Higa, H., ... Kuriyam.a, M. (2005). Autoant.ibodies against the amino terminal of alpha-enolase are a useful diagnostic marker of Hashimoto's encephalopathy. *Journal of Neuroimmunology*, *162*(1–2), 130–136. doi:10.1016/j.jneuroim.2005.02.004 PMID:15833368

Fujii, A., Yoneda, M., Ito, T., Yamamura, O., Satomi, S., Higa, H., ... Kuriyama, M. (2005). Autoantibodies against the amino terminal of enolase are a useful diagnostic marker of Hashimoto's encephalopathy. *Journal of Neuroimmunology*, *162*(1-2), 130–136. doi:10.1016/j.jneuroim.2005.02.004 PMID:15833368

Ghika-Schmid, F., Ghika, J., Regli, F., Dworak, N., Bogousslavsky, J., Stadler, C., ... Desplan.d, D. A. (1996). Hashimo.to's myoclonic encephalopathy: An underdiagnosed treatable condition? *Movement Disorders*, *11*(5), 555–562. doi:10.1002/mds.870110511 PMID:8866497

Graham, B. R., Shiff, N., Nour, M., Hasal, S., Huntsman, R., & Almubarak, S. (2016). Hashimoto encephalopathy presenting with stroke-like episodes in an adolescent female: A case report and literature review. *Pediatric Neurology*, *59*, 62–70. doi:10.1016/j.pediatrneurol.2016.02.003 PMID:27033176

Graus, F., Titulaer, M. J., Balu, R., Benseler, S., Bien, C. G., Cellucci, T., ... Dalmau, J. (2016). A clini.cal approach to diagnosis of autoimmune encephalitis *Lancet. Neurology*, *15*(4), 391–404. PMID:26906964

Hammar, C. H., & Regli, F. (1975). Cerebellar ataxia due to hypothyroidism in adults (case report). *Deutsche Medizinische Wochenschrift*, *100*(28), 1504–1506. doi:10.1055-0028-1106608 PMID:1137948

Hannan, M. A., Sarker, I., Fariduddin, M., Begum, A., Hossain, S., & Sultana, N. (2016). Recurrent cerebellar ataxia in a young lady with Hashimoto's thyroiditis. *The American Journal of Case Reports*, *4*(6), 204–207.

Hilberath, J. M., Schmidt, H., & Wolf, G. K. (2014). Steroid-responsive encephalopathy associated with autoimmune thyroiditis (SREAT): Case report of reversible coma and status epilepticus in an adolescent patient and review of the literature. *European Journal of Pediatrics*, *173*(10), 1263–1273. doi:10.100700431-014-2391-6 PMID:25084973

Hommet, C., Mondon, K., Huc, M., Jeffredo, S., Constans, T., de Toffol, B., & Camus, V. (2007). Atypical neuropsychiatric symptoms revealing Hashimoto's encephalopathy. *Journal of the American Geriatrics Society*, *55*(7), 1144–1146. doi:10.1111/j.1532-5415.2007.01219.x PMID:17608897

Hosoi, Y., Kono, S., Terada, T., Konishi, T., & Miyajima, H. (2013). Hashimoto's encephalopathy associated with an elevated intrathecal IgG4 level. *Journal of Neurology*, *260*(4), 1174–1176. doi:10.100700415-013-6878-2 PMID:23471612

Lee, H. J., Jeon, K., Lee, J. Y., Lee, J. E., Bae, D. W., Oh, Y. S., ... Kim, W. (2015). Ocular flutter and ataxia without cognitive impairment associated with steroid-responsive encephalopathy associated with autoimmune thyroiditis (SREAT). *Journal of the Neurological Sciences*, *359*(1–2), 86–87. doi:10.1016/j.jns.2015.10.037 PMID:26671092

Marshall, G. A., & Doyle, J. J. (2006). Long-term treatment of Hashimoto's encephalopathy. *The Journal of Neuropsychiatry and Clinical Neurosciences*, *18*(1), 14–20. doi:10.1176/jnp.18.1.14 PMID:16525066

Matsunaga, A., Ikawa, M., Fujii, A., Nakamoto, Y., Kuriyama, M., & Yoneda, M. (2013). Hashimoto's encephalopathy as a treatable adult-onset cerebellar ataxia mimicking spinocerebellar degeneration. *European Neurology*, *69*(1), 14–20. doi:10.1159/000342217 PMID:23128836

Moodley, K., Botha, J., Raidoo, D. M., & Naidoo, S. (2011). Immunolocalisation of anti-thyroid antibodies in adult human cerebral cortex. *Journal of the Neurological Sciences*, *302*(1-2), 114–117. doi:10.1016/j.jns.2010.11.027 PMID:21196016

Pari, E., Rinaldi, F., Premi, E., Codella, M., Rao, R., Paghera, B., ... Padovani, A. (2014). A follow-up ^{18}F-FDG brain PET study in a case of Hashimoto's encephalopathy causing drug-resistant status epilepticus treated with plasmapheresis. *Journal of Neurology*, *261*(4), 663–667. doi:10.100700415-013-7228-0 PMID:24390201

Payer, J., Petrovic, T., Lisy, L., & Langer, P. (2012). Hashimoto Encephalopathy: A Rare Intricate Syndrome. *International Journal of Endocrinology and Metabolism*, *10*(2), 506–514. doi:10.5812/ijem.4174 PMID:23843812

Pinelli, P., Pisano, F., & Miscio, G. (1990). Ataxia in myxoedema: A neurophysiological reassessment. *Journal of Neurology*, *237*(7), 405–409. doi:10.1007/BF00314730 PMID:2273408

Ihejirika, D.F. (2014). *PASS Program Course Notes:*PreparationUSMLE. Lulu.com.

Salpietro, V., Mankad, K., Polizzi, A., Sugawara, Y., Granata, F., David, E., ... Ruggieri, M. (2014). Pediatric Hashimoto's encephalopathy with peripheral nervous system involvement. *Pediatrics International*, *56*(3), 413–416. doi:10.1111/ped.12262 PMID:24894926

Sawka, A. M., Fatourechi, V., Boeve, B. F., & Mokri, B. (2002). Rarity of encephalopathy associated with autoimmune thyroiditis: A case series from Mayo Clinic from 1950 to 1996. *Thyroid*, *12*(5), 393–398. doi:10.1089/105072502760043477 PMID:12097200

Selim, M., & Drachman, D. (2001). Ataxia associated with Hashimoto's disease: Progressive non-familial adult onset cerebellar degeneration with autoimmune thyroiditis. *Journal ofNeurology, Neurosurgery, and Psychiatry*, *71*(1), 81–87. doi:10.1136/jnnp.71.1.81 PMID:11413268

Seo, S. W., Lee, B. I., Lee, J. D., Park, S. A., Kim, K. S., Kim, S. H., & Yun, M. J. (2003). Thyrotoxic autoimmune encephalopathy: A repeat positron emission tomography study. *The Journal of Neuropsychiatry and Clinical Neurosciences*, *74*(4), 504–506. PMID:12640074

Shah, S. D., & Murali, H. (2011). Steroid-responsive encephalopathy and autoimmune thyroiditis in a young boy. *Pediatric Neurology*, *45*(2), 132–134. doi:10.1016/j.pediatrneurol.2011.04.002 PMID:21763957

Sinharay, R. (2002). Hypothyroidism mimicking intra-abdominal malignancy. *British Medical Journal*, *325*(7370), 946–950. doi:10.1136/bmj.325.7370.946 PMID:12399347

Striano, P., Pagliuca, M., Andreone, V., Zara, F., Coppola, A., & Striano, S. (2006). Unfavourable outcome of Hashimoto encephalopathy due to status epilepticus. One autopsy case. *Journal of Neurology*, *253*(2), 248–249. doi:10.100700415-005-0925-6 PMID:16328109

Tang, Y., Chu, C., Lin, M. T., Wei, G., Zhang, X., & Da, Y. (2011). Hashimoto's encephalopathy mimicking spinocerebellar ataxia. *Journal ofNeurology*, 258.

Termsarasab, P., Pitakpatapee, Y., Frucht, S. J., & Srivanitchapoom, P. (2018). Steroid-responsive encephalopathy associated with autoimmune thyroiditis (SREAT) presenting with pure cerebellar ataxia. *Tremor and Other Hyperkinetic Movements (New York, N.Y.)*, *8*, 585. PMID:30191089

Varrasi, C., Vecchio, D., Magistrelli, L., Strigaro, G., Tassi, L., & Cantello, R. (2017). Auditory seizures in autoimmune epilepsy: A case with anti-thyroid antibodies. *Epileptic Disorders*, *19*(1), 99–103. doi:10.1684/epd.2017.0904 PMID:28287071

Yoneda, M., Fujii, A., Ito, A., Yokoyama, H., Nakagawa, H., & Kuriyama, M. (2007). High prevalence of serum autoantibodies against the amino terminal of α-enolase in Hashimoto's encephalopathy. *Journal of Neuroimmunology*, *185*(1-2), 195–200. doi:10.1016/j.jneuroim.2007.01.018 PMID:17335908

Yu, H., Lee, J., Seo, D., & Lee, M. (2014). Clinical manifestations and treatment response of steroid in pediatric Hashimoto encephalopathy. *Journal of Child Neurology*, *29*(7), 938–942. doi:10.1177/0883073813499823 PMID:24056154

Chapter 10
Hashimoto's Ophthalmopathy

ABSTRACT

Thyroid-associated ophthalmopathy is a self-limiting autoimmune disease associated mainly with Graves' disease, but also with Hashimoto's thyroiditis (HT) and euthyroid states. There are two distinct stages of the disease, an active inflammatory stage followed by inactive quiescent stage. Eye disease activity/severity is independent of gender, age, thyroid function, or smoking. There are no effective means of preventing the disease or reliably altering its course. Current therapeutic options include local supportive measures, corticosteroids, external beam radiation and steroid-sparing immunosuppressive agents for reducing the inflammation during active disease and surgery for correcting the residual abnormalities secondary to fibrosis in the inactive state of the disease. This chapter explores Hashimoto's ophthalmopathy.

INTRODUCTION

Autoimmune thyroid diseases comprise two main clinical presentations: Graves' disease (hyperthyroidism) and Hashimoto's thyroiditis (HT) (hypothyroidism), both characterized by antibodies that attack the thyroid. Indeed, these disorders are the opposite ends of the same underlying cause. Thyroid eye disease, also known as thyroid-associated ophthalmopathy or orbitopathy (TAO), is an autoimmune disorder of the extra-ocular muscles and surrounding orbital connective tissue. It is usually associated with Graves' disease, affecting approximately 25% of these patients, but can also

DOI: 10.4018/978-1-5225-9655-4.ch010

be associated with HT occurring in nearly 6% of those patients (Boulos, 2004; Yamada, 2000; Maheshwari, 2012; Dagi, 2010; El-Kaissi, 2004).

The close clinical relationship between hyper-thyroidism (Graves' disease), Graves' ophthalmopathy, and thyroid dermopathy (peritibial myxedema) suggests that these conditions arise from a single underlying systemic process with variable expression in the thyroid gland, eyes, and skin.

Bilateral ocular disease and hyperthyroidism usually occur simultaneously or within 18 months of each other, although occasionally Graves' ophthalmopathy precedes or follows the onset of hyperthyroidism by many years (Wiersinga, Smit, van der Gaag, & Koornneef, 1988). Approximately, 50% of patients with Graves' hyper-thyroidism have symptoms of Graves' ophthalmopathy. Thes include a dry and gritty ocular sensation, photophobia, excessive tearing, double vision, and a pressure sensation behind the eyes. The most common Typical signs include upper eyelid retraction, periorbital oedema, proptosis, and Typical clinical signs include upper eyelid retraction, periorbital edema and erythema, proptosis (Figure 1), and impairment of eye motility (Bahn, 2010). Approximately 3%-5% of patients with Graves' ophthalmopathy have severe disease with intense pain, inflammation, and sight-threatening corneal ulceration or compressive optic neuropathy (Wiersinga, & Bartalena, 2002). Subclinical eye involvement is common as revealed by magnetic resonance imaging (MRI) or computed tomographic (CT) scanning that show extraocular-muscle enlargement (Enzmann, Donaldson, & Kriss, 1979), in approximately 70% of adult patients with Graves' hyperthyroidism. Although clinically unilateral Graves' ophthalmopathy is not common, orbital imaging generally confirms the presence of asymmetric bilateral disease (Wiersinga, Smit, van der Gaag, Mourits, & Koornneef 1989).

Thyroid Dermopathy (nodular or diffuse thickening of pretibial skin) sometimes progresses to a debilitating disease. Although diagnosed on physical

Figure 1. A lady with thyroid associated ophthalmopathy showing proptosis, periorbital edema, chemosis, and conjunctivitis

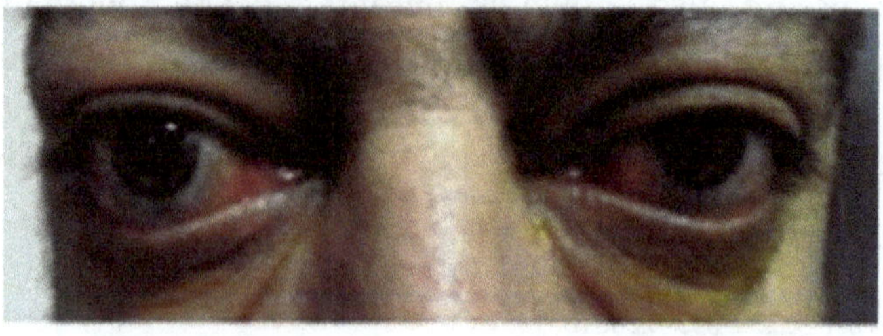

examination in only 13% of patients with severe Graves' ophthalmopathy, subclinical involvement of the skin of the legs and other regions of the body occurs more commonly (Fatourechi, 2005). Approximately 20% of patients with thyroid dermopathy have thyroid acropachy, manifesting as clubbing of fingers and toes.

Prevalence of Hashimoto's Ophthalmopathy

Thyroid associated Orbitopathy or ophthalmopathy (TAO) may occur simultaneously with the manifestations of hyperthyrdism (Graves' disease) or later (approximately 70%), before the manifestation of hypothyroidism (approximately 25%), in the euthyroid state (<5%) and in hypothyroidism (3-5%) (Shirakawa, Amemiya, & Kasagi, 1981). Ocular lesions in autoimmune thyroid diseases occur five times more often in women than in men (respectively, 16 and 2.9 cases per 100,000 annually); however, their course and prognosis is so far worse in men (Krassas, & Wiersinga, 2005).

Although numerous studies have been reported about the prevalence of Graves' ophthalmopathy, similar studies about the prevalence of Hashimato's ophthalmopathy are sparse. The first study about the prevalence of ophthalmopathy in HT was reported by Tjiang et al. (2010). They studied 91 patients with HT and reported that the overall prevalence of any eye signs was 34% and about one-third of patients had upper eyelid retraction. In addition to 2 patients who had eye muscle dysfunction, about a third of the patients had severe inflammatory changes such as periorbital swelling, chemosis, conjunctival injection, and proptosis.

In 2014, Kan and colleagues studied the prevalence of ophthalmopathy in 110 HT for eye signs and compared them with healthy controls. They reported that the prevalence of eye signs was significantly ($p=0.002$) higher then that of control subjects (22.7% versus 4.0%, respectively). In patients with Hashimoto's disease, 11.8% had upper eyelid retraction, 6.4% had proptosis and 5.5% had ocular myopathy (Kan, Kan, & Ecemis, 2014).

The levator palpebrae superioris and extra-ocular muscle involvement in Hashimoto's thyroiditis is rather common and has been emphasized in some studies. Grzesiuk et al. (2008) reported a 36-year-old man with Hashimoto's thyroiditis who had enlargement of the medial and inferior rectus muscles bilaterally, with eye pain, conjunctivitis, edema of the eyelid and exophthalmos. Hiraga et al. (2008) reported a 76-year-old woman with HT suffering from diplopia due to limitations of upper gaze in the right eye.

She had enlargement of inferior rectus muscle unilaterally. In another study published in 2011 by Yoshihara and colleagues, they reported two patients with HT thyroiditis with a high Clinical Activity Score (CAS). Their MRI images showed enlargement of the extra-ocular muscles and both patients required systemic glucocorticoid therapy and orbital irradiation to manage the thyroid associated ophthalmopathy (Yoshihara, 2011).

Pathophysiology

Although the pathophysiology of thyroid associated ophthalmopathy remains unclear, yet sensitized T-cells and autoantibodies against thyroid stimulating hormone receptor (TSH-r) located on thyroid cells (thereby stimulate excess production of thyroid hormone), orbit muscles and fibroblasts are targeted in patients developing ophthalmopathy (Fatourechi, 2005, Gahn, 2003). They may trigger an inflammatory process in the orbit tissues. As a result, leukocytes secrete cytokines, which stimulate fibroblasts to secrete and accumulate glycosamino-glycans, resulting in the swelling of extra-ocular tissues (Khoo and Bahn, 2007).

Thus, the presence of anti–TSH-r antibodies in almost all patients with Graves' ophthalmopathy suggests that an immune reaction thyrotropin (TSH) receptor underlies both Graves' ophthalmopathy and hyper-thyroidism (Khoo et al., 2000). Furthermore, levels of anti–TSH-r antibodies correlate positively with the clinical features of Graves' ophthalmopathy (Gerding et al., 2000), and influence also the prognosis (Eckstein et al., 2006); these antibody levels are particularly elevated in patients with thyroid dermopathy (Morris, Hay, Nelson, & Jiang, 1988).

However, the TSH-r hypothesis cannot explain TAO in Hashimoto's thyroiditis, because patients with Hashimoto's thyroiditis are usually negative for TSH-r (Wall et al., 1993). They generally have low titers of anti–thyrotropin-receptor antibodies, which are difficult to detect in some assays (Eckstein et al., 2009). Although a few cases have been reported, the spectrum of eye signs and their prevalence in Hashimoto's thyroiditis are not well documented.

Immunological cross-reactivity of sensitized T- lymphocytes and/or autoantibodies against thyroid and orbit may trigger the inflammatory process (Iyer and Bahn, 2012). In both conditions, Graves' disease and HT, anti-thyroglobulin (Tg) and anti-thyroid peroxidase (TPO) antibodies are detected in addition to the long-acting thyroid stimulator protector (LATS-P). Therefore a transformation of Graves' disease into HT disease and the reverse is also known and is probably related to altered number of the respective blocking and stimulating antibodies (Wall et al., 2009).

Specific antibodies against eye muscle antigens such as calsequestrin, collagen XIII flavoprotein (Fp) and G2s, which are also shown to be good markers of eye muscle damage in Graves' patients may be an alternative explanation for eye muscle damage in HT (Wescombe, 2010; Gopinath, 2009; Gopinath, 2006; Gopinath, 2007). Gopinath et al. (2007) reported that calsequestrin and collagen XIII antibodies are also associated with chronic upper eyelid retraction as a dominant feature of ophthalmopathy in patients with Graves' disease and HT In another study, Gopinath et al. (2007) evaluated 11 patients with HT for the presence of antibodies aganist eye muscle antigens and found that 7 patients were positive for at least one antibody with calsequestrin and Fp antibodies being the most frequently detected. Five of these seven patients developed ophthalmopathy. Moreover, a euthyroid lady with chronic upper eyelid retraction and positive calsequestrin and collagen XIII antibodies has been reported (Gopinath, Ma, Lahoot, & Wall, 2007). She developed HT and hypothyroidism 22 months later. Since the importance of eye muscle antibodies, particularly calsequestrin, were stated in the majority of the studies, it is conceivable that they may be used as indicators for prediction of the onset of eye muscle involvement, with the possibility of early treatment. A routine ophthalmical examination for patients with HT seems reasonable to avoid missing diagnosis of the associated ophthalmopathy.

Some researchers claim that the occurrence of TAO depends on gender and genetic predisposition and does not require the presence of antibodies stimulating the TSH receptor (Ludgate, 2000). This discovery could explain the occurrence of ophthalmic symptoms in euthyroid state or in hypothyroidism associated with HT. On account of differences between the immune systems of people and animals (mice), one should be careful in the interpretion of the results of these studies (Ludgate, 2002).

Clinical Implications

The records of 700 consecutive patients followed at the endocrine outpatient clinic and at the Joint Thyroid–Eye Clinic of the Johannes Gutenberg University Medical Center in Mainz, Germany with a diagnosis of HT were reviewed by Kahaly et al. (2016). All patients were screened for thyroid-associated eye disease, which was classified as clinically active or inactive, and as mild, moderate-to-severe, or sight-threatening. For comparison, a group of 53 patients with Graves' disease (26 without and 27 with eye disease) and 302 healthy control subjects were also included making a total of 1055 subjects studied.

Thyroid-associated eye disease (thyroid associated ophthalmopathy – TAO) was present in 44 (6%) of the 700 patients with HT. Compared to the patients without thyroid-associated eye disease, those with Hashimoto's disease and TAO had higher levels of THS-r Ab and were more likely to be smokers ($p=0.032$). They also tended to be older (49.3 years *versus* 35.2 years, $p<0.001$); have a longer duration of HT (2.4 years *versus* 0.9 years), and were less likely to have another associated autoimmune disease i.e. thyroid disease only (75% *versus* 52.6%, $p=0.005$). Associated type 1 diabetes mellitus was significantly less among those with Hashimoto's disease and TAO (2.3% *versus* 16.3%).

Moreover, TAO was inactive (i.e. non-inflammatory) and mild (i.e. not requiring glucocorticoid or radiation therapy) in two-thirds of HT patients. Eye disease activity/severity was independent of gender, age, thyroid function, and smoking. No differences were noted in the prevalence of hypothyroidism or rate of levothyroxine replacement.

Regarding immune reactivity, all healthy controls were TSH-r Ab negative. In contrast, serum was TSH-r Ab positive in 30/44 (68.2%) and 36/656 (5.5%) patients with and HT only, respectively ($P<0.001$). Compared to patients with HT, serum TSH-r Ab levels were significantly higher in patients with HT and TAO ($p<0.001$). Highest TSH-r Ab levels were noted in patients with active and severe TAO as compared to those with mild and inactive TAO ($p<0.001$).

In conclusion, TSH-r Ab is strongly associated with thyroid associated ophthalmopathy in HT and may contribute to the pathophysiology of the eye disease.

Assessment

One of the challenges in the management of TAO is to classify and grade its various clinical manifestations. Dolman and Rootman devised a classification system based on four disease end-points that can be used in the office setting to record changes and to guide and assess therapy (Dolmann and Rootman, 2006). These include Vision, Inflammation, Strabismus, and Appearance (VISA)/exposure, which help direct appropriate management in a logical sequence as shown in Table 1.

Vision

The primary goal of this section is to rule out optic neuropathy in which the patient presents with episodes of graying out with and without color desaturation. On examination, abnormalities in visual acuity, color vision assessment, relative afferent papillary defect, or peripheral visual field assessment may be detected.

Inflammation

The Clinical Activity Score (CAS) includes pain, redness, swelling, and impaired visual function, which may signal acute inflammation. It is inexpensive and can be done instantly in a clinic. The CAS consists of two conjunctival signs, two eyelid signs, and two orbital signs. Each sign is assigned points depending on the severity at presentation with a maximum score of 8. The worst scores from any of the 4 eyelids are recorded. A score of 3 or less is considered as "inactive" and 4 or more is "active" eye disease and thus is supposedly more likely to respond to immunosuppression.

Strabismus

The symptoms of strabismus include a progression from no diplopia, diplopia in horizontal or vertical gaze, intermittent diplopia in primary gaze, and constant diplopia in primary gaze. Strabismus can be measured objectively by prism cover testing in different gaze directions.

Table 1. Suggested sequential treatment of TAO according to disease severity and activity

Occular Involvement	Activity	Treatment
Non-severe	Active	Supportive measures
Non-severe	Inactive	Supportive measures
Severe	Active	- Glucocorticoids - Orbital radiotherapy - Orbital decompression*
Severe	Inactive	- Orbital decompression* - Strabismus surgery - Eyelid retraction surgery

*Only of compressive optic neuropathyhas not resolved with maximal medical treatment.
(Bartalena, Pinchera, & Marcoocci, 2000)

Appearance/Exposure

Objective measures of appearance change include eyelid retraction, proptosis, redundant skin and fat prolapse. Measures of exposure include corneal staining or ulceration.

Orbital Imaging

Computerized tomography (CT) scan is the most commonly utilized imaging technique for evaluating TAO. It is more sensitive than magnetic resonance imaging (MRI) in identifying enlarged extraocular muscles (Polito and Leccisotti, 1995). Findings on CT scanning may include muscle belly enlargement that typically spares the tendinous insertions, an apparent increase in orbital fat volume, and crowding of the optic nerve at the orbital apex. Imaging studies may be particularly helpful when radiation therapy or decompressive surgery is planned, as they define the degree of extraocular muscle and orbital fat involvement and delineate clearly sinus and skull base anatomy before intervention.

Treatment

General Considerations

From the endocrine perspective, the goal of treatment of patients with TAO is the achievement of a euthyroid state. In addition, patients should be counseled regarding the risks of smoking and benefits of cessation. The decision of treatment relies on activity and severity of the disease as mentioned before in Table 1. *Vision* dysfunction from optic neuropathy is the first priority and, depending on whether inflammation is present, might be treated with corticosteroids, radiotherapy, and/or orbital decompression. *Inflammation* is the next priority and may be treated with conservative measures, corticosteroids, steroid-sparing immunosuppressives and/or radiotherapy. *Strabismus* and appearance changes are usually managed medically and expectantly (with patching or Fresnel prisms) until signs of inflammation and disease progression have subsided. Strabismus can then be managed with ground-in prisms or surgery, whereas proptosis, eyelid retraction, dermatochalasis, and fat prolapse can be managed surgically.

Most patients with Hashimoto's disease have mild ocular manifestation. Simple local supportive measures are usually sufficient to obtain symptomatic relief.

Glucocorticoids

Glucocorticoids are employed for their anti-inflammatory and immunosuppressive actions (Bartalena, Marocci, Bogazzi, Bruno-Bossio, & Pinchera, 1991). In a review by Rajendram et al, the response to glucocorticoids ranged from 63% to 77% (Rajendram et al., 2008). Intravenous (IV) glucocorticoids have become the mainstay of treatment owing to their higher effectiveness and fewer side effects as compared to oral glucocorticoids (Kahaly, 2005; Macchia, 2001). The cumulative dose of IV steroids should not exceed 6-8 g (Wiersinga and Kahaly, 2007). Routine liver assessment during treatment to rule out liver toxicity is recommended by some centers. Recurrences are not infrequent, thus repeated dosing is often required.

Radiation Therapy

The rationale for the use of radiotherapy for TAO resides both in its non-specific anti-inflammatory effect and in the high radio-sensitivity of lymphocytes infiltrating the orbit (Kahaly et al., 1999). Orbital radiotherapy is effective in patients who have active eye disease with recent progression. Patients with inactive TAO do not respond to irradiation (Bartalena, Marcocci, & Pinchera, 2004). The most common delivered dose is 20 Gy per eye; fractionated over a two-week period. Side effects include transient exacerbations of inflammation, but this can be avoided with glucocorticoid coverage. With modern techniques, there seems to be no increased risk of cataract, or secondary malignancies, and only a remote risk of retinopathy (Marcocci et al., 2003). In patients with diabetes mellitus, irradiation should be considered as a relative contraindication. Even though the efficacy of radiation therapy has been recently questioned, it remains widely used (Bartly and Gorman, 2002).

Steroid-Sparing Immunosuppressive Drugs

Cyclosporine affects both cell-mediated and humoral immune reactions; however, its effect when given as a monotherapy was inferior to prednisone. Several controlled studies reported that the use of cyclosporine in combination with prednisone was more effective than prednisone alone (Kahaly, 1986; Prummel, 1989). Regular monitoring for side effects during the course of cyclosporine treatment is required. *Methotrexate* is given in doses of 5-25 mg once per week and may prove to be promising (Smith and Rosenbaum, 2001).

Surgical Treatment

Indications of surgical intervention in TAO include optic neuropathy, diplopia, corneal exposure, and cosmesis. *Surgical procedures* may be directed toward orbital decompression, strabismus repair, and the correction of eyelid abnormality. Traditionally, orbital decompression, if required, is performed initially, followed by strabismus surgery and then eyelid repair. This is because the nature and degree of strabismus may change after orbital surgery, and lid position may be altered following strabismus repair.

The *timing of surgery* is important. Decompression may be necessary urgently for compressive optic neuropathy or severe proptosis with corneal ulceration refractory to other treatment measures. Yet, most decompression surgery is performed when a patient has been stable in the inactive state for at least 6-8 months (Wiersinga and Kahaly, 2007).

Orbital Decompression

Any surgical procedure that enlarges the bony orbit and/or removes the orbital fat is defined as orbital decompression. At present, the medial wall, the orbital floor, and/or the lateral wall continue to be addressed during bony decompression surgery (Wiersinga and Kahaly, 2007). Preserving the medial orbital strut between the ethmoid cavity and the orbital floor may minimize the risk of globe dystopia and diplopia (Goldberg, Shorr, & Cohen, 1992). The combination of bony decompression and fat removal has gained popularity due to the low risks associated with fat decompression (Goldberg, 1998; Unal, 2003).

Eye Muscle Surgery

Ocular motility disorders in TAO are typically due to a restrictive myopathy, and extra-ocular muscle involvement is characterized by accumulation of inflammatory cells and fluid. Later, the muscle is replaced by fibrous tissue, which makes the muscle stiff and inextensible. Due to the often incomitant nature of stabismus, surgery in TAO is often aimed at resolution of diplopia in primary position and downgaze. Surgery should be performed on a patient who does not have active thyroid disease for at least 6 months, and typically involves release of the restricted muscle by recession rather than resection.

Eyelid Surgery

The most common indication for lid surgery is upper lid retraction. Treatment consists of a graded Muller's and levator aponeurosis weakening. Criterion for successful correction is covering of 1-2 mm of the superior cornea. Lower lid lengthening is indicated in lower lid retraction. Recession of lower lid retractors alone is insufficient to correct more than 1 mm of lid retraction and an interposition graft or spacer is needed if there is significant lower lid retraction.

Blepharoplasty

Blepharoplasty is the final surgical procedure in the rehabilitation of the TAO patient. Skin excision in the lower lid should be done carefully to avoid ectropion and/or lower lid retraction.

REFERENCES

Bahn, R. S. (2003). Clinical review 157: Pathophysiology of Graves' ophthalmopathy: the cycle of disease. *The Journal of Clinical Endocrinology and Metabolism*, *88*(5), 1939–1946. doi:10.1210/jc.2002-030010 PMID:12727937

Bahn, R. S. (2010). Graves' ophthalmopathy. *The New England Journal of Medicine*, *362*(25), 726–738. doi:10.1056/NEJMra0905750 PMID:20181974

Bartalena, L., Marcocci, C., & Pinchera, A. (2004). Orbital radiotherapy for Graves' ophthalmopathy. *The Journal of Clinical Endocrinology and Metabolism*, *89*(1), 13–14. doi:10.1210/jc.2003-031769 PMID:14715819

Bartalena, L., Marocci, C., Bogazzi, F., Bruno-Bossio, G., & Pinchera, A. (1991). Glucocorticoid therapy of Graves' ophthalmopathy. *Experimental and Clinical Endocrinology*, *97*(02/03), 320–327. doi:10.1055-0029-1211086 PMID:1915650

Bartalena, L., Pinchera, A., & Marcoocci, G. (2000). Management of Grave's ophthalmopathy: Reality and perspectives. *Endocrine Reviews*, *21*(2), 168–199. PMID:10782363

Bartley, G. B., & Gorman, C. A. (2002). Perspective – Part 1: Then Mayo orbital radiotherapy for Graves' ophthalmopathy (ORGO) study: Lessons learnt. *Ophthalmic Plastic and Reconstructive Surgery*, *18*, 170–172. doi:10.1097/00002341-200205000-00002 PMID:12021644

Boulos, P. R., & Hardy, I. (2004). Thyroid-associated orbitopathy: A clinicopathologic and therapeutic review. *Current Opinion in Ophthalmology*, *15*(5), 389–400. doi:10.1097/01.icu.0000139992.15463.1b PMID:15625899

Dagi, L. R., Elliott, A. T., Roper-Hall, G., & Cruz, O. A. (2010). Thyroid eye disease: Honing your skills to improve outcomes. *Journal of the American Assciation for Pediatric Ophthalmology and Strabismus*, *14*(5), 425–431. doi:10.1016/j.jaapos.2010.07.005 PMID:21035070

Dolman, P. J., & Rootman, J. (2006). VISA Classification for Graves' orbitopathy. *Ophthalmic Plastic and Reconstructive Surgery*, *22*(5), 319–324. doi:10.1097/01.iop.0000235499.34867.85 PMID:16985411

Eckstein, A. K., Lösch, C., Glowacka, D., Schott, M., Mann, K., Esser, J., & Morgenthaler, N. G. (2009). Euthyroid and primarily hypothyroid patients develop milder and significantly more asymmetrical Graves' ophthalmopathy. *The British Journal of Ophthalmology*, *93*(8), 1052–6105. doi:10.1136/bjo.2007.137265 PMID:19221109

Eckstein, A. K., Plicht, M., Lax, H., Neuhäuser, M., Mann, K., Lederbogen, S., ... Morgent.haler, N. G. (2006). Thyrotr.opin receptor autoantibodies are independent risk factors for Graves' ophthalmopathy and help to predict severity and outcome of the disease. *The Journal of Clinical Endocrinology and Metabolism*, *91*(9), 3464–3470. doi:10.1210/jc.2005-2813 PMID:16835285

El-Kaissi, S., Frauman, A. G., & Wall, J. R. (2004). Thyroid-associated ophthalmopathy: A practical guide to classification, natural history and management. *International Medical Journal, 34*(8), 482–491. doi:10.1111/j.1445-5994.2004.00662.x PMID:15317547

Enzmann, D. R., Donaldson, S. S., & Kriss, J. P. (1979). Appearance of Graves' disease on orbital computed tomography. *Journal of Computer Assisted Tomography, 3*(6), 815–819. doi:10.1097/00004728-197903060-00019 PMID:583152

Fatourechi, V. (2005). Pretibial myxedema: Pathophysiology and treatment options. *American Journal of Clinical Dermatology, 6*(5), 295–309. doi:10.2165/00128071-200506050-00003 PMID:16252929

Gerding, M. N., van der Meer, J. W., Broenink, M., Bakker, O., Wiersinga, W. M., & Prummel, M. F. (2000). Association of thyrotrophin receptor antibodies with the clinical features of Graves' ophthalmopathy. *Horumon To Rinsho, 52*(3), 267–271. doi:10.1046/j.1365-2265.2000.00959.x PMID:10718823

Goldberg, R. A. (1998). The evolving paradigm of orbital decompression surgery. *Archives of Ophthalmology, 116*(1), 95–96. doi:10.1001/archopht.116.1.95 PMID:9445215

Goldberg, R. A., Shorr, N., & Cohen, M. S. (1992). The medical orbital strut in the prevention of postdecompression dystopia in dysthyroid ophthalmopathy. *Ophthalmic Plastic and Reconstructive Surgery, 8*(1), 32–34. doi:10.1097/00002341-199203000-00005 PMID:1554650

Gopinath, B., Adams, C. L., Musselman, R., Tani, J., & Wall, J. R. (2007). Antibodies against calsequestrin and type XIII collagen are good markers for chronic upper eyelid lag and retraction. *Ocular Immunology and Inflammation, 15*(2), 81–88. doi:10.1080/09273940701299362 PMID:17558832

Gopinath, B., Ma, G., Lahooti, H., & Wall, J. R. (2007). A Case of Hashimoto's Thyroiditis Presenting with Chronic Upper eye Lid Retraction and Positive Calsequestrin and Collagen XIII Antibodies. *International Journal of Endocrinology and Metabolism, 6*(2), 34–37.

Gopinath, B., Ma, G., & Wall, J. R. (2007). Eye signs and serum eye muscle and collagen XIII antibodies in patients with transient and progressive thyroiditis. *Thyroid, 17*(11), 1123–1129. doi:10.1089/thy.2007.0054 PMID:17887926

Gopinath, B., Musselman, R., Beard, N., Tani, J., Adams, C., & Wall, J. R. (2006). Antibodies targeting the calcium binding skeletal muscle protein calsequestrin are sensitive and specific markers of ocular myopathy in patients with Graves' disease. *Clinical and Experimental Immunology*, *145*(1), 56–62. doi:10.1111/j.1365-2249.2006.03110.x PMID:16792674

Gopinath, B., Wescombe, L., Nguyen, B., & Wall, J. R. (2009). Can autoimmunity against calsequestrin explain the eye and eyelid muscle inflammation of thyroid eye disease? *Orbit (Amsterdam, Netherlands)*, *28*(4), 256–261. doi:10.1080/01676830903104629 PMID:19839885

Grzesiuk, W., Szydlarska, D., Pragacz, A., & Bar-Andziak, E. (2008). Thyroid associated orbitopathy in patients with Hashimoto's thyroiditis: A case report. *Polish Archives of Internal Medicine*, *118*(5), 318–321. doi:10.20452/pamw.400 PMID:18619184

Hiraga, A., Mimura, M., & Kamitsukasa, I. (2008). Isolated inferior rectus muscle myopathy due to Hashimoto's thyroiditis. *International Medicine*, *47*(13), 1283–1284. doi:10.2169/internalmedicine.47.1003 PMID:18591859

Iyer, S., & Bahn, R. (2012). Immunopathogenesis of Graves' ophthalmopathy: The role of the TSH receptor. *Best Practice & Research. Clinical Endocrinology & Metabolism*, *26*(3), 281–289. doi:10.1016/j.beem.2011.10.003 PMID:22632365

Kahaly, G., Schrezenmeir, J., Krause, U., Schweikert, B., Meuer, S., Muller, W., ... Beyer, J. (1986). … Beyer, J. (1986). Cyclosporine and prednisone v. prednisone in treatment of Graves' ophthalmopathy: A controlled, randomized and prospective study. *European Journal of Clinical Investigation*, *16*(5), 415–422. doi:10.1111/j.1365-2362.1986.tb01016.x PMID:3100309

Kahaly, G. J., Diana, T., Glang, J., Kanitz, M., Pitz, S., & König, J. (2016). Stimulating Antibodies Are Highly Prevalent in Hashimoto's Thyroiditis and Associated Orbitopathy. *The Journal of Clinical Endocrinology and Metabolism*, *101*(5), 1998–2004. doi:10.1210/jc.2016-1220 PMID:26964732

Kahaly, G. J., Pitz, S., Hommel, G., & Dittmar, M. (2005). Randomized, single blind trial of intravenous versus oral steroid monotherapy in Graves' orbitopathy. *The Journal of Clinical Endocrinology and Metabolism*, *90*(9), 5234–5240. doi:10.1210/jc.2005-0148 PMID:15998777

Kahaly, G. J., Roesler, H. P., Kutzner, J., Kutzner, J., Pitz, S., & Müller-Forell, W. (1999). Radiotherapy for thyroid-associated orbitopathy. *Experimental and Clinical Endocrinology & Diabetes*, *107*(Suppl 5), S201–S207. doi:10.1055-0029-1212186 PMID:10614923

Kan, E., Kan, E. K., & Ecemis, G. (2014). Presence of thyroid-associated ophthalmopathy in Hashimoto's thyroiditis. *International Journal of Ophthalmology*, *7*(4), 644–647. PMID:25161935

Khoo, D. H., Eng, P. H., Ho, S. C., Tai, E. S., Morgenthaler, N. G., Seah, L. L., ... Aw, S. E. (2000). Graves' ophthalmopathy in the absence of elevated free thyroxine and triiodothyronine levels: Prevalence, natural history, and thyrotropin receptor antibody levels. *Thyroid*, *10*(12), 1093–1000. doi:10.1089/thy.2000.10.1093 PMID:11201855

Khoo, T. K., & Bahn, R. S. (2007). Pathogenesis of Graves' ophthalmopathy: The role of autoanti-bodies. *Thyroid*, *17*(10), 1013–1018. doi:10.1089/thy.2007.0185 PMID:17935483

Krassas, G. E., & Wiersinga, W. M. (2005). Thyroid eye disease: Current concepts and the EUGOGO perspective. *Thyroid International*, *4*, 3–4.

Ludgate, M. (2000). Animals models of Graves' disease. *European Journal of Endocrinology*, *142*, 1–8. doi:10.1530/eje.0.1420001 PMID:10633214

Ludgate, M. E. (2002). Animal models of thyroid-associated ophthalmopathy. *Thyroid*, *12*(3), 205–208. doi:10.1089/105072502753600142 PMID:11952040

Macchia, P. E., Bagattini, M., Lupoli, G., Vitale, M., Vitale, G., & Fenzi, G. (2001). High-dose intravenous corticosteroid therapy for Graves' ophthalmopathy. *Journal of Endocrinological Investigation*, *24*(3), 152–158. doi:10.1007/BF03343835 PMID:11314743

Maheshwari, R., & Weis, E. (2012). Thyroid associated orbitopathy. *Indian Journal of Ophthalmology*, *60*(2), 87–93. doi:10.4103/0301-4738.94048 PMID:22446901

Marcocci, C., Bartalena, L., Rocchi, R., Marino, M., Menconi, F., Morabito, E., ... Pichera, A. (2003). Long te.rm safety of orbital radiotherapy for Grave's ophthalmopathy. *The Journal of Clinical Endocrinology and Metabolism*, *88*(8), 3561–3566. doi:10.1210/jc.2003-030260 PMID:12915636

Morris, J. C. III, Hay, I. D., Nelson, R. E., & Jiang, N. S. (1988). Clinical utility of thyrotropin-receptor antibody assays: Comparison of radioreceptor and bioassay methods. *Mayo Clinic Proceedings*, *63*(7), 707–717. doi:10.1016/S0025-6196(12)65533-5 PMID:2898572

Polito, E., & Leccisotti, A. (1995). MRI in Graves' orbitopathy: Recognition of enlarged muscles and prediction of steroid response. *Ophthalmologica*, *209*(4), 182–186. doi:10.1159/000310609 PMID:8545089

Prummel, M. F., Mourits, M. P., Berghout, A., Krenning, E. P., van der Gaag, R., Koornneef, L., & Wiersinga, W. M. (1989). Prednisone and cyclosporine in the treatment of severe Graves' ophthalmopathy. *The New England Journal of Medicine*, *321*(20), 1353–1359. doi:10.1056/NEJM198911163212002 PMID:2519530

Rajendram, R., Lee, R. W., Potts, M. J., Rose, G. E., Jain, R., Olver, J. M., ... Uddin, J. M. (2008). Protoco.l for the combined immunosuppression and radiotherapy in thyroid eye disease (CIRTED) trial: A multi-centre, double-masked, factorial randomised controlled trial. *Trials*, *9*(1), 6. doi:10.1186/1745-6215-9-6 PMID:18237441

Shirakawa, H., Amemiya, T., & Kasagi, K. (1981). Hashimoto disease with hyperthyroid ocular signs. *Metabolic and Pediatric Ophthalmology*, *5*, 213–218. PMID:6895539

Smith, J. R., & Rosenbaum, J. T. (2001). A role for methotrexate in the management of non-infectious orbital inflammatory disease. *The British Journal of Ophthalmology*, *85*(10), 1220–1224. doi:10.1136/bjo.85.10.1220 PMID:11567968

Tjiang, H., Lahooti, H., McCorquodale, T., Parmar, K. R., & Wall, J. R. (2010). Eye and eyelid abnormalities are common in patients with Hashimoto's thyroiditis. *Thyroid*, *20*(3), 287–290. doi:10.1089/thy.2009.0199 PMID:20146657

Unal, M., Leri, F., Konuk, O., & Hasanreisoglu, B. (2003). Balanced orbital decompression combined with fat removal in Graves' ophthalmopathy: Do we really need to remove the third wall? *Ophthalmic Plastic and Reconstructive Surgery*, *19*(2), 112–118. doi:10.1097/01.IOP.0000056145.71641.F5 PMID:12644756

Wall, J. R., Bernard, N., Boucher, A., Salvi, M., Zhang, Z. G., Kennerdell, J., ... Genovese, C. (1993). Pathogenesis of thyroid-associated ophthalmopathy: An autoimmune disorder of the eye muscle associated with Graves' hyperthyroidism and Hashimoto's thyroiditis. *Clinical Immunology and Immunopathology*, *68*(1), 1–8. doi:10.1006/clin.1993.1087 PMID:8513588

Wescombe, L., Lahooti, H., Gopinath, B., & Wall, J. R. (2010). The cardiac calsequestrin gene (CASQ2) is up-regulated in the thyroid in patients with Graves' ophthalmopathy--support for a role of autoimmunity against calsequestrin as the triggering event. *Horumon To Rinsho*, *73*(4), 522–528. PMID:20039900

Wiersinga, W. M., & Bartalena, L. (2002). Epidemiology and prevention of Graves' ophthalmopathy. *Thyroid*, *12*(10), 855–860. doi:10.1089/105072502761016476 PMID:12487767

Wiersinga, W. M., & Kahaly, G. J. (2007). *Graves' orbitopathy: A multidisciplinary approach*. Basel: Karger. doi:10.1159/isbn.978-3-8055-8343-5

Wiersinga, W. M., Smit, T., van der Gaag, R., & Koornneef, L. (1988). Temporal relationship between onset of Graves' ophthalmopathy and onset of thyroidal Graves' disease. *Journal of Endocrinal Investigation*, *11*, 615619. PMID:2907524

Wiersinga, W. M., Smit, T., van der Gaag, R., Mourits, M., & Koornneef, L. (1989). Clinical presentation of Graves' ophthalmopathy. *Ophthalmic Research*, *21*(2), 73–82. doi:10.1159/000266782 PMID:2786616

Yamada, M., Wu Li, A., & Wall, J. (2000). Thyroid-associated ophthalmopathy: Clinical features, pathogenesis, and management. *Critical Reviews in Clinical Laboratory Sciences*, *37*(6), 523–549. doi:10.1080/10408360091174303 PMID:11192331

Yoshihara, A., Yoshimura, J., Nakachi, A., Ohye, H., Sato, S., Sekiya, K., ... Ito, K. (2011). Severe thyroid associated orbitopathy in Hashimoto's thyroiditis. Report of 2 cases. *Endocrine Journal*, *58*(5), 343–348. doi:10.1507/endocrj.K11E-019 PMID:21427503

Chapter 11
Anxiety and Depression

ABSTRACT

It is an established entity that thyroid hormones play an important role in mood, behavior, and cognition. Autoimmune thyroiditis, including Hashimoto's thyroiditis (HT), can lead to depression and anxiety disorders. It is thus important to enhance awareness among physicians about this connection to accelerate the diagnostic process. In patients with depression and anxiety disorders, a test for autoimmune thyroiditis should be performed, and in patients with autoimmune thyroiditis, a screening for psychiatric symptoms is necessary. Thus, patients presenting with anxiety or depression disorders should be treated and monitored by both an endocrinologist and a psychiatrist in liaison with each other so as to optimize their management. Moreover, an early recognition of an endocrine condition will help minimize psychiatric morbidity and hence improve health. This chapter explores anxiety, depression, and Hashimoto's disease.

INTRODUCTION

Autoimmune thyroiditis (AIT) is considered a major health problem with implications for both patients and physicians as it causes somatic and psychiatric disorders the extent of which is not fully known so far.

Hashimoto's thyroiditis denotes an autoimmune thyroid condition in which the thyroid gland is attacked by the immune system resulting in impaired thyroid function (hypothyroidism). During destruction of thyroid gland cells, it is possible to experience increase in hormone levels temporarily resulting

DOI: 10.4018/978-1-5225-9655-4.ch011

in transient hyperthyroidism (Hashitoxicosis or thyrotoxicosis). When the high level of hormones is managed by the body, the thyroid function starts to decline resulting in hypothyroidism, which causes depression and anxiety.

Carta et al. (2004) suggested that people with thyroid autoimmunity are at increased risk of anxiety and mood related disorders. It indicated that both conditions are caused by the same aberrancy present in the immuno-endocrinal center, which is difficult to correct.

Effect of Thyroid Hormone on the Central Nervous System

Thyroid hormone affects and governs the central nervous system both during the development phase and also during the entire life. It regulates gene expression in myelination, differentiation of neuronal and glial cells, and neuronal viability and function. The effect of thyroid hormones on serotonin (5-hydroxytryptamine [5-HT]) is explained by desensitization of 5-HT1A auto-receptor at the site of raphe nuclei, which probably results in an increase in the release of serotonin from the raphe neurons (Bauer, 2002; Smith, 2002; Bernal, 1995).

The mechanism of thyroid hormone activity in the brain is unclear due to the complexity of neuro-transmission interaction with the thyroid. One hypothesis stated that thyroid hormone modulates postsynaptic beta-adrenergic receptors in the cerebral cortex and cerebellum, while others stated that the modulation of 5-HT and its receptors is responsible, which happens due to inhibition caused by the TH at the raphe, causing reduction in 5-HT levels (Atlerwillw, 2008; Belmaker, 2008).

Both the hyper- and hypo-thyroid states have co-morbidity with psychiatric conditions. Similarly, patients of mood disorders also show derangement in TSH and thyrotropin releasing hormone whereas T3 and T4 may remain normal. (Bauer, 2002; Smith, 2002; Linkowski, 1981; Loosen, 1985).

Prevalence

Autoimmune thyroiditis is a common disease with a prevalence of approximately 4% to 13% in the United States (Forman-Hoffman, 2006; Hollowell, 2002). It generally affects more women than men and its frequency increases with age, reaching up to 20% among elderly women (Canaris, 2000; Sarks, 2004; Chaudhary, 2014).

Depression and anxiety disorders are pervasive psychiatric diseases with prevalence rates of 6.6% for depression (Pies, 1995; Kessler, 2003). and 18.1% for anxiety disorders (Kessler et al., 2003) in the United States. Thus, approximately 23.8% of patients with AIT experience depression and nearly 41.6% of patients with AIT experience anxiety disorders. That implies that 3% of the US population (approximately 9.7 million people) has depression and 5.4% (approximately 17.5 million people) has anxiety disorders concomitantly with AIT. This also implies that about 45.5% of depressive disorders and 29.8% of anxiety disorders are associated with this endocrine disease.

Prevalence rates for autoimmune thyroiditis in Europe vary between 5% and 14% (Kessler, 2005; Bjoro, 2000), emphasizing the global nature of the disease. Assuming that depression and anxiety disorders are illnesses that often appear together (Vanderpump, 2011) with a co-morbidity of up to 57.5% (Sartorius, Ustün, Lecrubier, & Wittchen, 1996), patients with AIT have a high risk of suffering from both depression and anxiety (e.g. depression and panic disorder) (Belzer & Schneier, 2004).

Link between Autoimmune Thyroiditis and Psychiatric Disorders

Recently, the connection between autoimmunity and psychiatric disorders has been discovered for various autoimmune diseases including Hashimoto's thyroiditis. For example, N-methyl-D-aspartate receptor hypo-function caused by immunoglobulin antibodies has been reported to be associated with the development of schizophrenia and psychoses (Joffe, 1992; Pollak, 2014). Tic disorders were also found to be associated with a significant increase in anti-streptolysin O titers (Coyle, Tsai, & Goff, 2003). Furthermore, bipolar disorders (Pozzi et al., 2014) and Alzheimer disease (Eaton, Pedersen, Nielsen, & Mortensen, 2010) could be explained by autoimmune explanatory approaches.

Autoimmune thyroiditis results in hypothyroidism, which leads to alterations in cardiovascular function such as hypertension due to increased systemic vascular resistance (Nagele, Han, Demarshall, Belinka, & Nagele, 2011). and advanced atherosclerosis, Furthermore, it contributes to a higher risk of infertility and early miscarriage (Biondi & Cooper, 2008), in addition to weight gain even after treatment with thyroxine (Poppe, Velkeniers, & Glinoer, 2008).

Less is known about specific psychiatric burden of symptoms in AIT patients. Several authors reported a cumulative occurrence of mood disorders and symptoms of depression among hypothyroid patients, as well as frequent thyroid diseases among patients with depression (Kong, 2002; Iltermann, 2015; Hage, 2012; Kirim, 2012; Pegner, 2015). Moreover, many studies described symptoms of anxiety in patients with AIT (Kong, 2002; Pegner, 2015; Yalcin, 2017; Hall, 1999; Engum, 2005). in addition to other neuropsychological symptoms such as attentional and executive disturbances (Aslan, Ersoy, Kuruoglu, Karakoc, & Cakir, 2005), fatigue, or general reduction in the quality of life (Constant, 2006; Bianchi, 2004).

Association between Hashimoto's Disease and Anxiety / Depression Disorders

Autoimmune thyroid disease may be linked to depression (Gulseren et al., 2006) and anxiety *(Fountoulakis, Iacovides, & Grammaticos, 2004).* However, there are only a few qualitative reviews (and no quantitative studies) describing an association between Hashimoto's thyroiditis and the development of depression and anxiety disorders (Pollak, 2014; Iltermann, 2015; Hage, 2012; Kirim, 2012).

There are several papers suggesting that the thyroid function of depressed patients is within the normal range, and that the presence of subtle thyroid function abnormalities does not have an impact on treatment outcome (Carta, 2002; Fava, 1995; Joffe, 1990; Haggerty, 1997; Pop, 1988; Harris, 1989). However, there are even more papers supporting the idea of a subclinical thyroid dysfunction possibly of an autoimmune origin (Joffe, 1987; Howland, 1993; Raoe, 1989; Nemeroff, 1989; Maes, 1994; Bunevicius, 1994; Banki, 1985; Rupprecht, 1989; Gewirtz, 1988; Marchesi, 1988; Nemeroff, 1985; Kjellman, 1985) suggesting that subclinical hypothyroidism may lower the threshold for the occurrence of depression (Haggerty et al., 1993), or generally to any mental disorder (Haggerty, 1990; O'Donnell, 1988; Stein, 1989). *It has been reported that* depressed patients have higher Thyroid Binding Inhibitory Immunoglobulins (TBII), which is suggestive of the presence of an underlying autoimmune process in depression. It is also believed that depression is accompanied by various indicators of a moderate activation of the inflammatory response system, especially in the frame of the stress-response activity. Increased production of proinflammatory cytokines, such as interleukin-1, interleukin-6 and interferon (IFN gamma), may play a crucial role in the immune and acute phase response in depression (Loosen, 1985).

A recent meta-analysis by Siegmann et al. (2018) reviewed psychiatric disorders among patients with hypothyroidism. The study examined 19 studies with a total of 36,174 participants. Results showed that patients with AIT have a higher chance to show symptoms of depression and anxiety, irrespective of gender and age, compared with healthy controls (Scolari et al., 2005).

Marangell and Callahan (1998) described the first studies investigating a link between the thyroid disease and the brain using positron emission tomography (PET) paradigms and Hendrick et al (1998) reported a high occurrence of hypothyroidism among depression patients resistant to treatment. Despite these indications, no direct association between particular alterations in brain regions because of AIT and the development of a *depressive disorder* was found (Ittermann, 2015; Mussig, 2013). Regarding *anxiety,* the first symptoms among patients with hypothyroidism are often generalized agitation or extreme restlessness. As some of the symptoms of hypothyroidism are caused by hypertension and sensations of nightly tachycardia (Shojaie, & Eshraghian, 2008), it is presumable that this condition leads to a facilitated development of generalized anxiety disorder.

How Hypothyroidism Triggers Anxiety / Depression

Thyroid hormone exerts direct control over several major neurotransmitters including norepinephrine, serotonin and GABA receptors. In fact, the hormone is involved in creation of these neurotransmitters. In case of hypothyroidism, these neurotransmitters do not function properly resulting in ***anxiety*** and panic attacks. Physical symptoms associated with hypothyroidism further increases anxiety, not due to the hormone defect, but by the fear triggered by the symptoms.

A slight reduction in thyroid hormone secretion such as that found in subclinical hypothyroidism may affect cognition and mood (Schenck, Rizvi, & Lin, 2006). At variance with other tissues which mainly rely on peripherally generated Tri-iodothyronine (T3), the brain utilizes preferentially circulating thyroxine (T4) directly secreted by the thyroid gland and may become hypothyroid before other organs (Haggerty, 1995; Harris, 2002).

However, it must be emphasized that despite being reported in hypothyroidism, panic attacks and anxiety are seen more prevalently in hyperthyroidism, where excessive amount of thyroid hormone is secreted. In hypothyroidism, the most common symptoms may be fatigue and depression instead of anxiety.

The link between thyroid autoimmunity and ***depression*** may however, involve other mechanisms related to the autoimmune pathogenesis of thyroid disease rather than hypothyroidism. Since several neuroendocrine secretory systems are involved in the control of immune reaction, a common neuroendocrine dys-regulation involving cytokines might concur towards the pathogenesis of both affective disorders and autoimmune disease. Recent studies suggested that thyroid autoimmunity may be affected by the Hypothalamic-Pituitary-Adrenal axis (HPA) through the balance of pro-inflammatory and anti-inflammatory cytokines *(Engum, Bjero, Myketun, & Dahl, 2002).* In accordance with this view, the increased frequency of post-partum depression, contributed to the fact that pregnancy would seem to be a "protected" period, could explain at least in part the consequences on thyroid autoimmunity elicited by HPA-related modifications to the immunitary axis. Indeed, similar phenomena are observed in rheumatoid arthritis and multiple sclerosis (Elekov, 2002; Elenkov, 2001).

Clinical Implications

The current terminology concerning autoimmune thyroiditis is depicted in Table 1. Psychiatric manifestations usually appear first in cases of hypothyroidism. They form about 2-12% of the initial symptoms in about all of the reported cases. Initially, it starts with anxiety, memory lapses, progressive mental slowing, and speech deficits (Biondi, 1977; Hall, 1986). In cases of acute hypothyroidism, anxiety disorders occur in about 30-40% of patientsPatients with subclinical hypothyroidism (SCH) can present with anxiety, irritability, poor concentration, slow information processing, and poor learning in comparison to normal subjects (Popkin, 1980; Haug, 2004; Hall, 1983; Whybrow, 1969).

Hypothyroidism impacts certain aspects of cognitive functioning (slowed information processing speed, reduced efficiency in executive functions, and poor learning) and mood. More severe hypothyroidism can mimic melancholic depression and dementia, thus causing reduction in health-related quality of life. Before prescribing any antidepressant, physicians must go for thyroid function tests. Even mild cases of hypothyroid state can cause depression (Haggerty, 1990; Davidoff, 1977). Although the results are inconsistent, data do suggest that the neuropsychiatric symptoms tend to improve with treatment for both overt hypothyroidism and SCH and normalization to a euthyroid state Gold, Pottash, & Extein, 1981).

Treatment

Societal and economic costs caused by depression and anxiety disorders are high (Gold, 1981; Davis, 2007) and can be lowered by appropriate and early treatment. By awareness of the association between these disorders and AIT, proper thyroid and antidepressant treatment can be implemented beyond psychotherapy. Furthermore, screening tests for symptoms of depression and anxiety in patients with AIT and for AIT in patients with depression and anxiety could be established.

Patients often seek medical attention owing to psychiatric symptoms but are unaware of autoimmune thyroiditis. As AIT is a chronic disease (Lepine, 2002), so are symptoms of depression and anxiety associated with it. Both anxiety and depression have persistent courses owing to, among other factors, helplessness (Singer et al., 1995) and classical fear conditioning (Maier, & Seligman, 1976). Autoimmune thyroiditis, however, can appear in phases (hyperthyroid versus hypothyroid) (Lissek et al., 2005) and is thus not always traceable as the root cause of these symptoms, which impedes proper diagnoses and appropriate therapy.

Depression and anxiety disorders associated with a Hashimoto's thyroiditis require different treatment than usual. Occasionally, there are conditions when a *thyroidectomy* is indicated such as persistence of significant pain,

Table 1. Current terminology concerning autoimmune thyroiditis

Term	Definition
Hashimoto's thyroiditis	- Elevated TSH values - FT4 within normal range - Presence of thyroid peroxidase antibodies (TPO-Ab)
Autoimmune thyroiditis	- Elevated TSH values - FT4 within normal range - Presence of TPO-Ab comprising Hashimoto's and atrophic thyroiditis
Subclinical hypothyroidism	- Elevated TSH values - FT4 within normal range
Latent hypothyroidism	- Elevated TSH values - FT4 within normal range
Overt hypothyroidism	- Elevated TSH values

FT4, serum free T4; TSH, thyroid stimulating hormone

cosmetic symptoms, or pressure complaints after a fair trial of thyroid therapy (Chiovato et al., 1990).

Regarding *pharmacotherapy*, an extension of possible medication must be taken into consideration. Besides typical levothyroxine (LT4) treatment, selenium supplementation can help to reduce the amount of thyroid antibodies and improve mood or well-being (Pisanu, Piu, Lois, & Uccheddy, 2003).

Iodine plays an important role in mental health. The iodine provided by the thyroid hormone ensures the energy metabolism of the cerebral cells. The demonstration of a relationship between selenium deficiency and thyroid destruction in myxedematous cretinism and in rat experimental models underlined the importance of selenium (Se) in thyroiditis (Toulis, 2010; Goyens, 1987).

Several studies have suggested that selenium treatment reduces antibodies levels (Contempre, Denef, Dumont, & Many, 1993). allows lower dosage of LT_4 supplementation and may provide other beneficial effects (e.g. on mood and health-related quality of life; HRQoL) in patients with Hashimoto's thyroiditis (Gärtner, Gasnier, Dietrich, Krebs, & Angstwurm, 2002).

In a large review, Dr. David Benton. (2002) of the university of Wales identified at least five studies, which indicate that low selenium intake is associated with lowered mood status. Intervention studies with selenium with other patient populations reveal that selenium improves mood and diminishes anxiety.

Furthermore, an early administration of anti-depressants could be indicated to attenuate the chronic course of AIT. Thyroid metabolism is associated with the brain serotonin system (Short-Bosner et al., 2003), thus, selective serotonin reuptake inhibitors are appropriate medications to treat depression in patients with AIT (Duntas, Mantzou, & Koutras, 2003).

Classical, tricyclic anti-depressants, however, are not suited for patients with hypothyroidism. On the one hand, patients with hypothyroidism do not respond as well to tricyclic anti-depressants as patients with depression who are euthyroid and, on the other hand, typical adverse effects of tricyclic anti-depressants such as weight gain already occur in patients with hypothyroidism and can be further enhanced. Thus, it is important to administer modern anti-depressants with a neutral effect on weight (deCarvalho, Bahls, Boeving, & Graf, 2009).

A study by Bathla et al. (2016) revealed the difficulties associated with the presence of anxiety and depression symptoms in hypothyroid patients. This study used Hamilton scale for measuring anxiety and depression on 100 patients with hypothyroidism and showed that if thyroid hormone treatment is not working for hypothyroid patients, they should be checked for presence of anxiety and depression symptoms and the symptoms managed accordingly. Likewise, in case of patients who are under treatment for anxiety or depression, if the anti-anxiety or anti-depressive medications do not work they should be screened for thyroid disorder. The study suggested that even in euthyroid cases, the use of thyroxine could alleviate anxiety and depression.

Moreover, patients with AIT and no symptoms of depression or anxiety must be aware of the vulnerability to develop psychiatric issues. As a consequence, both a *screening* for psychiatric symptoms is advisable in patients with AIT and a test for AIT is recommended in patients with depression and anxiety disorders. This test must not be narrowed down to thyroid stimulating hormone (TSH) (thyrotropin) levels and free triiodothyronine (FT3) and free thyroxine (FT4) but should comprise thyroid peroxidase antibodies (TPO) as well. In population-based studies, only 4% to 5% of patients show elevated TSH levels, whereas 13% to 23% are positive for TPO antibodies (Fuman-Hoffman, 2006; Hollowell, 2002; Bjoro, 2000; Shinkov, 2014). If only the TSH level is measured, the clinician will miss many patients with AIT detectable by assessment of TPO antibodies and ultrasonography.

REFERENCES

Aslan, S., Ersoy, R., Kuruoglu, A. C., Karakoc, A., & Cakir, N. (2005). Psychiatric symptoms and diagnoses in thyroid disorders: A cross-sectional study. *International Journal of Psychiatry*, *9*(3), 187–192. PMID:24937789

Atterwill, C. K., Bunn, S. J., Atkinson, D. J., Smith, S. L., & Heal, D. J. (2008). Effects of thyroid status on presynaptic alpha 2-adrenoceptor function and beta-adrenoceptor binding in the rat brain. *Journal of Neural Transmission (Vienna, Austria)*, *84*(59), 43–55. PMID:6325592

Banki, C. M., Vojnik, M., Arato, M., Papp, Z., & Kovacs, Z. (1985). Dexamethasone suppression and multiple hormonal responses (TSH, prolactin and growth hormone) to TRH in some psychiatric disorders. *European Archives of Psychiatry and Neurological Sciences*, *235*(1), 32–37. doi:10.1007/BF00380966 PMID:3930250

Bathla, M., Singh, M., & Relan, P. (2016). Prevalence of anxiety and depressive symptoms among patients with hypothyroidism. *Indian Journal of Endocrinology and Metabolism*, *20*(4), 468–474. doi:10.4103/2230-8210.183476 PMID:27366712

Bauer, M., Heinz, A., & Whybrow, P. C. (2002). Thyroid hormones, serotonin and mood: Of synergy and significance in the adult brain. *Molecular Psychiatry*, *7*(2), 140–156. doi:10.1038j.mp.4000963 PMID:11840307

Belmaker, R. H., & Agam, G. (2008). Mechanisms of Disease: Major depressive disorder. *The New England Journal of Medicine*, *358*(1), 55–68. doi:10.1056/NEJMra073096 PMID:18172175

Belzer, K., & Schneier, F. R. (2004). Comorbidity of anxiety and depressive disorders: Issues in conceptualization, assessment, and treatment. *Journal of Psychiatric Practice*, *10*(5), 296–306. doi:10.1097/00131746-200409000-00003 PMID:15361744

Benton, D. (2002). Selenium Intake, mood and other aspects of psychological functioning. *Nutritional Neuroscience*, *5*(6), 363–374. doi:10.1080/1028415021000055925 PMID:12509066

Bernal, J., & Nunez, J. (1995). Thyroid hormones and brain development. *European Journal of Endocrinology*, *133*(4), 390–398. doi:10.1530/eje.0.1330390 PMID:7581959

Bianchi, G. P., Zaccheroni, V., Solaroli, E., Vescini, F., Cerutti, R., Zoli, M., & Marchesini, G. (2004). Health-related quality of life in patients with thyroid disorders. *Quality of Life Research: An International Journal of Quality of Life Aspects of Treatment, Care and Rehabilitation*, *13*(1), 45–54. doi:10.1023/B:QURE.0000015315.35184.66 PMID:15058786

Biondi, B., & Cooper, D. S. (2008). The clinical significance of subclinical thyroid dysfunction. *Endocrine Reviews*, *29*(1), 76–131. doi:10.1210/er.2006-0043 PMID:17991805

Biondi, M., & Zannino, L. G. (1997). Psychological stress, neuro-immunomodulation, and susceptibility to infectious diseases in animals and man: A review. *Psychotherapy and Psychosomatics*, *66*(1), 3–26. doi:10.1159/000289101 PMID:8996711

Bjoro, T., Holmen, J., Krüger, O., Jin, R., Koretz, D., Merikangas, K. R., ... Wang, P. S. (2000). The Hea.lth Study of Nord-Trondelag (HUNT) Prevale. nce of thyroid disease, thyroid dysfunction and thyroid peroxidase antibodies in a large, unselected population Eurpean. *The Journal of Endocrinology*, *143*(5), 639–647. PMID:11078988

Bunevicius, R., Kazanavicius, G., & Telksnys, A. (1994). Thyrotropin response to TRH stimulation in depressed patients with autoimmune thyroiditis. *Biological Psychiatry*, *36*(8), 543–547. doi:10.1016/0006-3223(94)90618-1 PMID:7827217

Canaris, G. J., Manowitz, N. R., Mayor, G., & Ridgway, E. C. (2000). The Colorado Thyroid Disease Prevalence Study. *Archives of Internal Medicine*, *160*(4), 526–534. doi:10.1001/archinte.160.4.526 PMID:10695693

Carta, M. G., Hardoy, M. C., Boi, M. F., Mariotti, S., Carpiniello, B., & Usai, P. (2002). Association between panic disorder, major depressive disorder and celiac disease. A possible role of thyroid autoimmunity. *Journal of Psychosomatic Research*, *53*(3), 789–793. doi:10.1016/S0022-3999(02)00328-8 PMID:12217453

Carta, M. G., Loviselli, A., Hardoy, M. C., Massa, S., Cadeddu, M., Sardu, C., ... Mariotti, S. (2004). The link between thyroid autoimmunity (antithyroid peroxidase autoantibodies) with anxiety and mood disorders in the community: A field of interest for public health in the future. *BMC Psychiatry*, *4*(1), 25–33. doi:10.1186/1471-244X-4-25 PMID:15317653

Chaudhary, R., Chabra, S., Singla, M., Mishra, B. P., & Sharma, A. (2014). Psychiatric morbidity among hypothyroid patients – A hospital based study. *Delhi Psychiatry Journal*, *4*(17), 35–38.

Chiovato, L., Vitti, P., Santini, F., Lopez, G., Mammoli, C., Bassi, P., ... Pinchera, A. (1990). Incidence of antibodies blocking thyrotropin effect in vitro in patients with euthyroid or hypothyroid autoimmune thyroiditis. *The Journal of Clinical Endocrinology and Metabolism*, *71*(1), 40–45. doi:10.1210/jcem-71-1-40 PMID:2164529

Constant, E. L., Adam, S., Seron, X., Bruyer, R., Seghers, A., & Daumerie, C. (2006). Hypothyroidism and major depression: A common executive dysfunction? *Journal of Clinical and Experimental Neuropsychology*, *28*(5), 790–807. doi:10.1080/13803390591000990 PMID:16723325

Contempre, B., Denef, J. F., Dumont, J. E., & Many, M. C. (1993). Selenium deficiency aggravates the necrotizing effects of a high iodide dose in iodine deficient rats. *Endocrinology*, *132*(4), 1866–1868. doi:10.1210/endo.132.4.8462484 PMID:8462484

Coyle, J. T., Tsai, G., & Goff, D. (2003). Converging evidence of NMDA receptor hypofunction in the pathophysiology of schizophrenia. *Annals of the New York Academy of Sciences*, *1003*(1), 318–327. doi:10.1196/annals.1300.020 PMID:14684455

Davidoff, F., & Gill, J. (1977). Myxedema madness: Psychosis as an early manifestation of hypothyroidism. *Connecticut Medicine*, *41*, 618–621. PMID:913091

Davis, J. D., & Tremont, G. (2007). Neuropsychiatric aspects of hypothyroidism and treatment reversibility. *Minerva Endocrinologica*, *32*, 49–65. PMID:17353866

deCarvalho, G. A., Bahls, S. C., Boeving, A., & Graf, H. (2009). Effects of selective serotonin reuptake inhibitors on thyroid function in depressed patients with primary hypothyroidism or normal thyroid function. *Thyroid*, *19*(7), 691–697. doi:10.1089/thy.2008.0261 PMID:19583486

Degner, D., Haust, M., Meller, J., Rüther, E., & Reulbach, U. (2015). Association between autoimmune thyroiditis and depressive disorder in psychiatric outpatients. *European Archives of Psychiatry and Clinical Neuroscience*, *265*(1), 67–72. doi:10.100700406-014-0529-1 PMID:25193677

Duntas, L. H., Mantzou, E., & Koutras, E. A. (2003). Effects of a six month treatment with selenomethionine in patients with autoimmune thyroiditis. *European Journal of Endocrinology*, *148*, 389–393. doi:10.1530/eje.0.1480389 PMID:12656658

Eaton, W. W., Pedersen, M. G., Nielsen, P. R., & Mortensen, P. B. (2010). Autoimmune diseases, bipolar disorder, and non-affective psychosis. *Bipolar Disorders*, *12*(6), 638–646. doi:10.1111/j.1399-5618.2010.00853.x PMID:20868462

Elenkov, I. J., & Chrousos, G. P. (2002). Stress hormones, proinflammatory and anti-inflammatory cytokines, and autoimmunity. *Annals of the New York Academy of Sciences*, *966*(1), 290–303. doi:10.1111/j.1749-6632.2002.tb04229.x PMID:12114286

Elenkov, I. J., Wilder, R. L., Bakalov, V. K., Dimitrov, M. A., Fisher, S., Crane, M., ... Chrousos, G. P. (2001). IL-12, TNF-alpha, and hormonal changes during late pregnancy and early postpartum: Implications for autoimmune disease activity during these times. *The Journal of Clinical Endocrinology and Metabolism*, *86*, 4033–4038. PMID:11600565

Engum, A., Bjero, T., Myketun, A., & Dahl, A. A. (2002). An association between depression, anxiety and thyroid function a clinical fact or an artifact? *Acta Psychiatrica Scandinavica*, *106*(1), 27–34. doi:10.1034/j.1600-0447.2002.01250.x PMID:12100345

Engum, A., Bjøro, T., Mykletun, A., & Dahl, A. A. (2005). Thyroid autoimmunity, depression and anxiety; are there any connections? An epidemiological study of a large population. *Journal of Psychosomatic Research*, *59*(5), 263–268. doi:10.1016/j.jpsychores.2005.04.002 PMID:16253615

Fava, M., Labbate, L. A., Abraham, M. E., & Rosenbaum, J. F. (1995). Hypothyroidism and hyperthyroidism in major depression revisited. *The Journal of Clinical Psychiatry*, *56*, 186–192. PMID:7737957

Forman-Hoffman, V., & Philibert, R. A. (2006). Lower TSH and higher T4 levels are associated with current depressive syndrome in young adults. *Acta Psychiatrica Scandinavica*, *114*(2), 132–139. doi:10.1111/j.1600-0447.2005.00703.x PMID:16836601

Fountoulakis, K. N., Iacovides, A., & Grammaticos, P. (2004). Thyroid function in clinical subtypes of major depression. *BMC Psychiatry*, *4*(6). PMID:15113438

Gärtner, R., Gasnier, B. C., Dietrich, J. W., Krebs, B., & Angstwurm, M. W. (2002). Selenium supplementation in patients with autoimmune thyroiditis decreases thyroid peroxidase antibodies concentrations. *The Journal of Clinical Endocrinology and Metabolism*, *87*(4), 1687–1691. doi:10.1210/jcem.87.4.8421 PMID:11932302

Gewirtz, G. R., Malaspina, D., Hatterer, J. A., Feureisen, S., Klein, D., & Gorman, J. M. (1988). Occult thyroid dysfunction in patients with refractory depression. *The American Journal of Psychiatry*, *145*(8), 1012–1014. doi:10.1176/ajp.145.8.1012 PMID:3394853

Gold, M. S., Pottash, A. L., & Extein, I. (1981). Hypothyroidism and depression. Evidence from complete thyroid function evaluation. *Journal of the American Medical Association*, *245*(19), 1919–1922. doi:10.1001/jama.1981.03310440019016 PMID:7230383

Goyens, P., Golstein, J., Nsombola, B., Vis, H., & Dumont, J. E. (1987). Selenium deficiency as a possible factor in the pathogenesis of myxoedematous endemic cretinism. *Acta Endocrinologica*, *114*(4), 497–502. doi:10.1530/acta.0.1140497 PMID:3577581

Gulseren, S., Gulseren, L., Hekimsoy, Z., Cetinay, P., Ozen, C., & Tokatlioglu, B. (2006). Depression, anxiety, health-related quality of life, and disability in patients with overt and subclinical thyroid dysfunction. *Archives of Medical Research*, *37*(1), 133–139. doi:10.1016/j.arcmed.2005.05.008 PMID:16314199

Hage, M.P., & Azar, S.T. (2012). The link between thyroid function and depression. *J Thyroid Res*, 590-648.

Haggerty, J. J. Jr, Evans, D. L., Golden, R. N., Pedersen, C. A., Simon, J. S., & Nemeroff, C. B. (1990). The presence of antithyroid antibodies in patients with affective and nonaffective psychiatric disorders. *Biological Psychiatry*, *27*(1), 51–60. doi:10.1016/0006-3223(90)90019-X PMID:2297552

Haggerty, J. J. Jr, Garbutt, J. C., Evans, D. L., Golden, R. N., Pedersen, C., Simon, J. S., & Nemeroff, C. B. (1990). Subclinical hypothyroidism: A review of neuropsychiatric aspects. *International Journal of Psychiatry in Medicine*, *20*(2), 193–208. doi:10.2190/ADLY-1UU0-1A8L-HPXY PMID:2203696

Haggerty, J. J. Jr, & Prange, A. J. Jr. (1995). Borderline hypothyroidism and depression. *Annual Review of Medicine*, *46*(1), 37–46. doi:10.1146/annurev.med.46.1.37 PMID:7598471

Haggerty, J. J., Silva, S. G., Marquardt, M., Mason, G. A., Chang, H. Y., Evans, D. L., ... Pederse.n, C. (1997). Prevale.nce of antithyroid antibodies in mood disorders. *Depression and Anxiety*, *5*(2), 91–96. doi:10.1002/(SICI)1520-6394(1997)5:2<91::AID-DA5>3.0.CO;2-8 PMID:9262939

Haggerty, J. J., Stern, R. A., Mason, G. A., Beckwith, J., Morey, C. E., & Prange, A. J. (1993). Subclinical hypothyroidism: A modifiable risk factor for depression? *The American Journal of Psychiatry*, *150*(3), 508–510. doi:10.1176/ajp.150.3.508 PMID:8434671

Hall, R. C. (1983). Psychiatric effects of thyroid hormone disturbance. *Psychosomatics*, *24*(1), 7–22. doi:10.1016/S0033-3182(83)73255-X PMID:6338551

Hall, R. C., Stickney, S., & Beresford, T. P. (1986). Endocrine disease and behaviour. *Integrative Psychiatry*, *4*, 122–135.

Hall, R. C. W., & Hall, R. C. (1999). Anxiety and endocrine disease. *Seminars in Clinical Neuropsychiatry*, *4*(2), 72–83. PMID:10378951

Harris, B., Fung, H., Johns, S., Kologlu, M., Bhatti, R., McGregor, A. M., ... Hall, R. (1989). Transie.nt post-partum thyroid dysfunction and postnatal depression. *Journal of Affective Disorders*, *17*(3), 243–249. doi:10.1016/0165-0327(89)90006-2 PMID:2529292

Harris, B., Oretti, L., Lazarus, J., Parkes, A., John, R., Richards, C., ... Hall, R. (2002). Randomised trial of thyroxine to prevent postnatal depression in thyroid antibody positive Women. *The British Journal of Psychiatry*, *180*(4), 327–330. doi:10.1192/bjp.180.4.327 PMID:11925355

Haug, T. T., Mykletun, A., & Dahl, A. A. (2004). The association between anxiety, depression, and somatic symptoms in a large population: The Hunt-II study. *Psychosomatic Medicine*, *66*(6), 845–851. doi:10.1097/01.psy.0000145823.85658.0c PMID:15564348

Hendrick, V., Altshuler, L., & Whybrow, P. (1998). Psychoneuroendocrinology of mood disorders: The hypothalamic-pituitary-thyroid axis. *The Psychiatric Clinics of North America*, *21*(2), 277–292. doi:10.1016/S0193-953X(05)70005-8 PMID:9670226

Hollowell, J. G., Staehling, N. W., Flanders, W. D., Hannon, W. H., Gunter, E. W., Spencer, C. A., & Braverman, L. E. (2002). Serum TSH, T4, and thyroid antibodies in the United States population (1988 to 1994): National Health and Nutrition Examination Survey (NHANES III). *The Journal of Clinical Endocrinology and Metabolism*, *87*(2), 489–499. doi:10.1210/jcem.87.2.8182 PMID:11836274

Howland, R. H. (1993). Thyroid dysfunction in refractory depression: Implications for pathophysiology and treatment. *The Journal of Clinical Psychiatry*, *54*, 47–54. PMID:8444820

Ittermann, T., Völzke, H., Baumeister, S. E., Appel, K., & Grabe, H. J. (2015). Diagnosed thyroid disorders are associated with depression and anxiety. *Social Psychiatry and Psychiatric Epidemiology*, *50*(9), 1417–1425. doi:10.100700127-015-1043-0 PMID:25777685

Joffe, R., Segal, Z., & Singer, W. (1996). Change in thyroid hormone levels following response to cognitive therapy for major depression. *The American Journal of Psychiatry*, *153*(3), 411–413. doi:10.1176/ajp.153.3.411 PMID:8610831

Joffe, R. T. (1987). Antithyroid antibodies in major depression. *Acta Psychiatrica Scandinavica*, *76*(5), 598–599. doi:10.1111/j.1600-0447.1987.tb02925.x PMID:3434332

Joffe, R. T., & Levitt, J. (1992). Major depression and subclinical (grade 2) hypothyroidism. *Psychoneuroendocrinology*, *17*(2-3), 215–221. doi:10.1016/0306-4530(92)90060-K PMID:1438646

Kessler, R. C. (2012). The costs of depression. *The Psychiatric Clinics of North America*, *35*(1), 1–14. doi:10.1016/j.psc.2011.11.005 PMID:22370487

Kessler, R. C., Berglund, P., Demler, O., Jin, R., Koretz, D., Merikangas, K. R., ... Wang, P. S. (2003). Nationa.l Comorbidity Survey Replication The epi. demiology of major depressive disorder: Results from the National Comorbidity Survey Replication (NCS-R). *Journal of the American Medical Association, 289*(23), 3095–3105. doi:10.1001/jama.289.23.3095 PMID:12813115

Kessler, R. C., Chiu, W. T., Demler, O., Merikangas, K. R., & Walters, E. E. (2005). Prevalence, severity, and comorbidity of 12-month DSM-IV disorders in the National Comorbidity Survey Replication. *Archives of General Psychiatry, 62*(6), 617–627. doi:10.1001/archpsyc.62.6.617 PMID:15939839

Kirim, S., Keşkek, Ş. Ö., Köksal, F., Haydardedeoğlu, F. E., Bozkirli, E., & Toledano, Y. (2012). Depression in patients with euthyroid chronic autoimmune thyroiditis. *Endocrine Journal, 59*(8), 705–708. doi:10.1507/endocrj.EJ12-0035 PMID:22673294

Kjellman, B. F., Ljunggren, J. G., Beck-Friis, J., & Wetterberg, L. (1985). Effect of TRH on TSH and prolactin levels in affective disorders. *Psychiatry Research, 14*(4), 353–363. doi:10.1016/0165-1781(85)90103-9 PMID:3927333

Kong, W. M., Sheikh, M. H., Lumb, P. J., Freedman, D. B., Crook, M., Doré, C. J., & Finer, N. (2002). A 6-month randomized trial of thyroxine treatment in women with mild subclinical hypothyroidism. *The American Journal of Medicine, 112*(5), 348–354. doi:10.1016/S0002-9343(02)01022-7 PMID:11904108

Lépine, J. P. (2002). The epidemiology of anxiety disorders: Prevalence and societal costs. *The Journal of Clinical Psychiatry, 63*(suppl 14), 4–8. PMID:12562112

Linkowski, P., Brauman, H., & Mendlewicz, J. (1981). Thyrotrophin response to thyrotrophin-releasing hormone in unipolar and bipolar affective illness. *Journal of Affective Disorders, 3*(1), 9–16. doi:10.1016/0165-0327(81)90014-8 PMID:6455462

Lissek, S., Powers, A. S., McClure, E. B., Phelps, E. A., Wolehawariat, G., Grillon, C., & Pine, D. (2005). Classical fear conditioning in the anxiety disorders: A meta-analysis. *Behaviour Research and Therapy, 43*(11), 1391–1424. doi:10.1016/j.brat.2004.10.007 PMID:15885654

Loosen, P. T. (1985). The TRH-induced TSH response in psychiatric patients: A possible neuroendocrine marker. *Psychoneuroendocrinology*, *10*(3), 237–260. doi:10.1016/0306-4530(85)90002-2 PMID:2865765

Loosen, P. T. (1985). The TRH-induced TSH response in psychiatric patients: A possible neuroendocrine marker. *Psychoneuroendocrinology*, *10*(3), 237–260. doi:10.1016/0306-4530(85)90002-2 PMID:2865765

Maes, M., D'Hondt, P., Blockx, P., & Cosyns, P. (1994). A further investigation of basal HPT axis function in unipolar depression: Effects of diagnosis, hospitalization, and dexamethasone administration. *Psychiatry Research*, *51*(2), 185–201. doi:10.1016/0165-1781(94)90038-8 PMID:8022953

Maier, S. F., & Seligman, M. E. (1976). Learned helplessness: Theory and evidence. *Journal of Experimental Psychology. General*, *105*(1), 3–46. doi:10.1037/0096-3445.105.1.3

Marangell, L. B., & Callahan, A. M. (1998). Mood disorders and the thyroid axis. *Current Opinion in Psychiatry*, *11*(1), 67–70. doi:10.1097/00001504-199801000-00023

Marchesi, C., Chiodera, P., DeRisio, C., Dassò, L., Govi, A. M., DeFerri, A., ... Gnudi, A. (1988). Dopamin.ergic control of TSH secretion in endogenous depression. *Psychiatry Research*, *25*(3), 277–282. doi:10.1016/0165-1781(88)90098-4 PMID:3141942

Müssig, K., & Leyhe, T. (2013). Kognitive und affektive störungen bei autoimmunthyreoiditis. *Der Nuklearmediziner*, *36*(4), 250–255.

Nagele, E., Han, M., Demarshall, C., Belinka, B., & Nagele, R. (2011). Diagnosis of Alzheimer's disease based on disease-specific autoantibody profiles in human sera. *PLoS One*, *6*(8), e23112. doi:10.1371/journal.pone.0023112 PMID:21826230

Nemeroff, C. B., Simon, J. S., Haggerty, J. J., & Evans, D. L. (1985). Antithyroid antibodies in depressed patients. *The American Journal of Psychiatry*, *142*(7), 840–843. doi:10.1176/ajp.142.7.840 PMID:4014506

Nemeroff, C.B. (1989). Clinical significance of psychoneuro-endocrinology in psychiatry: focus on the thyroid and adrenal. *Journal of Clinical Psychiatry*, *50*, 13-20.

O'Donnell, M., Silove, D., & Wakefield, D. (1988). Current perspectives on immunology and psychiatry. *The Australian and New Zealand Journal of Psychiatry*, *22*(4), 66–382. doi:10.3109/00048678809161345 PMID:3071320

Ott, J., Promberger, R., Kober, F., Neuhold, N., Tea, M., Huber, J. C., & Hermann, M. (2001). Hashimoto's thyroiditis affects symptom load and quality of life unrelated to hypothyroidism: A prospective case-control study in women undergoing thyroidectomy for benign goiter. *Thyroid*, *21*(2), 161–167. doi:10.1089/thy.2010.0191 PMID:21186954

Pies, R. W. (1995). Women, mood, and the thyroid. *Women Psychiatry Health*, *4*, 4–10.

Pisanu, A., Piu, S., Cois, A., & Uccheddu, A. (2003). Coexisting Hashimoto's thyroiditis with differentiated thyroid cancer and benign thyroid diseases: Indications for thyroidectomy. *Chirurgia Italiana*, *55*(3), 365–372. PMID:12872571

Pollak, T. A., McCormack, R., Peakman, M., Nicholson, T. R., & David, A. S. (2014). Prevalence of anti–N-methyl-D-aspartate (NMDA) receptor antibodies in patients with schizophrenia and related psychoses: A systematic review and meta-analysis. *Psychological Medicine*, *44*(12), 2475–2487. doi:10.1017/S003329171300295X PMID:24330811

Pop, V. J., Maartens, L. H., Leusink, G., vanSon, M. J., Knottnerus, A. A., Ward, A. M., ... Weetman, A. P. (1988). Are autoimmune thyroid dysfunction and depression related? *The Journal of Clinical Endocrinology and Metabolism*, *83*, 3194–3197. PMID:9745425

Popkin, M. K., & Mackenzie, T. B. (1980). Psychiatric presentations of endocrine dysfunction. In R. C. Hall (Ed.), *Psychiatric Presentations of Medical Illness* (pp. 142–143). New York, NY: Spectrum Books. doi:10.1007/978-94-011-7677-4_9

Poppe, K., Velkeniers, B., & Glinoer, D. (2008). The role of thyroid autoimmunity in fertility and pregnancy. *Nature Clinical Practice. Endocrinology & Metabolism*, *4*(7), 394–405. doi:10.1038/ncpendmet0846 PMID:18506157

Pozzi, M., Pellegrino, P., Carnovale, C., Perrone, V., Antoniazzi, S., Perrotta, C., ... Clementi, E. (2014). On the connection between autoimmunity, tic disorders and obsessive-compulsive disorders: A meta-analysis on anti-streptolysin O titres. *Journal of Neuroimmune Pharmacology*, *9*(5), 606–614. doi:10.100711481-014-9561-1 PMID:25091468

Rao, M. L., Vartzopoulos, D., & Fels, K. (1989). Thyroid function in anxious and depressed patients. *Pharmacopsychiatry*, *22*(02), 66–70. doi:10.1055-2007-1014580 PMID:2497474

Rupprecht, R., Rupprecht, C., Rupprecht, M., Noder, M., & Mahlstedt, J. (1989). Triiodothyronine, thyroxine, and TSH response to dexamethasone in depressed patients and normal controls. *Biological Psychiatry*, *25*(1), 22–32. doi:10.1016/0006-3223(89)90143-1 PMID:2912508

Sartorius, N., Ustün, T. B., Lecrubier, Y., & Wittchen, H. U. (1996). Depression comorbid with anxiety: Results from the WHO study on psychological disorders in primary health care. *The British Journal of Psychiatry*, *30*(30), 38–43. doi:10.1192/S0007125000298395 PMID:8864147

Schenck, J. B., Rizvi, A. A., & Lin, T. (2006). Severe primary hypothyroidism manifesting with torsades de pointes. *The American Journal of the Medical Sciences*, *331*(3), 154–156. doi:10.1097/00000441-200603000-00008 PMID:16538077

Scolari, A., Pozzi, M., Bellia, V., Apale, P., Santamaria, G., Bordoni, T., ... Roffi, L. (2005). Interferon-induced depression: Prevalence and management. *Digestive and Liver Disease*, *37*(2), 102–107. doi:10.1016/j.dld.2004.09.018 PMID:15733522

Shinkov, A., Borissova, A., Vlahov, J., Dakovska, L., & Blajeva, E. (2014). Male gender differences in the thyroid ultrasound features, thyroid peroxidase antibodies and thyroid hormone levels: A large population-based study. *Journal of Endocrinological Investigation*, *37*(3), 269–276. doi:10.100740618-013-0024-y PMID:24615363

Shojaie, M., & Eshraghian, A. (2008). Primary hypothyroidism presenting with torsades de pointes type tachycardia: A case report. *Cases Journal*, *1*(1), 298–301. doi:10.1186/1757-1626-1-298 PMID:18990220

Shor-Posner, G. R., Miguez, M. J., Miguez, M.-T., Moreno-Black, G., Zhnag, G., Rodriguez, N., ... Wilkie, F. (2003). Psychol.ogical burden in the era of HAART: Impact of selenium therapy. *International Journal of Psychiatry in Medicine*, *33*(1), 55–69. doi:10.2190/PFFD-D920-V041-N5KD PMID:12906343

Siegmann, E. M., Müller, H. H., Luecke, C., Philipsen, A., Kornhuber, J., & Grömer, T. W. (2018). Association of Depression and Anxiety Disorders with Autoimmune Thyroiditis: A Systematic Review and Meta-analysis. *Journal of the American Medical Association of Psychiatry*, *75*(6), 577–584. PMID:29800939

Singer, P. A., Cooper, D. S., Levy, E. G., Ladenson, P. W., Braverman, L. E., Daniels, G., ... Nikolai, T. F. (1995). Treatme.nt guidelines for patients with hyperthyroidism and hypothyroidism: Standards of Care Committee, American Thyroid Association. *Journal of the American Medical Association*, *273*(10), 808–812. doi:10.1001/jama.1995.03520340064038 PMID:7532241

Smith, J. W., Evans, A. T., Costall, B., & Smythe, J. W. (2002). Thyroid hormones, brain function and cognition: A brief review. *Neuroscience and Biobehavioral Reviews*, *26*(1), 45–60. doi:10.1016/S0149-7634(01)00037-9 PMID:11835983

Stein, M. B., & Uhde, T. W. (1989). Autoimmune thyroiditis and panic disorder. *The American Journal of Psychiatry*, *146*(2), 259–260. doi:10.1176/ajp.146.2.259 PMID:2912271

Surks, M. I., Ortiz, E., Daniels, G. H., Saein, C. T., Col, N. F., Cobin, R. H., ... Wessman, N. J. (2004). Subclinical thyroid disease: Scientific review and guidelines for diagnosis and management. *Journal of the American Medical Association*, *291*(2), 228–238. doi:10.1001/jama.291.2.228 PMID:14722150

Toulis, K. A., Anastasilakis, A. D., Tzellos, T. G., Goulis, D. G., & Kouvelas, D. (2010). Selenium supplementation in the treatment of Hashimoto's thyroiditis: A systematic review and a meta-analysis. *Thyroid*, *20*(10), 1163–1173. doi:10.1089/thy.2009.0351 PMID:20883174

Vanderpump, M. P. J. (2011). The epidemiology of thyroid disease. *British Medical Bulletin*, *99*(1), 39–51. doi:10.1093/bmb/ldr030 PMID:21893493

Whybrow, P. C., Prange, A. J. Jr, & Treadway, C. R. (1969). Mental changes accompanying thyroid gland dysfunction. A reappraisal using objective psychological measurement. *Archives of General Psychiatry*, *20*(1), 48–63. doi:10.1001/archpsyc.1969.01740130050004 PMID:4387067

Yalcin, M. M., Altinova, A. E., Cavnar, B., Bolayir, B., Akturk, M., Arslan, E., ... Toruner, F. B. (2017). Is thyroid autoimmunity itself associated with psychological well-being in euthyroid Hashimoto's thyroiditis? *Endocrine Journal*, *64*(4), 425–429. doi:10.1507/endocrj.EJ16-0418 PMID:28260699

Chapter 12
Differential Diagnosis

ABSTRACT

Diseases that should be considered in the differential diagnosis of Hashimoto's thyroiditis (HT) include subacute thyroiditis and Reidle's thyroiditis, Graves' disease, euthyroid sick syndrome, goiter, hypopituitarism, lithium-induced goiter, simple (non-toxic) goiter, thyroid lymphoma, toxic nodular goiter, and types I and II polyglandular autoimmune syndrome. The characteristic diagnostic clinical, biochemical, imaging (sonographic), and histological/cytological features of HT will help make a differential diagnosis. This chapter explores the differential diagnosis of Hashimoto's disease.

THYROIDITIS

Hashimoto's thyroiditis should be distinguished from other forms of ***thyroiditis***.

- *Subacute granulomatous thyroiditis:* It is a self-limiting painful disorder of the thyroid. Clinical examination, elevated erythrocyte sedimentation rate (ESR), elevated thyroglobulin (Tg) level and decreased radioactive iodine (RAI) uptake confirms the diagnosis.
- *Acute suppurative thyroiditis*: It is a rare infectious condition of the thyroid.
- *Reidle's thyroiditis*: It is a fibrosing disorder of thyroid characterized by hypothyroidism and hypocalcemia, and diagnosis is made by histo-pathology.

DOI: 10.4018/978-1-5225-9655-4.ch012

MULTINODULAR GOITER (MNG)

Hashimoto's thyroiditis is to be also distinguished from non-toxic nodular goiter or Graves' disease. The presence of gross nodularity is strong evidence against Hashimoto's thyroiditis, but differentiation on this basis is not reliable. In *multinodular goiter* (MNG), thyroid function test results are usually normal, and the patient is only rarely clinically hypothyroid. Thyroid auto-antibodies tend to be absent or titers are low, and the scan result is typical. Fine-needle aspiration (FNA) can resolve the question but is usually unnecessary. In fact, the two conditions quite commonly occur together in adult women. Whether this is a co-incidence, or due to the effect of thyroid growth stimulating antibodies (or other causes) is still unknown.

Moderately and diffusely enlarged thyroid glands in teen-agers are usually the result of thyroiditis, but some may be true adolescent goiters; that is, the enlargement may result from moderate hyperplasia of the thyroid gland in response to a temporarily increased demand for hormone. This condition is more often diagnosed than proved. Thyroid function test results should be normal. Antibody assays may resolve the issue. The diagnosis can be settled with certainty only by a biopsy disclosing normal or hyperplastic thyroid tissue and absence of findings of thyroiditis. The possibility of ***colloid goiter*** may also be entertained in the differential diagnosis. Colloid goiter is a definite pathologic entity. Presumably it is the resting phase after a period of thyroid hyperplasia.

THYROID NEOPLASM

A thyroid tumor must also be considered in the differential diagnosis of Hashimoto's disease, particularly if there is rapid growth of the gland or persistent pain. The diffuse nature of autoimmune thyroiditis, the characteristic hypothyroidism and involvement of the pyramidal lobe are usually sufficient for differentiation. It is still uncertain whether FNA is indicated. However, it must be remembered that lymphoma or a small-cell carcinoma of the thyroid can be and has been mistaken for Hashimoto's thyroiditis. Clusters of nodes at the upper poles strongly suggesting *papillary thyroid carcinoma* (PTC) may disappear when thyroid hormone replacement therapy is given. However, a sufficient number of patients with both thyroiditis and tumor have been recorded. Thus, one diagnosis in no way excludes the other. Papillary thyroid carcinoma with Hashimoto's thyroiditis is characterized by female predominance, multi-focality, no extra-thyroid extension, no lymph node metastasis and better recurrence-free survival (Zhang, 2012; Fiore, 2011; Krysiak, 2011). Thyroid *lymphoma* must always be considered if there is continued (especially asymmetric) enlargement of a Hashimoto's gland, or if pain, tenderness, hoarseness, or nodes develop. Thyroiditis is a risk factor for thyroid lymphoma, although the incidence is very low. Distinguishing thyroid lymphoma from Hashimoto's thyroiditis is sometimes quite difficultin cytology. Flow cytometry, immune histochemistry or polymerase chain reaction (PCR) should aid in diagnosis (wozniak, 1999; Miller, 1991). Reverse transcription-polymerase chain reaction (RT-PCR) detecting the mono-clonality of immunoglobulin heavy chain mRNA is useful for differentiation between the two (Tanako et al., 2000).

THYROTOXICOSIS

Occasionally, the picture of Hashimoto's thyroiditis blends rather imperceptibly into that of *thyrotoxicosis*, and some patients have symptoms of mild thyrotoxicosis, but then develop typical Hashimoto's thyroiditis. In fact, it is best to think of Graves' disease and Hashimoto's thyroiditis as two very closely related syndromes produced by thyroid autoimmunity. Categorization depends on associated *eye findings* and the *metabolic* level, but the pathogenesis, histologic picture, and function may overlap. Some patients may have a mixture of Hashimoto's thyroiditis and subacute thyroiditis, with goiter, positive thyroid auto-antibodies, and normal or low FT4.

AMYLOIDOSIS

A form of painful chronic thyroiditis with *amyloid* infiltration has also been described, and is probably etiologically distinct from Hashimoto's thyroiditis (McConahey, Woolner, Black, & Keating, 1959).

OTHER AUTOIMMUNE DISEASES

Other autoimmune diseases like Addison's disease, diabetes mellitus type-1, rheumatoid arthritis, systemic lupus erythymatosus or viteligo can co-exist with Hashimoto's thyroiditis.

Diseases that should be considered in the differential diagnosis of Hashimoto's thyroiditis are summarized in Table 1.

The characteristic diagnostic clinical, biochemical, imaging (sonographic) and histological/cytological features of Hashimoto's thyroiditis were depicted in "Table 1 in Chapter 7, pages 148-149". These characteristic features will help make a differential diagnosis.

Table 1. Differential diagnosis of Hashimoto's disease

• Subacute thyroiditis and Reidle's thyroiditis. • Diffuse Toxic Goiter (Graves' Disease) • Euthyroid Sick Syndrome • Goiter • Hypo-pituitarism (Pan-hypopituitarism) • Lithium-Induced Goiter • Nontoxic Goiter • Thyroid Lymphoma • Toxic Nodular Goiter • Type I Polyglandular Autoimmune Syndrome • Type II Polyglandular Autoimmune Syndrome

REFERENCES

Fiore, E., Rago, T., Latrofa, F., Provenzale, M. A., Piaggi, P., Delitala, A., ... Vitti, P. (2011). Hashimoto's thyroiditis is associated with papillary thyroid carcinoma: Role of TSH and treatment with L-thyroxine. *Endocrine-Related Cancer, 18*(4), 429–437. doi:10.1530/ERC-11-0028 PMID:21565972

Krysiak, R., & Okopien, B. (2011). The Effect of Levothyroxine and Selenomethionine on Lymphocyte and Monocyte Cytokine Release in Women with Hashimoto's Thyroiditis. *The Journal of Clinical Endocrinology and Metabolism, 96*(7), 2206–2215. doi:10.1210/jc.2010-2986 PMID:21508145

McConahey, W. M., Woolner, L. B., Black, B. M., & Keating, F. R. Jr. (1959). Effect of desiccated thyroid in lymphocytic (Hashimoto's) thyroiditis. *The Journal of Clinical Endocrinology and Metabolism, 19*(1), 45–49. doi:10.1210/jcem-19-1-45 PMID:13620732

Miller, B. S., & Paul, G. (1991). Image in endocrinology: Thyroid Lymphoma Arising from Hashimoto's Thyroiditis. *The Journal of Clinical Endocrinology and Metabolism, 10*, 3711–3712.

Takano, T., Miyauchi, A., Matsuzuka, F., Yoshida, H., Kuma, K., & Amino, N. (2000). Diagnosis of thyroid malignant lymphoma by reverse transcription-polymerase chain reaction detecting the monoclonality of immunoglobulin heavy chain messenger ribonucleic acid. *The Journal of Clinical Endocrinology and Metabolism, 85*, 671–675. PMID:10690874

Wozniak, R., Beckwith, L., Ratech, H., & Surks, M. I. (1999). Maltoma of the Thyroid in a Man with Hashimoto's Thyroiditis. *The Journal of Clinical Endocrinology and Metabolism, 4*, 84–88. PMID:10199754

Zhang, L., Li, H., Ji, Q., Zhu, Y., Wang, Z., Wang, Y., ... Wu, Y. (2012). Clinica.l features of papillary thyroid cancer in ht patients from an area with a high prevalence of Hashimoto's disease. *BMC Cancer, 12*, 610–615. doi:10.1186/1471-2407-12-610 PMID:23256514

Chapter 13
Association with Papillary Thyroid Carcinoma

ABSTRACT

There is a close relationship between Hashimoto's thyroiditis (HT) and papillary thyroid carcinoma (PTC). As the incidence of HT is increased in PTC patients, careful clinical monitoring for the patients with HT and meticulous histopathological examination of surgical specimens from these patients are required. The PTCs with Hashimoto's thyroiditis are characterized by female predominance, multi-focality, no extra-thyroidal extension, no lymph node metastasis, and better recurrence-free survival outcomes. Occurrence of HT with PTC is not related to age of the patient or size of the tumor. This chapter explores Hashimoto's disease's association with papillary thyroid carcinoma.

INTRODUCTION

No consensus exists on the association between Hashimoto's thyroiditis and papillary thyroid carcinoma (PTC), which is the most prevalent form of thyroid cancer, comprising about 80% of all diagnosed thyroid cancers. Hashimoto's thyroiditis (chronic lymphocytic thyroiditis or autoimmune thyroiditis) is a well-defined clinico-pathological entity and its incidence has increased over the past 50 years (Antonaci, Consorti, Mardente, & Giovannone, 2009). It is characterized by hypothyroidism, the presence of serum anti-thyroglobulin and anti-peroxidase antibodies, and widespread lymphocytic infiltration with depletion of follicular cells. In addition to the classical Hashimoto's

DOI: 10.4018/978-1-5225-9655-4.ch013

thyroiditis, recent studies have proposed that IgG 4-related thyroiditis may be considered as a variant of the disease (Ahmed, Al-Shaikh, & Akhtar, 2012).

The association between Hashimoto's thyroiditis and PTC has been a subject of long and ongoing debate((Antonaci, 2009; Ahmed, 2012). Hashimoto's thyroiditis has shown a wide range of occurrence from 5% to 85% in thyroid specimens resected for PTC. In addition, the clinico-pathological characteristics of PTC with concomitant Hashimoto's thyroiditis have not been definitely proposed.

This chapter aims at clarifying the relationship between Hashimoto's thyroiditis (histologically- proven) and PTC and identifying the clinico-pathological features of PTC with coexistent Hashimoto's thyroiditis.

META-ANALYSIS

A total of 38 articles satisfied the eligibility criteria for this meta-analysis. (Kim, 2011; Consorti, 2010; Mazokopakis, 2010; Fiori, 2009; Kurukahvecioglu, 2007; Matsumoto, 2006; Cipolla, 2005; Tamimi, 2002; O,Hanlon, 1997; Okayaso, 1995; McLeod, 1988; Huang, 2011; Repplinger, 2008; Van Savell, 2004; Herach, 2002; Loh, 1999; Singh, 1999; Schaffler, 1998; Mancini, 1993; Baroni, 1983; Peterson, 1957; Yoon, 2012; Muzza, 2010; Kim, 2010, Fernch, 2010; Kim 2009a; Kim, 2009b; Bruland, 2009; Onak, 2009; Ohmori, 2007; Neuhold, 2001; Kebebew, 2001; Kashima, 1998; Asanuma, 1998; Gomez-Saez, 1997; Matsubayashi, 1985; Del Rio, 2008; Gul, 2010).

The number of patients in each study ranged from 6 to 1788, for a total of 10,648 PTC patients. Among the PTC patients, Hashimoto's thyroiditis was present in 2,471 (23.2%) cases.

Hashimoto's Thyroiditis in PTC *versus* Benign Lesions

Eleven studies compared the occurrences of HT in PTCs and in benign thyroid diseases such as nodular hyperplasia and follicular adenoma (Kim, 2011; Consorti, 2010; Mazokopakis, 2010; Fiori, 2009; Kurukahvecioglu, 2007; Matsumoto, 2006; Cipolla, 2005; Tamimi, 2002; O,Hanlon, 1997; Okayaso, 1995; McLeod, 1988). Hashimoto's thyroiditis was found in 938 (40.5%) of 2,317 PTC patients, whereas it was found in 634 (21%) of 3,019 benign thyroid diseases. Thus, the coexistence of HT was significantly associated with PTCs than benign lesions (P=0.001).

Hashimoto's Thyroiditis in PTC versus Other Carcinomas

Sixteen studies investigated the frequencies of HT in PTCs and in other carcinomas such as follicular thyroid carcinoma (FTC) and medullary thyroid carcinoma (FTC) (Kim, 2011; Mazokopakis, 2010; Matsumoto, 2006; Tamimi, 202; O'Hanlon, 1997; McLeod, 1988; Huang, 2011; Repplinger, 2008; Van Savell, 2004; Herach, 2002; Loh, 1999; Singh, 1999; Schaffler, 1998; Mancini, 1993; Baroni, 1983; Peterson, 1957). Hashimoto's thyroiditis was present in 797 (17.1%) of 4,664 PTC patients as compared to 57 (7.9%) of 725 other carcinoma patients. The coexistence of HT was thus significantly more related to PTCs than other thyroid carcinomas (P=0.001).

Clinico-Pathological Characteristics of PTCs with Hashimoto's Thyroiditis

Gender

The incidence of Hashimoto's thyroiditis in PTCs according to gender was compared in 23 studies (Kim, 2011; Consorti, 2010; Mazokopakis, 2010; Fiori, 2009; Kurukahvecioglu, 2007; Huang, 2011; Repplinger, 2008; Singh, 1999; Yoon, 2012; Muzza, 2010; Kim, 2010, Fernch, 2010; Kim 2009a; Kim, 2009b; Bruland, 2009; Onak, 2009; Ohmori, 2007; Neuhold, 2001; Kebebew, 2001; Kashima, 1998; Asanuma, 1998; Gomez-Saez, 1997; Matsubayashi, 1985). Hashimoto's thyroiditis in PTCs was observed in 1,677 of 7,346 (23%) female patients as compared to 180 of 573 (11%) male patients. On the basis of this finding, there was a highly significant association of HT in PTCs with females but not with males (P=0.001).

Age

Fourteen studies addressed the frequency of Hashimoto's thyroiditis in PTCs according to patients' mean age (Kim, 2011; Consorti, 2010; Mazokopakis, 2010; Huang, 2011; Repplinger, 2008; Van Savell, 2004; Herach, 2002; Loh, 1999; Singh, 1999; Schaffler, 1998; Mancini, 1993; Baroni, 1983; Peterson, 1957; Yoon, 2012). The mean age of PTC patients with Hashimoto's thyroiditis ranged from 39.5 to 69.0 years, whereas the mean age of PTC patients without HT ranged from 38.2 to 56.3 years. There was no association between the mean age of PTC patients and the incidence of Hashimoto's thyroiditis in PTC.

Tumor Size

Eleven studies identified the prevalence of Hashimoto's thyroiditis in PTCs according to average tumor size (Kim, 2011; Consorti, 2010; Huang, 2011; Yoon, 2012; Kim, 2009a; Ohmori, 2007; Neuhold, 2001; Asanuma, 1998; Gomez-Saez, 1997; Matsubayashi, 1985; Del Rio, 2008). The mean tumor size of PTCs with Hashimoto's thyroiditis ranged from 0.6 to 4.8 cm, whereas those of PTCs without HT ranged from 0.6 to 3.0 cm. Thus, the tumor size was not related to the frequency of Hashimoto's thyroiditis in PTC.

Tumor Extension

Eleven studies presented 4,128 PTCs *without* extra-thyroidal extension and 2,897 PTCs with extra-thyroidal involvement (Kim, 2011; Huang, 2011; Singh, 1999); Yoon, 2012; Fernch, 2010; Kim 2009a; Kim, 2009b; Kashima, 1998; Matsubayashi, 1985; Del Rio, 2008; Gul, 2010). Hashimoto's thyroiditis was found in 722 (17.5%) of 4,128 PTCs without extra-thyroidal extension and in 500 (17.2%) of 2,897 PTCs with extra-thyroidal extension. The coexistence of Hashimoto's thyroiditis in PTCs was not thus associated with extra-thyroidal involvement of PTC.

Lymph Node Metastasis

Sixteen studies reported 4,185 PTC patients without lymph node metastasis and 3,462 patients with lymph node metastasis (Kim, 2011; Consorti, 2010; Kurukahvecioglu, 2007; Huang, 2011; Singh, 1999; Yoon, 2012; Muzza, 2010; Fernch, 2010; Kim 2009a; Kim, 2009b; Bruland, 2009; Kashima, 1998; Gomez-Saez, 1997; Matsubayashi, 1985; Del Rio, 2008; Gul, 2010). Hashimoto's thyroiditis was seen in 746 (17.8%) of 4,185 PTC cases without lymph node metastasis as compared to 622 (17.9%) of 3,462 cases with lymph node metastasis. The difference between both Groups was statistically significant ($p=0.012$).

Multi-Focality

Twelve studies addressed the frequencies of Hashimoto's thyroiditis in single and multi-focal PTCs (Kim, 2011; Consorti, 2010; Kurukahvecioglu, 2007;

Yoon, 2012; Kim, 2010; Kim, 2009a; Neuhold, 2001; Kebebew, 2001; Asanuma, 1998; Gomez-Saez, 1997; Del Rio, 2008; Gul, 2010).

The studies included 1,378 patients with multi-focal PTC and 2,549 with single PTC. Hashimoto's thyroiditis was present in 359 (26%) of 1,378 multi-focal PTCs and in 541 (21%) of 2,549 single PTCs. Hashimoto's thyroiditis was significantly more often observed in multi-focal PTCs than in single PTCs (p=0.015).

Analysis of Survival

Four studies including 616 patients of PTC with Hashimoto's thyroiditis and 4,241 of PTC without Hashimoto's thyroiditis reported that Hashimoto's thyroiditis in PTCs was significantly associated with a long duration of recurrence-free survival (P=0.001) (Huang, 2011; Kim, 2009a; Kashima, 1998; Matsubayashi, 1985).

Significance of Presence of Hashimoto's Thyroiditis in Papillary Thyroid Carcinoma (PTC)

This meta-analysis showed that pathologically confirmed Hashimoto's thyroiditis is more often found in PTC than in benign thyroid diseases and in other carcinomas. Moreover, it revealed that PTCs with coexisting HT are associated with female gender, multi-focal involvement, the absence of extra-thyroidal extension or lymph node metastasis, as well as high recurrence-free survival rates.

The pooled analysis indicates that the frequency of Hashimoto's thyroiditis in PTCs was about 23%, (range 5-85%. The varying incidence rates of Hashimoto's thyroiditis in PTC may be due to several factors such as different diagnostic criteria for Hashimoto's thyroiditis, various surgical procedures, and heterogeneous patient characteristics. Most studies presented the incidence of Hashimoto's thyroiditis in surgically resected PTC cases. In cytology specimens of Hashimoto's thyroiditis patients, follicular cells often exhibit nuclear elongation, nuclear grooves, and even intra-nuclear inclusions, leading to a mis-diagnosis of PTC (Feldt-Rasmussen, 2010; Haberal, 2009). Therefore, the current meta-analysis included only the studies that presented cases of Hashimoto's thyroiditis confirmed by histo-pathological diagnosis.

The occurrence rate of Hashimoto's thyroiditis in PTC patients is 2.8 times higher than Hashimoto's thyroiditis HT patients in benign thyroid diseases.

In addition, the incidence of Hashimoto's thyroiditis in patients with PTC is 2.4 times higher than in those patients with other types of thyroid carcinoma. Some studies supported the tight association between Hashimoto's thyroiditis and PTC, based on the fact that RET/PTC rearrangements were found in about 90% of Hashimoto's thyroiditis cases (wirtschafter et al., 1997) and transgenic mice expressing RET/PTC developed Hashimoto's thyroiditis and PTCs (Powel et al., 1998).

Interestingly, this meta-analysis revealed that PTC patients with coexisting Hashimoto's thyroiditis had distinctive clinico-pathological characteristics such as female gender, multi-focality, no extra-thyroidal extension, no lymph node metastasis, and long recurrence-free survival. Considerable controversy exists concerning the prognostic significance of Hashimoto's thyroiditis in PTC patients. It has been reported that PTC with Hashimoto's thyroiditis was significantly associated with females and a lower incidence of extra-thyroidal invasion and lymph node metastasis (Loh, 1999; Yoon, 2012). Several studies reported that PTC with Hashimoto's thyroiditis had a tendency for multi-focal involvement (Kim, 2011; Consorti, 2010; Kim, 2010; Kebebew, 2001). On the contrary, other studies have failed to present any significant clinico-pathological characteristics in PTC with Hashimoto's thyroiditis (Mazokopakis, 2010; Muzza, 2010; Gul, 2010). Occurrence of Hashimoto's thyroiditis with PTC is not related to age of the patient or size of the tumor (Lee, Kim, Choi, & Kim, 2013).

There may be a possible tight link between Hashimoto's thyroiditis and the development of PTC rather than a chance occurrence of two relatively common diseases. Paradoxically, Hashimoto's thyroiditis in PTC patients appears to play a role in impeding cancer progression. Therefore, the cross-link of these two conditions may represent a cause and effect relationship or a predisposing factor. It is hypothesized that PTC is induced or facilitated by a pre-existing lymphocytic infiltration. Conversely, lymphocytic infiltration of Hashimoto's thyroiditis may be due to autoimmune thyroiditis and/or immune reaction to tumor-specific antigens from a pre-existing PTC (Kim, 2011).

REFERENCES

Ahmed, R., Al-Shaikh, S., & Akhtar, M. (2012). Hashimoto's thyroiditis: A century later. *Advances in Anatomic Pathology*, *19*(3), 181–186. doi:10.1097/PAP.0b013e3182534868 PMID:22498583

Antonaci, A., Consorti, F., Mardente, S., & Giovannone, G. (2009). Clinical and biological relationship between chronic lymphocytic thyroiditis and papillary thyroid carcinoma. *Oncology Research*, *17*(10), 495–503. doi:10.3727/096504009789735431 PMID:19725229

Asanuma, K., Sugenoya, A., Kasuga, Y., Itoh, N., Kobayashi, S., & Amano, J. (1998). The relationship between multiple intrathyroidal involvement in papillary thyroid carcinoma and chronic non-specific thyroiditis. *Cancer Letters*, *122*(1-2), 177–180. doi:10.1016/S0304-3835(97)00398-4 PMID:9464507

Baroni, C. D., Manente, L., Maccallini, V., & Di Matteo, G. (1983). Primary malignant tumors of the thyroid gland. Histology, age and sex distribution and pathologic correlations in 139 cases. *Tumori*, *69*(3), 205–213. doi:10.1177/030089168306900306 PMID:6868138

Bruland, O., Fluge, O., Akslen, L. A., Eiken, H. G., Lillehaug, J. R., Varhaug, J. E., & Knappskog, P. M. (2009). Inverse correlation between PDGFC expression and lymphocyte infiltration in human papillary thyroid carcinomas. *BMC Cancer*, *9*(1), 425–429. doi:10.1186/1471-2407-9-425 PMID:19968886

Cipolla, C., Sandonato, L., Graceffa, G., Fricano, S., Torcivia, A., Vieni, S., ... Latteri, M. A. (2005). Hashimo.to's thyroiditis coexistent with papillary thyroid carcinoma. *The American Surgeon*, *71*, 874–878. PMID:16468540

Consorti, F., Loponte, M., Milazzo, F., Potasso, L., & Antonaci, A. (2010). Risk of malignancy from thyroid nodular disease as an element of clinical management of patients with Hashimoto's thyroiditis. *European Surgical Research*, *45*(3-4), 333–337. doi:10.1159/000320954 PMID:21051899

Del Rio, P., Cataldo, S., Sommaruga, L., Concione, L., Arcuri, M. F., & Sianesi, M. (2008). The association between papillary carcinoma and chronic lymphocytic thyroiditis: Does it modify the prognosis of cancer? *Minerva Endocrinologica*, *33*, 1–5. PMID:18277374

Feldt-Rasmussen, U., & Rasmussen, A. K. (2010). Autoimmunity in differentiated thyroid cancer: Significance and related clinical problems. *Hormones*, *9*(2), 109–117. doi:10.14310/horm.2002.1261 PMID:20687394

Fiore, E., Rago, T., Scutari, M., Ugolini, C., Proietti, A., Di Coscio, G., ... Vitti, P. (2009). Papillary thyroid cancer, although strongly associated with lymphocytic infiltration on histology, is only weakly predicted by serum thyroid autoantibodies in patients with nodular thyroid diseases. *Journal of Endocrinological Investigation*, *32*(4), 344–351. doi:10.1007/BF03345725 PMID:19636204

French, J. D., Weber, Z. J., Fretwell, D. L., Said, S., Klopper, J. P., & Haugen, B. R. (2010). Tumor-associated lymphocytes and increased FoxP3C regulatory T cell frequency correlate with more aggressive papillary thyroid cancer. *The Journal of Clinical Endocrinology and Metabolism*, *95*(5), 2325–2333. doi:10.1210/jc.2009-2564 PMID:20207826

Gomez-Saez, J. M., Gomez-Arnaiz, N., Sahun de la Vega, M., & Soler Ramon, J. (1997). Prevalence and significance of lymphocyte infiltration in papillary carcinoma of the thyroid gland. *Anales de Medicina Interna (Madrid, Spain)*, *14*, 403–405. PMID:9376479

Gul, K., Dirikoc, A., Kiyak, G., Ersoy, P. E., Ugras, N. S., Ersoy, R., & Cakir, B. (2010). The association between thyroid carcinoma and Hashimoto's thyroiditis: The ultrasonographic and histopathologic characteristics of malignant nodules. *Thyroid*, *20*(8), 873–878. doi:10.1089/thy.2009.0118 PMID:20677997

Haberal, A. N., Toru, S., Ozen, O., Arat, Z., & Bilezikci, B. (2009). Diagnostic pitfalls in the evaluation of fine needle aspiration cytology of the thyroid: Correlation with histopathology in 260 cases. *Cytopathology*, *20*(2), 103–108. doi:10.1111/j.1365-2303.2008.00594.x PMID:18713250

Harach, H. R., Escalante, D. A., & Day, E. S. (2002). Thyroid cancer and thyroiditis in Salta, Argentina: A 40-yr study in relation to iodine prophylaxis. *Endocrine Pathology*, *13*(3), 175–181. doi:10.1385/EP:13:3:175 PMID:12446916

Huang, B. Y., Hseuh, C., Chao, T. C., Lin, K. J., & Lin, J. D. (2011). Well-differentiated thyroid carcinoma with concomitant Hashimoto's thyroiditis present with less aggressive clinical stage and low recurrence. *Endocrine Pathology*, *22*(3), 144–149. doi:10.100712022-011-9164-9 PMID:21647844

Kashima, K., Yokoyama, S., Noguchi, S., Murakami, N., Yamashita, H., Watanabe, S., ... Nakayam.a, I. (1998). Chronic thyroiditis as a favorable prognostic factor in papillary thyroid carcinoma. *Thyroid*, *8*(3), 197–202. doi:10.1089/thy.1998.8.197 PMID:9545105

Kebebew, E., Treseler, P. A., Ituarte, P. H., & Clark, O. H. (2001). Coexisting chronic lymphocytic thyroiditis and papillary thyroid cancer revisited. *World Journal of Surgery*, *25*(5), 632–637. doi:10.1007002680020165 PMID:11369991

Kim, E. Y., Kim, W. G., Kim, W. B., Kim, T. Y., Kim, J. M., Ryu, J. S., ... Shong, Y. K. (2009). Coexist.ence of chronic lymphocytic thyroiditis is associated with lower recurrence rates in patients with papillary thyroid carcinoma. *Horumon To Rinsho*, *71*(4), 581–586. doi:10.1111/j.1365-2265.2009.03537.x PMID:19222495

Kim, H. S., Choi, Y. J., & Yun, J. S. (2010). Features of papillary thyroid microcarcinoma in the presence and absence of lymphocytic thyroiditis. *Endocrine Pathology*, *21*(3), 149–153. doi:10.100712022-010-9124-9 PMID:20506003

Kim, K. W., Park, Y. J., Kim, E. H., Park, S. Y., Park, J., Ahn, S. H., ... Cho, B. Y. (2011). Elevated risk of papillary thyroid cancer in Korean patients with Hashimoto's thyroiditis. *Head & Neck*, *33*(5), 691–695. doi:10.1002/hed.21518 PMID:21484918

Kim, S. K., Song, K. H., Lim, S. D., Lim, Y. C., Yoo, Y. B., Kim, J. S., & Hwang, T. S. (2009). Clinical and pathological features and the BRAF (V600E) mutation. *Thyroid*, *19*(2), 137–141. doi:10.1089/thy.2008.0144 PMID:19014278

Kurukahvecioglu, O., Taneri, F., Yuksel, O., Aydin, A., Tezel, E., & Onuk, E. (2007). Total thyroidectomy for the treatment of Hashimoto's thyroiditis coexisting with papillary thyroid carcinoma. *Advances in Therapy*, *24*(3), 510–516. doi:10.1007/BF02848773 PMID:17660159

Lee, J. H., Kim, Y., Choi, J. W., & Kim, Y. S. (2013). The Association between Papillary Thyroid Carcinoma and Histologically Proven Hashimoto's Thyroiditis: A Meta-Analysis. *European Journal of Endocrinology*, *168*(3), 343–349. doi:10.1530/EJE-12-0903 PMID:23211578

Loh, K. C., Greenspan, F. S., Dong, F., Miller, T. R., & Yeo, P. P. (1999). Influence of lymphocytic thyroiditis on the prognostic outcome of patients with papillary thyroid carcinoma. *The Journal of Clinical Endocrinology and Metabolism*, *84*(2), 458463. doi:10.1210/jcem.84.2.5443 PMID:10022401

Mancini, A., Rabitti, C., Conte, G., Gullotta, G., & De Marinis, L. (1993). Lymphocytic infiltration in thyroid neoplasms. Preliminary prognostic assessments. *Minerva Chirurgica*, *48*, 1283–1288. PMID:8152558

Matsubayashi, S., Kawai, K., Matsumoto, Y., Mukuta, T., Morita, T., Hirai, K., ... Tamai, H. (1985). The cor.relation between papillary thyroid carcinoma and lymphocytic infiltration in the thyroid gland. *The Journal of Clinical Endocrinology and Metabolism*, *80*, 3421–3424. PMID:8530576

Matsumoto, F., Fujii, H., Abe, M., Kajino, K., Kobayashi, T., Matsumoto, T., ... Hino, O. (2006). A novel. tumor marker, Niban, is expressed in subsets of thyroid tumors and Hashimoto's thyroiditis. *Human Pathology*, *37*(12), 1592–1600. doi:10.1016/j.humpath.2006.06.022 PMID:16949643

Mazokopakis, E. E., Tzortzinis, A. A., Dalieraki-Ott, E. I., Tsartsalis, A. N., Syros, P. K., Karefilakis, C. M., ... Starakis, I. K. (2010). Coexistence of Hashimoto's thyroiditis with papillary thyroid carcinoma. A retrospective study. *Hormones*, *9*(4), 312–317. doi:10.14310/horm.2002.1282 PMID:21112862

McLeod, M. K., East, M. E., Burney, R. E., Harness, J. K., & Thompson, N. W. (1988). Hashimoto's thyroiditis revisited: The association with thyroid cancer remains obscure. *World Journal of Surgery*, *12*(4), 509–516. doi:10.1007/BF01655435 PMID:3420933

Muzza, M., Degl'Innocenti, D., Colombo, C., Perrino, M., Ravasi, E., Rossi, S., ... Fugazzola, L. (2010). The tight relationship between papillary thyroid cancer, autoimmunity and inflammation: Clinical and molecular studies. *Horumon To Rinsho*, *72*, 702–708. PMID:20447069

Neuhold, N., Kaiser, H., & Kaserer, K. (2001). Latent carcinoma of the thyroid in Austria: A systematic autopsy study. *Endocrine Pathology*, *12*(1), 23–31. doi:10.1385/EP:12:1:23 PMID:11478265

O'Hanlon, D. M., Little, M. P., Given, H. F., & Quill, D. S. (1997). Thyroid disease in the west of Ireland: An atypical incidence of neoplasia. *Irish Medical Journal*, *90*, 70–71. PMID:9105132

Ohmori, N., Miyakawa, M., Ohmori, K., & Takano, K. (2007). Ultrasonographic findings of papillary thyroid carcinoma with Hashimoto's thyroiditis. *International Medicine*, *46*(9), 547–550. doi:10.2169/internalmedicine.46.1901 PMID:17473486

Okayasu, I., Fujiwara, M., Hara, Y., Tanaka, Y., & Rose, N. R. (1995). Association of chronic lymphocytic thyroiditis and thyroid papillary carcinoma. A study of surgical cases among Japanese, and white and African Americans. *Cancer*, *76*(11), 2312–2318. doi:10.1002/1097-0142(19951201)76:11<2312::AID-CNCR2820761120>3.0.CO;2-H PMID:8635037

Onak, N. K., Barut, F., Keser, S., Karadayi, N., Bektas, S., Dogan Gu¨n, B. B., & O¨zdamar, S. O. (2009). Chronic lymphocytic thyroiditis and tumor-infiltrating lymphocytes combined in thyroid papillary carcinoma. *Turkish Journal of Oncology*, *24*, 172–176.

Peterson, C. A., & Shidler, F. P. (1957). Lymphocytic thyroiditis in 757 thyroid operations. *American Journal of Surgery*, *94*(2), 223–228. doi:10.1016/0002-9610(57)90649-9 PMID:13444540

Powell, D. J. Jr, Russell, J., Nibu, K., Li, G., Rhee, E., & Liao, M. (1998). The RET/PTC3 oncogene: Metastatic solid-type papillary carcinomas in murine thyroids. *Cancer Research*, *58*, 5523–5528. PMID:9850089

Repplinger, D., Bargren, A., Zhang, Y. W., Adler, J. T., Haymart, M., & Chen, H. (2008). Is Hashimoto's thyroiditis a risk factor for papillary thyroid cancer? *The Journal of Surgical Research*, *150*(1), 49–52. doi:10.1016/j.jss.2007.09.020 PMID:17996901

Schaffler, A., Palitzsch, K. D., Seiffarth, C., Hohne, H. M., Riedhammer, F. J., Hofstadter, F., ... Ruschoff, J. (1998). Coexistent thyroiditis is associated with lower tumour stage in thyroid carcinoma. *European Journal of Clinical Investigation*, *28*(10), 838–844. doi:10.1046/j.1365-2362.1998.00363.x PMID:9792998

Singh, B., Shaha, A. R., Trivedi, H., Carew, J. F., Poluri, A., & Shah, J. P. (1999). Coexistent Hashimoto's thyroiditis with papillary thyroid carcinoma: Impact on presentation, management, and outcome. *Surgery*, *126*(6), 1070–1076. doi:10.1067/msy.2099.101431 PMID:10598190

Tamimi, D. M. (2002). The association between chronic lymphocytic thyroiditis and thyroid tumors. *International Journal of Surgical Pathology, 10*(2), 141–146. doi:10.1177/106689690201000207 PMID:12075407

Van Savell, H. Jr, Hughes, S. M., Bower, C., & Parham, D. M. (2004). Lymphocytic infiltration in pediatric thyroid carcinomas. *Pediatric and Developmental Pathology, 7*(5), 487–492. doi:10.100710024-003-3028-3 PMID:15547772

Wirtschafter, A., Schmidt, R., Rosen, D., Kundu, N., Santoro, M., Fusco, A., ... Rothstein, J. L. (1997). Expression of the RET/PTC fusion gene as a marker for papillary carcinoma in Hashimoto's thyroiditis. *Laryngoscope, 107*(1), 95–100. doi:10.1097/00005537-199701000-00019 PMID:9001272

Yoon, Y. H., Kim, H. J., Lee, J. W., Kim, J. M., & Koo, B. S. (2012). The clinicopathologic differences in papillary thyroid carcinoma with or without co-existing chronic lymphocytic thyroiditis. *European Archives of Oto-Rhino-Laryngology, 269*(3), 1013–1017. doi:10.100700405-011-1732-6 PMID:21822854

Chapter 14
Management

ABSTRACT

Treatment of Hashimoto thyroiditis (HT) is mainly medical supplementing L-thyroxine (L-T4) for hypothyroidism. L-thyroxine has proved to reduce the volume of the thyroid gland in both hypothyroidism and euthyroid state. The dose of L-T4 is tailored according to the patient's needs; the standard dosage is 1.6-1.8 μ/kg/day. The level of TSH is frequently monitored for dose adjustment till euthyroid state is attained thereafter every 6-12 months. Thyroidectomy is considered in patients with cosmetic problem; with compressive symptoms (such as dysphagia, dyspnea, change of voice), suspicion of malignancy as papillary thyroid carcinoma is commonly associated. Surgery has a beneficial effect in cases of painful thyroiditis. Radioactive iodine treatment can be considered as a last option in elderly patients with large goiter who refuse surgery and their thyroiditis is not responding to L-T4 treatment. This chapter explores the management of Hashimoto's disease.

INTRODUCTION

Hypothyroidism caused by Hashimoto's thyroiditis is treated with thyroid hormone replacement agents such as levothyroxine (L-T4), tri-iodothyronine or desiccated thyroid extract. A tablet taken once a day, generally keeps the thyroid hormone levels normal. In most cases, the treatment needs to be taken for the rest of the person's life. In the event that hypothyroidism is caused by Hashimoto's thyroiditis, it is recommended that the TSH levels be kept below 3.0 mU/L.

DOI: 10.4018/978-1-5225-9655-4.ch014

No Treatment - Observation and Monitoring

Many patients with Hashimoto's disease require no treatment, for frequently the disease is *asymptomatic* and the goiter is small. This approach is justified by the old study of Vickery and Hamlin. (1961), who found, on both clinical and pathologic grounds, that the disease may remain static and the clinical condition unchanged over many years.

Medical Treatment

The treatment of choice for Hashimoto thyroiditis (or hypothyroidism from any cause) is thyroid hormone replacement. The drug of choice is orally administered levothyroxine (L-T4) sodium, usually for life.

L-Thyroine (L-T4) Replacement Therapy

Indications

If the goiter is problematic because of local pressure symptoms or disfigurement, *thyroid hormone therapy* is indicated. Thyroid hormone often causes a gratifying reduction in the size of the goiter after several months of treatment (McConahey, Woolner, Black, & Keating, 1959), particularly in young patients. It seems likely that in older patients there may be more fibrosis and therefore a less tendency for the thyroid to shrink. In young patients the response often occurs within 2-4 weeks, but in older ones the thyroid decreases in size more gradually. Recently, Aksoy et al. (2005) reported that "prophylactic" thyroid hormone treatment is associated with a decrease in thyroid size and in thyroid antibody levels 15 months after initiation of therapy.

Thyroid hormone in a full replacement dose is, of course, indicated if *hypothyroidism* is present. Therapy is probably indicated if the TSH level is elevated and the FT4 is low normal (subclinical hypothyroidism), since the onset of hypothyroidism is predictable in such patients. There is no evidence that thyroid replacement actually halts the ongoing process of thyroiditis, but in some patients receiving treatment, antibody levels gradually fall over many years (Papapetrou, MacSween, Lazarus, & Harden, 1972).

Dosage of L-T4

The dosage of thyroxine should normally be that required to bring the serum TSH level to the low normal range, such as 0.3-1 μU/ml. This is typically achieved with 1 μg L-T4/lb body weight/day, ranging from 75-125 μg/day in women, and 125-200 μg/day in men. Elderly patients and patients on androgens for various reasons usually require decreased levothyroxine replacement dosing. Patients who have undergone bowel resection and have short-bowel syndrome (or malabsorption for any reason) often require increased doses of levothyroxine to maintain the euthyroid state.

It is sensible to initiate therapy with a partial dose, since in some instances the thyroid gland may be non-suppressible even though functioning at a level below normal. Once thyroxine treatment is initiated, it is required indefinitely in most patients. However, it has been reported that up to 20% of initially hypothyroid individuals will later recover and have normal thyroid function if challenged by replacement hormone withdrawal. This may represent subsidence of cytotoxic antibodies, modulation of TSH-Ab, or some other mechanism (Okamura et al., 1990). These individuals can be identified by administration of TRH, which will induce an increase in serum T4 and T3 if the thyroid has recovered (Takasu, Komiya, Asawa, Nagasawa, & Yamada, 1990).

Replacement L-T4 therapy should be taken several hours before or after medications such as cholesterol-binding resins(cholestyramine), sucralfate, calcium carbonate, aluminium hydroxide and other antacids, in addition to ferrous sulfate (FeSO4) and iron-containing multivitamins, all of which can reduce absorption of L-T4. (Campbell, Hasinoff, Stalts, Rao, & Wong, 1992). Medications that enhance the metabolism and clearance of levothyroxine may necessitate an increase in the replacement dose. These medications include phenytoin, carbamazepine, and rifampin.

Autoimmune disease usually takes an ongoing process and Hashimoto's thyroiditis develops into hypothyroidism. Recent trial of prophylactic treatment with L-T4 (1.0-2.0μg/Kg/day) for one year in euthyroid patients with Hashimoto's thyroiditis showed decrease of anti-TPO antibodies and thyroid B-lymphocytes (Padberg, Heller, Usadel, & Schumm-Draeger, 2001), suggesting that prophylactic L-T4 therapy might be useful in stopping progression of the disease. The long-term clinical benefit should be established in the future. Whether or not *subclinical hypothyroidism* should be treated is still under debate. Cardiac dysfunction may be associated with subclinical hypothyroidism, even when serum TSH is still in the normal range. These abnormalities are reversible with L-T4 replacement therapy (Mariotti et al., 2008). In their study of 830 patients with Hashimoto thyroiditis, Tagami et al. (2010) reported that, following treatment with small doses of L-T4 in 32 of patients with subclinical hypothyroidism, significant decreases occurred in the patients' total cholesterol, low density lipids (LDL), and non-HDL levels, as well as in their LDL/HDL ratios.

Treatment of children and adolescents with 1.3μg/kg/day thyroxine for 24 months was shown in a recent study to cause significant reduction in thyroid size in patients with autoimmune thyroiditis, but not affect antibody levels, or significantly alter TSH or freeT4 (Karges et al., 2007).

Combination Therapy

One popular treatment, more so among patients than physicians, is the combined use of liothyronine (T3) and levothyroxine (L-T4) in an effort to mimic more closely thyroid hormone physiology. However, review of literature showed that out of 9 controlled clinical trials, only 1 indicated that combined therapy seemed to improve the mood, quality of life, and psychometric performance of patients more than did L-T4 alone (Escobar-Morreale, Botella-Carretero, Escobar del Rey, & de Escobar, 2005).

Until investigators can demonstrate a definite advantage to the administration of L-T4 plus T3, the use of *levothyroxine alone* should remain the treatment of choice for replacement therapy in hypothyroidism.

Replacement Therapy during Pregnancy

Pregnancy induces a state of increased need for levothyroxine. In women with hypothyroidism and in women with inadequate thyroid reserve from Hashimoto thyroiditis or partial thyroidectomy, this is manifested by an increase in the level of TSH and a decrease in the level of free T4 (overt hypothyroidism).

The increase in L-T4 requirement is thought to be due to increased levels of thyroid hormone–binding protein, increased use by the fetus, and increased metabolism of thyroxine by the feto-placental unit. The increase usually resolves and levothyroxine requirements return to the pre-pregnancy levels 6-8 weeks post-partum. The pregnancy-induced increased need for T4 occurs in the first trimester, usually within the first 8 weeks, and persists throughout pregnancy. Patients with hypothyroidism may require up to a 45-50% increase in L-T4 dose.

Patients who are diagnosed with Hashimoto thyroiditis or hypothyroidism from any cause during pregnancy should be started on a levothyroxine dose close to their replacement requirement, and the TSH level should be normalized as soon as possible. Untreated hypothyroidism carries increased maternal and fetal complications. The incidence of fetal loss is increased in patients who are TPO antibody positive.

Patients with hypothyroidism are best followed up by monitoring the TSH and free T4 levels. Upon becoming pregnant, patients should have the TSH and free T4 levels checked within 4-8 weeks and then every 6-8 weeks while dose adjustments are being made. Patients who are adequately dosed and who are in a clinically and biochemically euthyroid state should have thyroid function tests (TSH and free T4) every 8 weeks. Dose adjustments should be made to keep the free T4 and TSH within reference ranges.

A transient reduction in serum TSH levels occurs toward the end of the first trimester, owing to high circulating levels of human chorionic gonadotropin (hCG); this phenomenon is often confused with hyperthyroidism.

Levothyroxine Replacement for Myxedema Coma

Myxedema coma is a state of extreme hypothyroidism with a very high mortality rate (approaching 60%). Patients with this condition usually present with an acute precipitating condition, most often in the setting of long-standing, undiagnosed hypothyroidism, discontinuation of L-T4 replacement therapy, or failure to institute T4 replacement after radioactive iodine (RAI) ablation of the thyroid in Graves' disease or after total thyroidectomy. The usual precipitating causes include infection, cardiovascular accident, pulmonary infection, congestive cardiac failure, and drugs such as narcotics, sedatives, anesthetic agents, anti-depressants, and tranquilizers (all of which depress the respiratory drive).

Myxedema coma typically manifests in winter (or during extremely cold weather) in an elderly woman who has long-standing hypothyroidism. Hospitalized patients may have a history of sedating medication use. Typical clinical findings include hypothermia, obtundation or coma, hypoventilation, bradycardia, hyponatremia, hypoglycemia, and hypotension. Those patients have an elevated TSH level and may have undetectable free T4 levels.

Therapy should be conducted in an intensive care unit (ICU), where patients may require the following:

- Ventilatory support for hypoventilation and carbon dioxide retention
- Electrocardiographic monitoring and a Swan-Ganz catheter insertion for hemodynamic monitoring
- Judicious re-warming to avoid excessive vasodilatation, which would increase oxygen consumption and could lead to worsening of hypotension and vascular collapse
- Steroids, preferably hydrocortisone in stress doses
- Treatment of infection or any other precipitating causes
- Fluid restriction with or without hypertonic saline and lasix to promote water diuresis
- ***Levothyroxine***: L-T4 is administered intravenously (IV) in a loading dose of 4 μg/kg of lean body weight (approximately 300-600 mcg), which should be administered by rapid IV injection. The daily maintenance dose is 50-100 μg/d, administered IV until the patient can take it orally.

Glucocorticoids

In some instances, the acute onset of Hashimoto's disease, in association with pain, has prompted therapy with glucocorticoids. This treatment alleviates the symptoms and improves the associated biochemical abnormalities, and in some studies has been shown to increase plasma T3 and T4 levels by suppression of the autoimmune process (Yamada, Ikejiri, Kotani, & Kusakabe 1981). Blizzard et al. (1962) prescribed steroids for children with Hashimoto's disease over several months in an attempt at suppressing antibody production and possibly achieving a permanent remission. The adrenocortical hormones dramatically depress clinical activity of the disease and antibody titers, but all return to pre-therapy levels when treatment is withdrawn. *Steroid therapy is currently, not recommended for Hashimoto's thyroiditis* because of the undesirable side effects of the drug.

Chloroquine

Chloroquine has been reported in one study to reduce antibody titers (Ito, Tamura, & Nishikawa, 1968). However, because of toxicity of this drug, its use is *not advised*.

Selenium

In a randomized prospective controlled study, 77 TPO+ pregnant women received 200 μg *seleno-methionine* daily starting at the 12th week of pregnancy, and 74 TPO+ women received a placebo. The treated group had significantly lower TPO antibody levels at the end of pregnancy and during the post-partum while on treatment. The incidence of post-partum thyroiditis (PPT was reduced from 48.6 to 28.6% in the treated group, and the incidence of permanent hypothyroidism was equivalently reduced. However, thyroid hormone levels did *not* differ (Negro et al., 2007). Confirming earlier studies, in Hashimoto's patients, 200 mug Se in the form of L-seleno-methionine orally for 6 months caused a significant reduction of 21% in serum anti-TPO levels, but cessation caused an increase in the anti-TPO concentrations (Mazok et al., 2007).

A slightly opposing study, however, reported no immunological benefit of selenium in patients with moderate disease activity (in terms of TPO-Ab and cytokine production patterns) or those with high disease activity (Wichman, Winther, Bonnema, & Hegedüs, 2016). Selenium responsiveness may be different among patients with Hashimoto's thyroiditis. A systematic review and meta-analysis revealed that selenium supplementation reduced serum TPO-Ab levels after 3, 6, and 12 months in an LT4-treated Hashimoto's population, and after three months in an untreated population.(18) However, no effect of selenium supplementation on thyroid stimulating hormone, health-related quality of life or thyroid ultrasound was found in levothyroxine substitution-untreated individuals, and sporadic evaluation of clinically relevant outcomes in levothyroxine substitution-treated patients (Winther, Wichman, Bonnema, & Hegedüs, 2017).

Future well-powered randomized controlled trials (RCTs), evaluating disease progression or health-related quality of life, are warranted before determining the relevance of selenium supplementation in autoimmune thyroiditis. Further, combined treatment with *myo-inositol and selenium* was reported that the beneficial effects obtained by seleno-methionine treatment on patients affected by subclinical hypothyroidism were further improved by combination with myo-inositol (Nordio and Pajalich, 2013). Myo-inositol is an isomer of a C6 sugar alcohol and plays an important role in several cellular processes. In particular, it has been demonstrated that myo-inositol is the precursor for the synthesis of phosphor-inositides, which are part of the phosphatidyl-inositol (Ptd-Ins) signal transduction pathway. In one study, the administration of myo-inositol plus selenium has been reported to be effective in decreasing TSH, TPO-Ab, and Tg-Ab levels, as well as enhancing thyroid hormones and personal wellbeing, therefore restoring euthyroidism in patients diagnosed with Hashimoto's thyroiditis (Nordio and Basciani, 2017).

Anatabine

Anatabine, an alkaloid found in *Solanaceae plants* including tobacco, has been reported to ameliorate a mouse model of Hashimoto's thyroiditis (Cauregeli et al., 2012). In a double-blind, randomized, placebo-controlled multi-center study for three months, anatabine treated patients had a significant reduction in absolute serum Tg-Ab levels from baseline by study end relative to those on placebo (Schmaltz et al., 2014). Further studies are warranted to determine longer-term effects and possible actions of anatabine on the course of Hashimoto's thyroiditis.

SURGICAL TREATMENT

Indications

Surgery has been used as a method of therapy of Hashimoto's disease. This treatment, of course, removes the goiter but usually results in hypothyroidism. Generally, surgery is *not* indicated unless significant pain, cosmetic, or pressure symptoms remain after a fair trial of thyroid therapy. Among patients with post-partum thyroid dysfunction, the most common type is destructive thyrotoxicosis and simple symptomatic treatment, using beta-adrenergic--antagonists, is usually sufficient (Amino, Tada & Hidaka, 1996). In the case of post-partum hypothyroidism, replacement with a submaximal dose of T3 is useful to relieve symptoms more quickly and to predict spontaneous recovery which is detected by an increase of T4 level.

Some patients do not fit easily into the usual diagnostic categories; accordingly, choosing an appropriate course of therapy is more difficult.

Frequently, it is impossible to differentiate Hashimoto's thyroiditis from multinodular goiter (MNG) short of performing an open biopsy. In these cases, if there is *no suggestion of carcinoma*, it is logical to treat the patient with hormone replacement and to observe closely. A reduction in the goiter justifies continuation of the therapy, even in the absence of a diagnosis.

In some patients, especially teenagers, the examination discloses peri-thyroidal lymph nodes or an apparent discrete nodule, in addition to the diffusely enlarged thyroid of Hashimoto's thyroiditis. Such nodules should be evaluated by fine-needle aspiration cytology (FNAC), ultrasound and possibly scintiscan. Thyroid hormone treatment may cause regression of the nodes or the nodule. If after full evaluation uncertainty persists, if nodes remain present, or if a nodule grows, surgical exploration is indicated.

Indications of thyroidectomy for patients with HD (Hashimoto's thyroiditis) are summarized in Table 1.

Complications of Thyroidectomy

The morbidity associated with thyroid surgery is very low, but remains a matter of concern since thyroid disease often occurs in younger patients who have long life expectancy. Most complications can be avoided by an experienced endocrine surgeon.

General complications associated with thyroidectomy include cardiac and pulmonary problems, gastrointestinal dysfunction such as nausea, vomiting and ileus, and renal and urinary tract problems. *Local complications* common to all operations include post-operative bleeding, infection and keloid formation, while those specific to thyroidectomy include injury to the RLN, external branch of the superior laryngeal nerve, hypo-parathyroidism and airway obstruction. Other local complications such as injury to the esophagus, trachea, thoracic duct, internal jugular vein, carotid artery and spinal accessory nerve are extremely rare (Harnes, 2000; Luft, 1979; Hannan, 1989; Begg, 1998; Birkmeyer, 2002; Birkmeyer, 2001).

Table 1. Indications of surgery in HD

• A large goiter with obstructive symptoms (dysphagia, voice hoarseness, and stridor) (evaluation should include pulmonary function tests and a neck CT- scan). • Presence of a malignant nodule as found by FNAC. • Presence of a lymphoma diagnosed on FNA (thyroid lymphoma responds very well to radiotherapy - the treatment modality of choice) • Cosmetic reasons - For large, unsightly goiters

Bleeding

The thyroid gland is extremely vascular and bleeding can occur anywhere in the operative field. Special care must be taken with the superior thyroid vessels as these can retract and become difficult to control. Post-operative bleeding can be life-threatening by compromising the airway. Any post-operative respiratory distress can be thought of as attributable to a neck hematoma until proved otherwise. Most bleeding occurs within four hours of operation, and virtually all occur within 24 hours. Several studies have reported the successful use of bipolar vessel sealing systems (Manouras, 2008; Franko, 2006; Shen, 2005), or the harmonic scalpel (Cordon, 2005; Kilic, 2007) in shortening the length of thyroid surgery and reducing blood loss, while retaining a good hemostasis.

Drains do not prevent hemorrhage and are unlikely to prevent airway compromise since they are usually blocked by clot formation. If respiratory distress occurs, the wound should be opened immediately to release and drain the hematoma. If respiratory distress is not relieved, a tracheostomy should be performed. An alternative approach is to insert an endotracheal tube to secure the airway and then return the patient to the operating theatre to gain hemostasis. Seromas also occur after thyroidectomy, and most of them are small and do not pose any respiratory problem. They resolve spontaneously; though some must be aspirated (Kaplan, 2009; Kukora, 1981; Duddley, 1998).

Respiratory Distress

Respiratory distress does not only occur due to respiratory compression and/or laryngeal edema by bleeding and hematoma formation. It can also occur with tracheal collapse from chondromalacia or kinking of a soft tortuous trachea. These problems are quite rare and usually occur with long-standing large multinodular goiters. Tracheostomy is the standard treatment in such cases, although prolonged endotracheal intubation and external splinting of the trachea by custom made rings or Marlex mesh has been tried (Harness, Fung, Thompson, Burney, & McLeod, 1986).

Recurrent Laryngeal Nerve (RLN) Injury

Patients with a *single RLN injury* may remain asymptomatic, but are more likely to have temporary or permanent hoarseness. Injury of the RLN associated with thyroidectomy has progressively decreased but still occurs in 0.1-5% of patients. If the nerve is inadvertently transected, it should be re-anastomosed immediately, if recognized intra-operatively, to avoid permanent hoarseness (more than one year). In such cases, a number of measures can help lessen hoarseness. These include speech therapy, Teflon injection into the vocal cord, and nerve anastomoses. *Bilateral RLN injury* will cause respiratory distress and stridor since both vocal cords will assume a midline position. Patients will require reintubation or tracheostomy to secure an airway. A vocal cord lateralization procedure can be performed if the injury has been present for over a year (Roy van Zuidewijn, Songun, Kievit & Van de Velde, 1995).

External Branch of Superior Laryngeal Nerve Injury

Damage to the external branch of the superior laryngeal nerve occurs in 0.3-2% of patients undergoing thyroidectomy. The nerve may be injured when taking down the superior pole of the thyroid lobe. This will lead to. The patient will complain of voice weakness and a subtle loss of voice pitch. In case of *bilateral injury,* patients can experience swallowing disorders and be susceptible to aspiration (Songun, Kievit, van de Velde, 1997).

Other Nerve Injuries

Rarely the *cervical sympathetic trunk* may be injured during thyroidectomy, resulting in Horner's syndrome. This is a rare complication, but can occur with very large glands, invasive tumors or with recurrent goiters due to obliteration of normal tissue planes by scar tissue. Injury to the *spinal accessory nerve* can occur with neck dissections when combined with thyroidectomy but should not occur with thyroidectomy alone (Songun, Kievit, van de Velde, 1997).

Hypoparathyroidism

Transient asymptomatic hypocalcemia occurs in most patients undergoing thyroidectomy, but this complication has decreased dramatically with the increased understanding of the anatomy and physiology of the parathyroid glands. *Permanent hypo-parathyroidism* has been reported in <1-2% of patients. It occurs if all the parathyroid glands are removed, injured or rendered ischemic during thyroidectomy. Symptoms of acute post-operative hypocalcemia usually develop 1 to 7 days post-operatively. If untreated, carpal pedal spasm, tetany and life-threatening cardiac arrhythmias may occur (Olson, DeBenedetti, Baumann, & Wells, 1996).

For symptomatic patients, intravenous calcium gluconate must be administered. Asymptomatic patients with mild hypocalcemia should be treated with oral calcium supplements. If the total serum calcium is <8 mg/dl, vitamin D replacement therapy should be initiated with one alpha-hydroxy cholecalciferol. It is important to also measure serum phosphorous in these patients. If the serum phosphorous is low, the cause of hypocalcemia may be the "bone hunger" syndrome, but if the serum phosphorous is high, the cause of hypocalcemia is hypo-parathyroidism. If hypocalcemia and hyperphosphatemia remain after a year, permanent hyperparathyroidism is present and the patient will require long term therapy with oral calcium and vitamin D.

Permanent hypoparathyroidism can be prevented by giving special attention to identifying the parathyroid glands and preserving their blood supply during thyroidectomy by individually ligating the branches of the inferior thyroid artery. If a gland cannot be left in-situ with an intact vascular pedicle, it should be removed and auto-transplanted (after being confirmed by frozen section) into the ipsilateral sternocleidomastoid muscle or brachioradialis of the non-dominating hand.

Radioactive Iodine (RAI) Treatment

Tajiri (2006) conducted a retrospective cohort study to evaluate whether radioactive iodine (RAI) is effective for Hashimoto's patients with a large goiter. The study included 13 patients, 11 women and 2 men, with a mean age of 61.2±8.9 years (50-79 years). The goiter had been present for 12.0±7.9 year (4-33 years) before RAI. He recommended that RAI treatment can be considered as a *last option* in elderly patients with large goiter in whom thyroiditis is *not* responding to L-T4 and refusing surgery (Tajiri, 2006).

Long-Term Monitoring

Upon the initiation of the L-T4 replacement therapy, thyroid function tests, specifically TSH should be checked, initially every 6-8 weeks as dose adjustments are made. After the attainment of the clinical euthyroid state and a normal TSH level, patients and TSH levels may be checked every 6-12 months.

More frequent follow-up and TSH checks may need to be performed when patients start taking medications, such as ferrous sulfate, calcium supplementation, and multivitamins, that have the potential to impair the absorption of levothyroxine and therefore to affect the TSH level. Patients need to be advised to separate these medications from levothyroxine by at least 4 hours.

Follow-up care should include clinical evaluation for symptoms of hypothyroidism or iatrogenic hyperthyroidism. Physical examination should routinely include weight measurement, pulse and blood pressure determinations, and thyroid examination for the presence of nodules.

Patient Education

Patients should know that *thyroid replacement therapy* in Hashimoto thyroiditis is, except in very rare cases, *life-long*. Patients must be informed about the importance of *compliance* with their replacement therapy and must be instructed to *report* any symptoms suggestive of hyperthyroidism caused by over-replacement.

Patients must also be instructed to separate - by at least 4 hours - ingestion of L-T4 from ingestion of cholestyramine, ferrous sulfate, sucralfate, calcium carbonate, aluminum hydroxide (and other antacids), and iron-containing multivitamins, all of which impair the absorption of L-T4.

REFERENCES

Aksoy, D. Y., Kerimoglu, U., Okur, H., Canpinar, H., Karaagaoglu, E., Yetgin, S., ... Gedik, O. (2005). Effects. of prophylactic thyroid hormone replacement in euthyroid Hashimoto's thyroiditis. *Endocrine Journal*, *52*(3), 337–343. doi:10.1507/endocrj.52.337 PMID:16006728

Amino, N., Tada, H., & Hidaka, Y. (1996). The spectrum of postpartum thyroid dysfunction: Diagnosis, management, and long-term prognosis. *Endocrine Practice*, *2*, 406–412. doi:10.4158/EP.2.6.406 PMID:15251502

Begg, C. B., Cramer, L. D., & Hoskins, W. J. (1998). Impact of hospital volume on operative mortality for major cancer surgery. *Journal of the American Medical Association*, *280*(20), 1747–1751. doi:10.1001/jama.280.20.1747 PMID:9842949

Birkmeyer, J. D., Finlayson, E. V., & Birkmeyer, B. S. (2001). Volume standards for high-risk surgical procedures: Potential benefits of the Leapfrog initiative. *Surgery*, *130*(3), 415–422. doi:10.1067/msy.2001.117139 PMID:11562662

Birkmeyer, J. D., Siewers, A. E., Finlayson, E. V., Stukel, T. A., Lucas, F. L., Batista, I., ... Wennberg, D. E. (2002). Hospital volume and surgical mortality in the United States. *The New England Journal of Medicine*, *346*(15), 1128–1137. doi:10.1056/NEJMsa012337 PMID:11948273

Blizzard, R. M., Hung, M., Chandler, R. W., Aceto, T. Jr, Kyle, M., & Winship, T. (1962). Hashimoto's thyroiditis. Clinical and laboratory response to prolonged cortisone therapy. *The New England Journal of Medicine*, *267*, 1015–1019. doi:10.1056/NEJM196211152672004 PMID:13971663

Campbell, N. R., Hasinoff, B. B., Stalts, H., Rao, B., & Wong, N. C. (1992). Effect of ferrous sulfate on thyroid hormone replacement in hypothyroidism. *Annals of Internal Medicine*, *117*, 1010–1013. doi:10.7326/0003-4819-117-12-1010 PMID:1443969

Caturegli, P., De Remigis, A., Ferlito, M., Landek-Salgado, M. A., Iwama, S., Tzou, S. C., & Ladenson, P. W. (2012). Anatabine ameliorates experimental autoimmune thyroiditis. *Endocrinology*, *153*(9), 4580–4587. doi:10.1210/en.2012-1452 PMID:22807490

Cordon, C., Fajardo, R., Ramirez, J., & Herrera, M. F. (2005). A randomized, prospective, parallel group study comparing the harmonic scalpel to electrocautery in thyroidectomy. *Surgery*, *137*(3), 337–341. doi:10.1016/j.surg.2004.09.011 PMID:15746789

Dudley, H. A. F. (1998). Thyroid. In R. C. Williamson & B. P. Waxman (Eds.), *An aid to clinical surgery* (6th ed.; pp. 107–120). London: Churchill Livingstone.

Escobar-Morreale, H. F., Botella-Carretero, J. I., Escobar del Rey, F., & de Escobar, G. M. (2005). REVIEW: Treatment of hypothyroidism with combinations of levothyroxine plus liothyronine. *The Journal of Clinical Endocrinology and Metabolism*, *90*(8), 4946–4954. doi:10.1210/jc.2005-0184 PMID:15928247

Franko, J., Kish, K. J., Pezzi, C. M., Pak, H., & Kukora, J. S. (2006). Safely increasing the efficiency of thyroidectomy using a new bipolar electro-sealing device (LigaSure) versus conventional clamp-and tie technique. *The American Surgeon*, *72*(2), 132–136. PMID:16536242

Hannan, E. L., O'Donnell, J. F., Kilburn, H., Bernard, H. R., & Yazici, A. (1989). Investigation of the relationship between volume and mortality for surgical procedures performed in New York State hospitals. *Journal of the American Medical Association*, *262*(4), 503–510. doi:10.1001/jama.1989.03430040075029 PMID:2491412

Harness, J., Heerden, J., Lennquist, S., Rothmund, M., Barraclough, B. H., Goode, A. W., ... Proye, C. (2000). Future. of thyroid surgery and training surgeons to meet the expectations of 2000 and beyond. *World Journal of Surgery*, *24*(8), 976–982. doi:10.1007002680010168 PMID:10865044

Harness, J. K., Fung, L., Thompson, N. W., Burney, R. E., & McLeod, M. K. (1986). Total thyroidectomy: Complications and technique. *World Journal of Surgery*, *10*(5), 781–786. doi:10.1007/BF01655238 PMID:3776215

Ito, S., Tamura, T., & Nishikawa, M. (1968). Effects of desiccated thyroid, prednisolone and chloroquine on goiter and antibody titer in chronic thyroiditis. *Metabolism: Clinical and Experimental*, *17*(4), 317–322. doi:10.1016/0026-0495(68)90100-5 PMID:4171466

Kaplan, E. L. (2009). Thyroid and parathyroid. In S. I. Schwartz, C. T. Shires, F. O. Spencer, & E. U. Storer (Eds.), *Principles of surgery* (9th ed.; p. 1545). New York, NY: McGraw-Hill.

Karges, B., Muche, R., Knerr, I., Ertelt, W., Wiesel, T., Hub, R., ... Karges, W. (2007). Levothy.roxine in euthyroid autoimmune thyroiditis and type 1 diabetes: A randomized, controlled trial. *The Journal of Clinical Endocrinology and Metabolism*, *92*(5), 1647–1652. doi:10.1210/jc.2006-2493 PMID:17299067

Kilic, M., Keskek, M., Ertan, T., Yoldas, O., Bilgin, A., & Koc, M. (2007). A prospective randomized trial comparing the harmonic scalpel with conventional knot tying in thyroidectomy. *Advances in Therapy*, *24*(3), 632–638. doi:10.1007/BF02848788 PMID:17660174

Kukora, S. S., & Hardy, S. D. (1981). Complications of thyroid and parathyroid surgery. In J. D. Hardy (Ed.), *Complications in surgery and their management* (4th ed.; pp. 295–312). Philadelphia, PA: WB Saunders Co.

Luft, H. S., Bunker, J. P., & Enthoven, A. C. (1979). Should operations be regionalized? The empirical relation between surgical volume and mortality. *The New England Journal of Medicine*, *301*(25), 1364–1369. doi:10.1056/NEJM197912203012503 PMID:503167

Manouras, A., Markogiannakis, H., Koutras, A. S., Antonakis, P. T., Drimousis, P., Lagoudianakis, E. E., ... Bramis, I. (2008). Thyroid surgery: Comparison between the electrothermal bipolar vessel sealing system, harmonic scalpel, and classic suture ligation. *American Journal of Surgery*, *195*(1), 48–52. doi:10.1016/j.amjsurg.2007.01.037 PMID:18082542

Mariotti, S., Zoncu, S., Pigliaru, F., Putzu, C., Cambuli, V. M., Vargiu, S., … Mercuro, G. (2008). Cardiac effects of l-thyroxine administration in borderline hypothyroidism. International Journal of Cardiology, 126(2), 190-195.

Mazokopakis, E. E., Papadakis, J. A., Papadomanolaki, M. G., Batistakis, A. G., Giannakopoulos, T. G., Protopapadakis, E. E., & Ganotakis, E. S. (2007). Effects of 12 Months Treatment with l-Selenomethionine on Serum Anti-TPO Levels in Patients with Hashimoto's Thyroiditis. *Thyroid*, *17*(7), 609–612. doi:10.1089/thy.2007.0040 PMID:17696828

McConahey, W. M., Woolner, L. B., Black, B. M., & Keating, F. R. Jr. (1959). Effect of desiccated thyroid in lymphocytic (Hashimoto's) thyroiditis. *The Journal of Clinical Endocrinology and Metabolism*, *19*(1), 45–49. doi:10.1210/jcem-19-1-45 PMID:13620732

Negro, R., Greco, G., Mangieri, T., Pezzarossa, A., Dazzi, D., & Hassan, H. (2007). The influence of selenium supplementation on postpartum thyroid status in pregnant women with thyroid peroxidase autoantibodies. *The Journal of Clinical Endocrinology and Metabolism*, *92*(4), 1263–1268. doi:10.1210/jc.2006-1821 PMID:17284630

Nordio, M., & Basciani, S. (2017). Treatment with Myo-Inositol and Selenium Ensures Euthyroidism in Patients with Autoimmune Thyroiditis. *International Journal of Endocrinology*, *2549491*. doi:10.1155/2017/2549491 PMID:28293260

Nordio, M., & Pajalich, R. (2013). Combined treatment with Myo-inositol and selenium ensures euthyroidism in subclinical hypothyroidism patients with autoimmune thyroiditis. *Journal of Thyroid Research*, *13*, 4241–4263. PMID:24224112

Okamura, K., Sato, K., Yoshinari, M., Ikenoue, H., Kuroda, T., Nakagawa, M., ... Fujishima, M. (1990). Recovery of the thyroid function in patients with atrophic hypothyroidism and blocking type TSH binding inhibitor immunoglobulin. *Acta Endocrinologica*, *122*(1), 107–114. doi:10.1530/acta.0.1220107 PMID:1968305

Olson, J. A. Jr, DeBenedetti, M. K., Baumann, D. S., & Wells, S. A. Jr. (1996). Parathyroid autotransplantation during thyroidectomy. Results of long-term follow-up. *Annals of Surgery*, *223*(5), 472–478. doi:10.1097/00000658-199605000-00003 PMID:8651738

Padberg, S., Heller, K., Usadel, K. H., & Schumm-Draeger, P. M. (2001). One-year prophylactic treatment of euthyroid hashimoto's thyroiditis patients with levothyroxine: Is there a benefit? *Thyroid*, *11*(3), 249–255. doi:10.1089/105072501750159651 PMID:11327616

Papapetrou, P. D., MacSween, R. M., Lazarus, J. H., & Harden, R. (1972). Long-term treatment of Hashimoto's thyroiditis with thyroxine. *Lancet*, *2*, 7786–7789. PMID:4117375

Roy van Zuidewijn, D. B., Songun, I., Kievit, J., & Van de Velde, C. J. H. (1995). Complications of thyroid surgery. *Annals of Surgical Oncology*, *2*(1), 56–60. doi:10.1007/BF02303703 PMID:7834455

Schmeltz, L. R., Blevins, T. C., Aronoff, S. L., Ozer, K., Leffert, J. D., Goldberg, M. A., ... Wright, C. IV. (2014). Anatabine supplementation decreases thyroglobulin antibodies in patients with chronic lymphocytic autoimmune (Hashimoto's) thyroiditis: A randomized controlled clinical trial. *The Journal of Clinical Endocrinology and Metabolism*, *99*(1), E137–E142. doi:10.1210/jc.2013-2951 PMID:24178792

Shen, W. T., Baumbusch, M. A., Kebebew, E., & Duh, Q. Y. (2005). Use of the electro-thermal vessel sealing system versus standard vessel ligation in thyroidectomy. *Asian Journal of Surgery*, *28*(2), 86–89. doi:10.1016/S1015-9584(09)60268-2 PMID:15851359

Songun, I., Kievit, J., & van de Velde, C. J. H. (1997). Complications of thyroid surgery. In Textbook of Endocrine Surgery. Philadelphia, PA: WB Saunders.

Tagami, T., Tamanaha, T., Shimazu, S., Honda, K., Nanba, K., Nomura, H., ... Shimatsu, A. (2010). Lipid Profiles in the Untreated Patients with Hashimoto Thyroiditis and the Effects of Thyroxine Treatment on Subclinical Hypothyroidism with Hashimoto Thyroiditis. *Endocrine Journal*, *57*(3), 253–258. doi:10.1507/endocrj.K09E-315 PMID:20032565

Tajiri, J. (2006). Radioactive Iodine Therapy for Goitrous Hashimoto's Thyroiditis. *The Journal of Clinical Endocrinology and Metabolism*, *91*(11), 4497–4500. doi:10.1210/jc.2006-1163 PMID:16895949

Takasu, N., Komiya, I., Asawa, T., Nagasawa, Y., & Yamada, T. (1990). Test for recovery from hypothyroidism during thyroxine therapy in Hashimoto's thyroiditis. *Lancet*, *336*(8723), 1084–1086. doi:10.1016/0140-6736(90)92567-2 PMID:1977978

Vickery, A. L., & Hamlin, E. Jr. (1961). Struma lymphomatosa (Hasimoto's thyroiditis): Observations on repeated biopsies in 16 patients. *The New England Journal of Medicine*, *264*, 226–229. doi:10.1056/NEJM196102022640505 PMID:13781168

Wichman, J., Winther, K. H., Bonnema, S. J., & Hegedüs, L. (2016). Selenium Supplementation Significantly Reduces Thyroid Autoantibody Levels in Patients with Chronic Autoimmune Thyroiditis: A Systematic Review and Meta-Analysis. *Thyroid*, *26*(12), 1681–1692. doi:10.1089/thy.2016.0256 PMID:27702392

Winther, K. H., Wichman, J. E., Bonnema, S. J., & Hegedüs, L. (2017). Insufficient documentation for clinical efficacy of selenium supplementation in chronic autoimmune thyroiditis, based on a systematic review and meta-analysis. *Endocrine*, *55*(2), 376–385. doi:10.100712020-016-1098-z PMID:27683225

Yamada, T., Ikejiri, K., Kotani, M., & Kusakabe, T. (1981). An increase of plasma triiodothyronine and thyroxine after administration of dexamethasone to hypothyroid patients with Hashimoto's thyroiditis. *The Journal of Clinical Endocrinology and Metabolism*, *46*(5), 784–789. doi:10.1210/jcem-46-5-784 PMID:233634

Chapter 15
Dietary Management

ABSTRACT

The best diets for Hashimoto's thyroiditis (HT) patients are the gluten-free diet, paleo diet, and vegetarian and vegan diets. Micro-nutrients to integrate in diet for patients with HT are Iodine (150-290 µg/day), Selenium (55-75 µg/day), Zinc (34-40 mg/day), Vitamin D (1500-2500 IU/day), and Vitamin B12 (2.4-2.8 µg/day). The worst foods for patients with HT that should be avoided are gluten, goitrogens, alcoholic drinks, food additives, and supplements (gums, lecithin, and coffee and fiber supplements). This chapter explores the dietary management of Hashimoto's disease.

INTRODUCTION

Hashimoto's thyroiditis is part of the spectrum of chronic autoimmune thyroid diseases (AITD) and is associated with thyroid hypofunction, lymphocytic infiltration and production of thyroid auto-antibodies such as thyroid peroxidase antibodies (TPO-Ab) and thyroglobulin antibodies (Tg-Ab) (Caturegli, 2014; Mazokopakis, 2007a; Mazokopakis, 2010; Mazokopakis, 2007b; Mazokopakis, 2014). Although the exact mechanism of progressive thyroid tissue destruction is not clear, Hashimoto's thyroiditis is considered a disorder of T cell-mediated immunity, caused by an interaction between susceptibility genes and environmental factors, the research of which is still inconclusive (Mazokopakis and Kotsiris, 2014). In the majority of patients with Hashimoto's thyroiditis, life-long levothyroxine (LT4) substitution to achieve normal circulating thyrotropin (TSH) levels, is required (Topliss,

DOI: 10.4018/978-1-5225-9655-4.ch015

2016; Pearce, 2013) The additional role of diet for the management of Hashimoto's thyroiditis is usually overlooked and careful supplementation of possible deficiencies in Hashimoto's thyroiditis is recommended for the dietary management of these patients.

In addition, the co-existence of Hashimoto's thyroiditis with other organ-specific diseases (e.g. pernicious anemia, vitiligo, celiac disease, type 1 diabetes mellitus, autoimmune liver disease, primary biliary cirrhosis, myasthenia gravis, alopecia areata, sclerosis multiplex, Addison's disease), and non-specific non-endocrine autoimmune diseases (e.g. rheumatoid arthritis, systemic lupus erythematosus, Sjögren syndrome, systemic sclerosis), should be evaluated (Dillas, 2011; Boelaert, 2010).

The Best Diet for Hashimoto Disease

There are specific nutrients that should be regularly taken to maintain a healthy and functional thyroid. The top nutrients are *Iodine (I_2), Selenium (Se) and Zinc (Zn).* A diet optimizing these nutrients is vital to an overall recovery plan. The best way to get the daily requirement of these minerals and nutrients is to eat a balanced diet, but if this is not possible, supplements are available. Diets beneficial for patients with Hashimoto disease include paleo diet, gluten-free diet and vegetarian or vegan diet.

Iodine

Iodine is an essential micronutrient of the diet necessary for thyroid function and synthesis of thyroid hormones (Rohner et al., 2014). The amount of iodine found in food sources is small and depends on environmental factors like use of fertilizers and soil concentration (vegetables and fruits grown near coasts have higher iodine levels).

Recommended Iodine Intake

The recommended adult daily iodine intake is 150 μg, reaching up to 220 and 290 μg during pregnancy and lactation, respectively (Zimmermann and Boelaert, 2015). Daily iodine requirements according to life stage are summarized in Table 1.

Main Diet Iodine Sources

It is important to be conscious of the iodine in diet. Too little iodine can cause goiter and other clinical problems, while too much iodine can make hypothyroidism worse. *Main diet iodine sources* are sea vegetables (seaweed) and seafood (e.g. scallops, cod, sardines, shrimps, salmon and tuna), animal products (dairy products and eggs), fruits (prunes, cranberries and strawberries) and iodinated table salt

Iodized salt is the main source of iodine in our diet. It consists of table salt combined with minuscule amounts of iodine containing salts. Just one gram of salt provides the body with 77 µg of iodine and 0 calories.

The most reliable sources of *natural* iodine are sea vegetables (seaweed) and seafood. The other common sources are typically high in iodine because they were grown in iodine-rich soil, fed fish in their diet (i.e., chickens and eggs), or fortified (grains). Eggs contain iodine because commercially raised chickens are fed fish in their diets (Fordyces, 2003). Bread typically contains iodine because bread conditioners containing potassium iodate or calcium iodate are added; grains are *not* generally good sources of iodine (Fordyces, 2003).

The main diet Iodine sources are summarized in Table 2 (Wilde, 2018; Gropper, 2013; Chung, 2013; Food and Drug Administration, 2016; Tranvnicke, 2006; Medline Plus, 2018; Gastaldi, 2014; Zimmermann, 2015; Cerretani, 2014).

Table 1. Recommended dietary adequate intake of iodine

Life Stage	Recommended Iodine Intake
Infants - 0-6 months - 6-12 months	110 µg/d 130 µg/d
Children - 1-3 years - 4-8 years - 9-13 years	90 µg/d 90 µg/d 120 µg/d
Adults - Males - Females	150 µg/d 150 µg/d
Pregnancy	220 µg/d
Lactation	290 µg/d

(Institute of Medicine, Food and Nutrition Board, 2001)

Iodine Deficiency

Iodine deficiency manifests with a wide clinical range, from goiter to cretinism (Pearce, Andersson, & Zimmermann, 2013), but this problem was solved in many countries worldwide with *iodized salt* (IS) programs, and nowadays about

Table 2. Food rich in iodine, amount served and amount of iodine

Food	Amount Serving	I_2 Amount
Salt - Iodized table salt - Himalaya crystal salt	1 g 1/2 g	77 µg 250 µg
Sea Vegetables (Seaweed) - Nori (red algae of the genus *Porphyra*). - *Arame Kelp (*Eisenia bicyclis*):* - *Kombu Kelp (*Saccharina japonica*):* - *Wakame Kelp (*Undaria pinnatifida*):*	1 sheet 1 table-spoon 1-inch piece 1 table-spoon	16 µg 730 µg 1,450 µg 80 µg
Sea Food - Cod - Snapper (steamed). - Canned Salmon - Canned Albacore Tuna - Shrimp - Lobster	3 ounces 1 fillet (125 g) 3 ounces (small tin) 3 ounces (small tin) 3 ounces 3.5 ounces (100 g)	99 µg 50 µg 63 µg 17 µg 35 µg 100 µg
Animal Products - Turkey breast - Beef liver - Boiled eggs. - Dairy products • Milk. • Plain yoghurt • Cheese (cheddar)	3 ounces 2.5 ounces 1 medium 1 large 1 cup (250 ml) 1 cup 1 ounce	34 µg 32 µg 15 µg 24 µg 56 µg 90 µg 12 µg
Fruits / juice - Cape cod cranberries - Prunes (dried) - Strawberries - Apple (juice) - Fruit cocktail (canned) - Bannanas	1 ounce 5 prunes 1 cup 1 cup 1/2 cup 1 medium	100 µg 13 µg 13 µg 11 µg 42 µg 3 µg
Vegetables - Potatoes (organic). - Balck-eyed peas - Green peas - Corn (canned)*	1 medium 1/2 cup 1/2 cup 1/2 cup	60 µg 32 µg 3 µg 14 µg
Legumes - Navy beans - Lima beans.	4 ounces 1/2 cup	32 µg 8 µg
White bread	2 slices	45 µg
Macaroni (enriched, boiled)	1 cup	27 µg
Ice cream chocolate	1/2 cup	30 µg

*Corn is actually a vegetable, a whole grain and a fruit !

two thirds of the world's population (71%) uses IS (Zimmermann, 2009). On the other hand, most persons with thyroid disorders in *iodine-replete- areas*, have auto-immune thyroid disease (AITD) ranging from primary atrophic hypothyroidism, Hashimoto's thyroiditis to thyrotoxicosis (Graves' disease) (Vanderpump, 2011).

Other studies revealed the influence of dietary iodine intake on the *epidemiology of thyroid dysfunction* (Vanderpump, 2011). Autoimmune hypothyroidism and thyroid antibodies are more common in iodine-replete areas than in iodine deficient areas (Laurberg et al., 1998). Hypothyroidism induced by iodine in AITD may be due to a persistent inhibitory effect of iodine on thyroid hormone synthesis and secretion (*Wol-Chaiko effect* (Markou, Georgopoulos, Kyriazopoulou, & Vagenakis, 2001). Patients with Hashimoto's thyroiditis may have inadequate thyroid hormone synthesis, may be unable to escape from the acute Wolf Chaiko effect, and can develop iodine-induced hypothyroidism.

Iodine Excess

Several studies reported that moderate or even mild iodine excess (median urinary iodine 220 μg per 24 hours) is associated with a more frequent occurrence of hypothyroidism, especially in elderly subjects, the exact mechanism of which has not been clarified (Lauerberg, 2001; Bjergred, 2012). Furthermore, a cross-sectional study from south China showed that high iodine intake was likely to lead to the occurrence of thyroid diseases, such as Hashimoto's thyroiditis, nodular goiter, and hyperthyroidism, through a long-term process (Zhao et al., 2014). Pedersen et al. (2011) reported an increased prevalence of thyroid antibodies, 4-5 years after a cautious salt iodization program, supporting the view that even a small increase in iodine supplementation may be associated with increased thyroid autoimmunity. The underlying mechanism for this association is yet to be elucidated.

A recent study by Xu et al. (2016) suggested that the apoptosis of thyroid follicular cells seen in Hashimoto's thyroiditis is probably caused by suppression of autophagy activity, which is induced by iodine excess. This process is mediated through transforming growth factor-1 down-regulation, activation of the Akt/mTOR signaling pathway and enhanced reactive oxygen species (ROS) production. Another potential mechanism could be that iodine excess increases intra-thyroid infiltrating Th17-cells and inhibits T-regulatory (TREG) cells development, while it triggers an abnormal expression of tumor necrosis factor (TNF) related apoptosis-inducing ligand (TRAIL) in thyrocytes, thus inducing apoptosis and parenchymal destruction (Duntas, 2015). The fact that excessive iodine plays a significant role in inducing thyroid autoimmunity is also strongly supported in genetically predisposed animals by increasing the immunogenicity of thyroglobulin (Tg) (Caraynniotis, 2007. This phenomenon may be explained by the fact that Tg is the only self-antigen that undergoes post-translational modification as a consequence of the environmental supply of iodine, with the exposure of previously hidden epitopes (Dai, 2002; Li, 2007; Jiang, 2007; Shi, 2014; Flore, 2015). Thus, high iodine supplementation in Hashimoto's thyroiditis should be discouraged, and should be considered as "not beneficial" and "possibly harmful". Discouraging iodine *over-supplementation* must not preclude its appropriate supplementation in pregnancy to a total intake of 250 g/day (Topliss, 2016).

The US Food and Nutrition Board (2001) has established iodine upper limits for food and supplement intakes (Table 3). In most people, iodine intakes from foods and supplements are unlikely to exceed the UL.

Selenium

Selenium (Se) is an essential micronutrient of diet with many pleiotropic effects ranging from anti-oxidant and anti-inflammatory to increasing active thyroid hormone production (Brown, 2001; Beckett, 2005; Duntas, 2006; Schomburg, 2016; Rayman, 2012). The thyroid has the highest Se content per gram of tissue in the entire body.

Among at least 30 selenoproteins, the *seleno-enzymes* such as glutathione peroxidases (GPX), thioredoxin reductases (TR), iodothyronine deiodinases and seleno-protein P, seem to play a unique role in thyroid function and thyroid

Table 3. Tolerable upper intake levels (TUL) of iodine (Institute of Medicine, Food and Nutrition Board, 2001)

Life Stage	TUL of I_2
- 1-3 years	200 µg
- 4-8 years	300 µg
- 9-13 years	600 µg
- 14-18 years	900 µg
- 19 years and older	1,100 µg
- Pregnant women 14-18 years	900 µg
- Pregnant women 19 years and older	1,100 µg
- Lactating women 14-18 years	909 µg

hormone homeostasis.[2,29,30] Selenium supplementation in patients with AITD, including Hashimoto's thyroiditis, seems to modify the inflammatory and immune responses, probably by enhancing plasma GPX and TR activity and by decreasing toxic concentrations of hydrogen peroxide and lipid hydroperoxides, resulting from thyroid hormone synthesis (Beckett, 2005; Duntas, 2006). When Se intake is adequate, the intra-cellular GPX and TR systems protect thyrocytes from these peroxides, as oxidative stress induces TR1 and GPX. The current recommended *dietary intake* of Se in adults, in order to achieve the maximal activity of GPX in plasma or in erythrocytes ranges from 55 to 75 µg/day (Rayman, 2012; Institute of Medicine, 2000; Mazokopakis, 2007). *Foods rich in Se* are Brazil nuts, oysters, tuna, whole-wheat bread, sunflower seeds, meat (pork, beef, lamb, turkey, chicken), mushrooms and rye. Studies have shown different results regarding the efficacy of Se supplementation in Hashimoto's thyroiditis patients (Toulis, 2010; Fan, 2014; Wichman, 2016).

Three meta-analysis studies confirmed that patients with Hashimoto's thyroiditis who receive selenium supplements have shown a decrease in the serum levels of antibodies (TPO-Ab and Tg-Ab) attacking the thyroid gland (Toulis, 2010; Fan, 2014; Wichman, 2016). The recently published systematic review and meta-analysis of Wichman et al. (2016) in particular showed that Se supplementation effectively reduces serum TPO-Ab levels at 3, 6, and 12 months and serum Tg-Ab at 12 months in LT4-treated populations, but not in non- treated ones. This meta-analysis also showed a significant decrease in serum TPO-Ab levels in patients receiving 200g seleno-methionine, but not in those receiving 200g sodium selenite. The difference might be related to absorption of selenite which is approximately two-thirds of the absorption of seleno-methionine (Mazokopakis, 2010). However, another meta-analysis in the Cochrane library concluded that the evidence to support or refute the efficacy of Se supplementation in patients with Hashimoto's thyroiditis is insufficient.[51] A most recent study from Italy showed that supplementation with L-seleno-methionine for 6 months had no effect on TPO-Ab (Esposito et al., 2017), but other studies have shown that Se supplementation for 12 months decreased TPO-Ab (Nacamulli et al., 2010).

A recent population-based study in China reported that the prevalence of thyroid diseases (except Graves' and nodular disease) was higher in a region of low Se intake (serum Se < 69 g/L) compared to a region of adequate Se intake (serum Se 69 g/L or more) (Wu et al., 2015)

However, long-term intake of large amounts of Se may have adverse effects on human health (Kaprara, 2006; Vinceti, 2001; Fan, 1990; Yang, 1983; Vinceti, 2010; Zldosary, 2012). Consumption of approximately 330 g of Se/

day could be toxic not only for growth hormones and insulin-like growth factor 1 metabolism but also in the synthesis of thyroid hormones (Kaprara, 2006; Vinceti, 2001). Possible major *side effcts* include nail and hair loss, anorexia, diarrhea, depression, hemorrhage, liver and kidney necrosis, blindness, ataxia and respiratory disturbances (Kaprara, 2006; Vinceti, 2001). There have also been reported cases of dermatitis and CNS disorders in an area with high Se content in Enshi, China (Yang, 1983). These signs and symptoms of Se toxicity are known as *selenosis*. A Se intake of 50-400 g/d is considered a safe range for adults, while 850-900 g could be allowed as minimum for Se toxicity (Parekh, Khan, Torres, & Kitto, (2008).

In order to predict whether a patient with Hashimoto's thyroiditis would benefit from Se supplementation, the clinician should first investigate the patient's iodine status by determining the urinary iodine excretion test in a 24-hour urine sample. It should be noted that excessive iodine may indicate dietary excess intake (Katagiri, Asakura, Uechi, Masayasu, & Sasaki, 2016), recent imaging contrast media exposure or use of drugs containing iodine (e.g. amiodarone). The effect of iodine-containing antiseptic solutions appears to be negligible (Michalaki, 2013; Markou, 2012). Selenium supplementation in the form of seleno-methionine would be beneficial in Hashimoto's thyroiditis patients with Se deficiency and adequate iodine intake.

Zinc

Zinc is an essential nutrient for thyroid health that assists in the conversion of T4 to T3. The hypothalamus requires zinc to accurately gauge thyroid hormone levels to increase production when levels are low. For these reasons, zinc deficiency is linked with decreased thyroid production and hypothyroidism. A 2010 study showed that taking zinc supplements increased thyroid hormone levels in patients with goiter. Furthermore, zinc supplementation improves thymic and immune functions in children with Down's syndrome (Ertek, Cicero, Caglar, & Erdogan, 2010). Zinc deficits, like iodine, are extremely uncommon in the developed world. The daily required dose of zinc in diet ranges between 34 and 40 mg for adults. The following foods are excellent sources: oysters and shellfish, beef, chicken, legumes such as lentils and beans, as well as cow's milk.

Vitamin D

Vitamin D is now considered as both a fat-soluble vitamin and a steroid hormone that plays a central role in the regulation of calcium/phosphate homeostasis and bone intensity (Caprio, Infante, Calanchini, 2016). It is synthesized within the body via skin exposure to sunlight and through dietary intake (Mazokopakis and Kotsiris, 2014). The *natural sources* that provide humans with large amounts of vitamin D3 are fish (cod liver oil, wild fresh salmon and sardines), milk and dairy products, cereal, orange juice, pork chops (with fat), and eggs (Mazokopakis and Kotsiris, 2014). Its serum normal ranges between 30 and 80 ng/mL.

Several studies showed the correlation between vitamin D deficiency and thyroid autoimmunity by demonstrating that cholecalciferol supplements are effective in reducing TPO-Ab among Hashimoto's thyroiditis patients with vitamin D deficiency, owing to its its anti-inflammatory and immuno-modulatory functions (Kivity, 2011; Sonmezgoz, 2016; Muscogiori, 2013; Bozkurt, 2013; Mazokopakis, 2015; Chaudhary, 2016).

The Endocrine Society of USA guidelines indicated that daily vitamin D intakes of 1500-2000 IU are needed to raise the blood level of 25(OH) D constantly above 30 ng/mL (Holick et al., 2011), while the Institute of Medicine of USA reported that the tolerable upper intake level, defined as the maximum daily intake above which the potential for adverse health effects may increase after chronic use, is 4000 IU per day (Institute of Medicine, 2011). Levels of 25(OH) D between 30 and 40 ng/mL that are adequate for avoiding metabolic and autoimmune disorders (Holick, 2011), in more than 97% of the population, can be achieved by an optimal dosage of approximately 2000 IU cholecalciferol daily, regardless of increased exposure to ultraviolet rays (Heaney, 2007). The main *side effects* of vitamin D over-treatment are hypercalcemia (calcium serum levels above 11 mg/dL) and nephrolithiasis. To avoid coronary artery calcification, which is an important predictor of cardiovascular disease, concomitant use of cholecalciferol with vitamin K2 (menaquinones) may be necessary (Beulens, Booth, van den Heuvel, & Stoecklin, 2013). Patients with renal disease cannot convert 25[OH] D to active 1,25 [OH] D2 and need to receive calcitriol instead of cholecalciferol. In addition, one must consider the potential interactions of some drugs with vitamin D supplements (Robien, Oppeneer, Kelly, Hamilton-Reevs, 2013).

Apart from cholecalciferol or calcitriol, a regular exposure to sunlight could contribute to the prevention and management of vitamin D deficiency in Hashimoto's thyroiditis patients. It is obvious that excessive sun exposure and sunburn should be avoided because of the high risk of skin cancer (particularly melanoma) (van der Rhee, de Vries, & Coebergh, 2016). Taking into consideration the low cost and the minimal side effects of vitamin D supplementation, screening for vitamin D deficiency and careful vitamin D supplementation with monthly monitoring of calcium and 25[OH] D levels, when required, may be recommended for patients with Hashimoto's thyroiditis (Caprio, Infante, Calanchini, 2016).

Vitamin B12

Vitamin B12 deficiency is observed in over 30% of people with autoimmune thyroid disease including Hashimoto's thyroiditis. The required daily dose of vitamin B12 is 2.4 μg, reaching up to 2.6 μg and 2.8 μg during pregnancy and lactation, respectively. Food sources of B12 include molluscs, sardines, salmon, and organ meats such as liver, muscle meat, and dairy products. The primary sources of vitamin B12 in vegan diets include fortified cereals and nutritional yeast (Sworczak & Wisniewski, 2001).

Gluten-free Diet

While foods containing gluten are not the cause of Hashimoto's disease, for some people, those foods can trigger an autoimmune response (Volta, De Franceschi, Molinaro, Tetta, & Bianchi, 1997). This results in inflammation and tissue destruction. Gluten is part of every wheat flour product and can hide in many different foods, which thus should be avoided by patients with Hashimoto's thyroiditis such as *wheat, barley, cookies, cakes, pizza and bread.* Gluten-free alternatives for common flour-based foods are available, though they can be expensive. Many healthy foods are naturally gluten-free, including fruits, vegetables, fresh meat, fish and poultry, legumes, certain whole grains, dairy products and oils.

Whereas it is not yet clear whether a gluten-free diet can prevent autoimmune diseases, it is worth mentioning that Hashimoto's thyroiditis patients (with or without celiac disease) benefit from a diet low in gluten as far as the progression and the potential disease complications are concerned (Lundin & Wijmenga, 2015). Still, a lifelong gluten-free diet is not easy to maintain, it could be very costly and the subject's quality of life may deteriorate (Collin, 2008).

Paleo Diet

The paleo diet (also known as *caveman diet*) focuses on eating what humans during the Paleolithic period of evolution ate. The focus is on "hunter-and-gatherer" style food. Because it eliminates foods that can trigger an autoimmune reaction (such as grains, dairy, and highly processed food), the paleo diet is a highly effective diet for Hashimoto's disease. The anti-inflammatory benefits of the paleo diet can be achieved by eating the following foods: lean meat, fish, seafood, fruit, vegetables (avoid starches such as potatoes), nuts and seeds (Limitiris & Mazokopakis, 2017).

Vegetarian and Vegan Diets

Vegetarians do not eat meat, and *vegans* donot eat any animal products, including milk, butter and eggs. These diets are said to help improve the autoimmune response involved in Hashimoto disease. They also reduce inflammation and promote gut health. However, vegetarian and vegan diets are deficient in important vitamins and minerals such as iron, B12 and vitamin D. Supplements should help balance the nutritional deficiencies found in this type of diet. The following whole, plant-based foods may improve thyroid and gut health: fruits, vegetables, nuts, seeds, vegetable oils, legumes like lentils and beans, vegetable proteins like tofu and tempeh. (Limitiris & Mazokopakis, 2017).

Worst Diet for Hashimoto Disease

In addition to foods that help the thyroid, there are specific foods in certain amounts that can have a negative impact on the thyroid. Gluten and goitrogens are the worst foods to have in diet of patients with Hashimoto's disease.

Gluten

Celiac disease is an immune-mediated disease characterized by chronic inflammation and destruction of the villous structure of the small intestine (Green, 2007; Tonutti, 2014). It is triggered by the ingestion of gluten, a protein complex, found in wheat and related grains, such as barley, rye and oat. Celiac disease is now considered a multi-organ disorder, often presenting with diarrhea, malabsorption syndrome and weight loss, and has been linked to a many diseases including autoimmune disorders (Green, 2007; Tonutti, 2014; Kaukinen, 1999; Freeman, 2016). According to the International Medical Bibliography, AITD and celiac disease are clearly associated (Freeman, 2016; Hadithi, 2007; Tuhan, 2016). This might be explained partly by the increased immuno-sensitivity of celiac disease patients, as part of an autoimmune polyglandular syndrom, by the deficiency of key elements such as Se and iodine due to malabsorption (Stazi, 2008; Stazi, 2010) or due to antibodies that affect both target-tissues (Naiyer et al., 2008).

Some authors reported that between 3.2% (Liberman, 2007) and 4.8% (Collin, Salmi, Hallstrom, Reunala, & Pasternack, 1994) of patients with autoimmune thyroid disorder tested positive for celiac disease. Valentino et a.l (2002) reported that 43% of Hashimoto's thyroiditis patients proved to have potential celiac disease. A study in 2003 examined 400 patients with either Grave's or Hashimoto's thyroiditis and found that 5.5% tested positive for IgA, indicating gluten sensitivity (Akcay & Akcay, 2003). More recently, another study published in 2015 reported that 29% of patients with positive gluten sensitivity developed autoimmune disorders, most commonly Hashimoto's thyroiditis over the course of the ten-year study (Carroccio et al., 2015). These findings all suggest that gluten plays a huge rule in autoimmune disorders, specifically related to Hashimoto's thyroiditis.

Patients with Hashimoto's thyroiditis must therefore, undergo celiac serological tests [serum IgA and IgG gliadin antibodies (AGA-IgA, AGA-IgG), IgA trans-glutaminase antibodies (TGA), and serum IgA endomysium antibodies (EMA)] (Freeman, 2016). If any of the celiac serological tests is positive, the patients must be investigated with gastro-duodenoscopy and duodenal biopsy (Roy et al., 2016).

Some authorss suggested that gluten intolerance can be largely attributed to all autoimmune disorders. If symptoms of patients with Hashimoto's thyroiditis do not improve with lifestyle change and medication, patients may try to avoid foods that include *wheat*, (common in breads, cookies, and crackers), barley (common in soups and stews) and rye (common in bread and whiskey). In conclusion, any patient suffering from Hashimoto's thyroiditis should most certainly eliminate gluten from their diet.

Goitrogens

Goitrogens are compounds that impair the function of thyroid gland and interfere with the production of thyroxin hormones. *Pro-goitrin* is a biochemical from the glucosinolate family that is found in some food. It is inactive but after ingestion is converted to *goitrin*, which interferes with iodine utilization in the synthesis of thyroid hormones. This has been reported to be of concern only when associated with an iodine deficiency (Felker, Bunch, & Leung, 2016). Pro-goitrin has been isolated in cabbage, cauliflower, pricoli, spinach, kale, peanuts, mustard and rapeseed oil. These foods do not pose much of a threat if eaten in small amounts. Moreover, heating cruciferous vegetables alters the potential goitrogenic effect.

While people with goiters should be especially wary of goitrogens, most patients with Hashimoto's disease will not negatively impact their symptoms unless they consume a large amount of these foods every day.

Soy, which comes from soybeans, is another potential goitrogen and the isoflavone and genistein in soy inhibited the synthesis of thyroxin which could result in goitre. Nonetheless, multiple studies revealed that hypothyroidism is not associated with soy intake in people with adequate amounts of iodine (Divia 1997; Messini, 2006).

Alcohol

Alcohol feeds negative bacteria, and can allow them to get into the bloodstream through tiny holes in the epithelial cells and create an autoimmune response even in very small amounts. For this reason, alcohol is best avoided. Cooking with alcohol is also best to avoid at least initially and may be consider it again after some healing has occurred (Bethesda, 2013).

Other Food Additives, Supplements and Chemicals

Gums such as guar and xanthin gum, lecithin, carrageenan, act as emulsifiers and thickeners in recipes and are hidden in a lot of prepared and canned foods. They are complex sugar molecules that are very hard to digest and therefore anyone suffering from leaky gut should avoid them.

Coffee and fiber supplements lower the absorption of thyroid medication (L-thyroxine) suggesting a one hour gap between the both with thyroid medication (Mazokopakis 2008; Benvenga, 2008). In addition, flavonoids in fruits, vegetables and exhibit a potential cardiovascular benefit; however, high-dosages of flavonoid supplements attenuate thyroid function (Egnet & Rimbach, 2011).

Table 4. Recommended diets for Hashimoto's thyroiditis patients

Recommended Diet	Main Sources
Gluten-free Diet	Fruits, vegetables, fresh meat, fish and poultry, legumes, certain whole grains, dairy products and oils.
Paleo Diet	Lean meat, fish, seafood, fruit, vegetables (avoid starches such as potatoes), nuts and seeds
*Vegentarean and Vegan Diet**	Fruits, vegetables, nuts, seeds, vegetable oils, legumes like lentils and beans, vegetable proteins like tofu and tempeh.

**Vegetarians* do not eat meat; *vegans* do not eat any animal products

Table 5. Recommended micro-nutirients for Hashimoto's thydoiditis patients

Micronutrients	Daily Dose	Main Sources
Iodine	- Adult: 150 µg - Pregnancy: 220 µg - Lactation: 290 µg	Seaweed) and seafood (e.g. cod, sardines, shrimps, salmon and tuna), animal products (dairy products and eggs), fruits (prunes, cranberries and strawberries) and iodinated table salt
Selenium	55-75 µg	Brazil nuts, oysters, tuna, whole-wheat bread, sunflower seeds, meat (pork, beef, lamb, turkey, chicken), mushrooms and rye
Zinc	34-40 mg	Oysters and shellfish, beef, chicken, legumes (e.g. lentils, beans), nuts and cow's milk.
*Vitamin D**	1500-2500 IU	Fish (cod, salmon, sardines), milk and dairy products, cereal, orange juice, pork chops (with fat), and eggs.
Vitamin B12	- Adult: 2.4 µg - Pregnancy: 2.6 µg - Lactation: 2.8 µg	Molluscs, sardines, salmon, meat, liver, dairy products, fortified cereals and nutritional yeast.

*Vitamin D is synthesized within the body via skin exposure to sunlight (main natural source)

Table 6. Foods and supplements to avoid in the diet for Hashimoto's thydoiditis patients

Foods to Avoid	Examples
Gluten	Wheat, barley, cookies, cakes, pizza and bread.
Goitorgens	Cabbage, cauliflower, pricoli, spinach, kale, peanuts, mustard and rapeseed oil.
Alcohololic Drinks	All drinks that contains ethanol, commonly known as alcohol (e.g.gin, whisky, vodka, wine, etc).
Food additives / supplements	Gums such as guar and xanthin gum, lecithin, carrageenan and coffee and fiber supplements

Summary

The best diets for Hashimoto's thyroiditis patients are summarized in Table 4. These are the gluten-ree diet, paleo diet and vegetarian and vegan diets Micro-nutrients to integrate in diet for patients with Hashimoto's thyroiditis are summarized in Table 5. The worst foods for patients with Hashimoto's thyroiditis that should be avoided are depicted in Table 6.

REFERENCES

Akcay, M., & Akcay, G. (2003). The presence of the antigliadin antibodies in autoimmune thyroid diseases. *Hepatogastroenterology*, *50*(2).

Aldosary, B. M., Sutter, M. E., Schwartz, M., & Morgan, B. W. (2012). Case series of selenium toxicity from a nutritional supplement. *Clinical Toxicology (Philadelphia, PA)*, *50*(1), 57–64. doi:10.3109/15563650.2011.641560 PMID:22165838

Beckett, G. J., & Arthur, J. R. (2005). Selenium and endocrine systems. *The Journal of Endocrinology*, *184*(3), 455–465. doi:10.1677/joe.1.05971 PMID:15749805

Benvenga, S., Bartolone, L., Pappalardo, M. A., Lapa, R. A., Giorgianni, G., & Trimarchi, F. (2008). Altered intestinal absorption of L-thyroxine cause by coffee. *Thyroid*, *18*(3), 293–301. doi:10.1089/thy.2007.0222 PMID:18341376

Beulens, J. W., Booth, S. L., van den Heuvel, E. G., Stoecklin, E., Baka, A., & Vermeer, C. (2013). The role of menaquinones (vitamin K) in human health. *British Journal of Nutrition*, *110*(8), 1357–1368. doi:10.1017/S0007114513001013 PMID:23590754

Bjergved, L., Jorgensen, T., Perrild, H., Carle, A., Cerqueira, C., Krejbjerg, A., ... Knudsen, N. (2012). Predict.ors of change in serum TSH after iodine fortification: An 11-year follow-up to the DanThyr study. *The Journal of Clinical Endocrinology and Metabolism*, *97*(11), 4022–4029. doi:10.1210/jc.2012-2508 PMID:22962423

Boelaert, K., Newby, P.R., Simmonds, M.J., Holder, R.L., Carr-Smith, J.D., Heward, J.M., … Franklyn, J.A. (2010). Prevalence and relative risk of other autoimmune diseases in subjects with autoimmune thyroid disease. *American Journal of Medicine*, *123*, 183.

Bozkurt, N. C., Karbek, B., Ucan, B., Sahin, M., Cakal, E., Ozbek, M., & Delibasi, T. (2013). The association between severity of vitamin D deficiency and Hashimoto's thyroiditis. *Endocrine Practice*, *19*(3), 479–484. doi:10.4158/EP12376.OR PMID:23337162

Brown, K. M., & Arthur, J. R. (2001). Selenium, selenoproteins and human health: A review. *Public Health Nutrition*, *4*(2b), 593–599. doi:10.1079/PHN2001143 PMID:11683552

Caprio, M., Infante, M., & Calanchini, M. (2016). Vitamin D: Not just the bone. Evidence for benecial pleiotropic extraskeletal effects. *Eating and Weight Disorders*. doi:10.100740519-016-0312-6 PMID:27553017

Carayanniotis, G. (2007). Recognition of thyroglobulin by T cells: The role of iodine. *Thyroid*, *17*(10), 963–973. doi:10.1089/thy.2007.0199 PMID:17900225

Carroccio, A., D'Alcamo, A., Cavataio, F., Soresi, M., Seidita, A., Sciume, C., & Mansueto, P. (2015). High proportions of people with non-celiac what sensitivity have autoimmune disease of anti-nuclear antibodies. *Gastroenterology, 149*(3). doi:.2015.05.040 doi:10.1053/j.gastro

Caturegli, P., De Remigis, A., & Rose, N. R. (2014). Hashimoto thyroiditis: Clinical and diagnostic criteria. *Autoimmunity Reviews*, *13*(4-5), 391–397. doi:10.1016/j.autrev.2014.01.007 PMID:24434360

Cerretani, L., Comandini, P., Fumanelli, D., Scazzia, F., & Chiavaro, E. (2014). Evaluation of iodine content and stability in recipes prepared with biofortified potatoes. *International Journal of Food Sciences and Nutrition*, *65*(7), 1–6. doi:10.3109/09637486.2014.917155 PMID:24828007

Chaudhary, S., Dutta, D., Kumar, M., Saha, S., Mondai, S. A., Kumar, A., & Mukhopashyay, S. (2016). Vitamin D supplementation reduces thyroid peroxidase antibody levels in patients with autoimmune thyroid disease: An open-labeled randomized controlled trial. *Indian Journal of Endocrinology and Metabolism*, *20*(3), 391–398. doi:10.4103/2230-8210.179997 PMID:27186560

Chung, J.H. (2013). *Low-Iodine Diet for Preparation for Radioactive Iodine therapy in differentiated thyroid cancer in Korea*. doi. doi:10.3803/EnM.2013.28.3.157

Collin, P. (2005). Should adults be screened for celiac disease? What are the benefits and harms of screening? *Gastroenterology*, *128*(4), S104–S108. doi:10.1053/j.gastro.2005.02.021 PMID:15825117

Collin, P., Salmi, J., Hallstrom, O., Reunala, T., & Pasternack, A. (1994). Autoimmune thyroid disorders and coeliac disease. *European Journal of Endocrinology*, *30*(2), 137–140. doi:10.1530/eje.0.1300137 PMID:8130887

Dai, Y. D., Rao, V. P., & Carayanniotis, G. (2002). Enhanced iodination of thyroglobulin facilitates processing and presentation of a crypticpathogenic peptide. *Journal of Immunology (Baltimore, Md.: 1950)*, *168*(11), 5907–5911. doi:10.4049/jimmunol.168.11.5907 PMID:12023396

Dilas, L. T., Icin, T., Paro, J. N., & Bajkin, I. (2011). Autoimmune thyroid disease and other non-endocrine autoimmune diseases. *Medicinski Pregled*, *64*(3-4), 183–187. doi:10.2298/MPNS1104183T PMID:21905597

Divia, R. L., Changa, H. C., & Doerge, D. R. (1997). Anti-thyroid isoflavones from soy bean: Isolation, characterization and mechanisms of action. *Biochemical Pharmacology*, *54*, 1087–1096. doi:10.1016/S0006-2952(97)00301-8 PMID:9464451

Duntas, L. H. (2006). The role of selenium in thyroid autoimmunity and cancer. *Thyroid*, *16*(5), 455–460. doi:10.1089/thy.2006.16.455 PMID:16756467

Duntas, L. H. (2015). The role of iodine and selenium in autoimmune thyroiditis. *Hormone and Metabolic Research. Hormon- und Stoffwechselforschung. Hormones et Metabolisme*, *47*(10), 721–726. doi:10.1055-0035-1559631 PMID:26361258

Egert, S., & Rimbach, G. (2011). Which sources of flavonoids: Complex diets or dietary supliments? *Advances in Nutrition*, *2*(1), 8–14. doi:10.3945/an.110.000026 PMID:22211185

Ertek, S., Cicero, A., Caglar, O., & Erdogan, G. (2010). Relationship between serum zinc levels, thyroid hormones andthyroid volume following successful iodine supplementation. *Hormones*, *9*(3), 263–268. doi:10.14310/horm.2002.1276 PMID:20688624

Esposito, D., Rotondi, M., Accardo, G., Vallone, G., Docimo, G., Selvaggi, F., ... Pasqual.i, D. (2017). Influen.ce of short term selenium supplementation on the natural course of Hashimoto's thyroiditis: Clinical results of a blinded placebo-controlled randomized prospective trial. *Journal of Endocrinological Investigation*, *40*(1), 83–89. doi:10.100740618-016-0535-4 PMID:27572248

Fan, A. M., & Kizer, K. W. (1990). Selenium. Nutritional, toxicologic and clinical aspects. *The Western Journal of Medicine*, *153*, 160–167. PMID:2219873

Fan, Y., Xu, S., Zhang, H., Cao, W., Wang, K., Chen, G., ... Liu, C. (2014). Selenium supplementation for autoimmune thyroiditis: A systematic review and meta-analysis. *International Journal of Endocrinology*, *14*, 904573. PMID:25574167

Felker, P., Bunch, R., & Leung, A. M. (2016). Concentrations of thiocyanate and goitrin in human plasma, their precursor concentrations in brassica vegetable and associated potential for hypothyroidism. *Nutrition Reviews*, *74*(4), 248–258. doi:10.1093/nutrit/nuv110 PMID:26946249

Fiore, E., Latrofa, F., & Vitti, P. (2015). Iodine, thyroid autoimmunity and cancer. *European Thyroid Journal*, *4*(1), 26–35. doi:10.1159/000371741 PMID:25960959

Fordyce, F. M. (2003). Database of the Iodine Content of Food and Diets Populated with Data from Published Literature. British Geological Survey, Natural Environment Research Council.

Freeman, H. J. (2016). Endocrine manifestations in celiac disease. *World Journal of Gastroenterology*, *22*(38), 8472–8479. doi:10.3748/wjg.v22.i38.8472 PMID:27784959

Gastaldi, R., Muraca, M., Beltramo, A., & Poggi, E. (2014). Iodine deficiency and its consequences for cognitive and psychomotor development of children. *Italian Journal of Pediatrics*, *40*(S1), A15. doi:10.1186/1824-7288-40-S1-A15

Green, P. H., & Cellier, C. (2007). Celiac disease. *The New England Journal of Medicine*, *357*(17), 1731–1743. doi:10.1056/NEJMra071600 PMID:17960014

Gropper, S. S., Smith, J. L., & Groff, J. L. (2013). *Advanced Nutrition and Human Metabolism* (6th ed.). Belmont, CA: Wadsworth Publishing Company.

Hadithi, M., de Boer, H., Meijer, J. W., Willekens, F., Kerckhaert, J. A., Heijmans, R., ... Mulder, C. J. (2007). Coeliac. disease in Dutch patients with Hashimoto's thyroiditis and vice versa. *World Journal of Gastroenterology*, *13*(11), 1715–1722. doi:10.3748/wjg.v13.i11.1715 PMID:17461476

Heaney, R. P. (2007). The case for improving vitamin D status. *The Journal of Steroid Biochemistry and Molecular Biology*, *103*(3-5), 635–641. doi:10.1016/j.jsbmb.2006.12.006 PMID:17222549

Holick, M. F. (2007). Vitamin D deficiency. *The New England Journal of Medicine*, *357*(3), 266–281. doi:10.1056/NEJMra070553 PMID:17634462

Holick, M. F., Binkley, N. C., Bischo-Ferrari, H. A., Gordon, C. M., Hanley, D. A., Heaney, R. P., ... Weaver, C. M. (2011). Evaluation, treatment, and prevention of vitamin D deficiency: An Endocrine Society clinical practice guideline. *The Journal of Clinical Endocrinology and Metabolism*, *96*(7), 1911–1930. doi:10.1210/jc.2011-0385 PMID:21646368

Hypothyroidism: National endocrine and metabolic diseases information service. (2013). Department of Health and Human Services, NIH Publication.

Institute of Medicine. (2000). *Dietary Reference Intakes for Vitamin C, Vitamin E, Selenium, and Carotenoids*. National Academic Press.

Institute of Medicine. (2011). Dietary Reference Intakes for Calcium and Vitamin D. Washington, DC: National Academic Press (US).

Institute of Medicine, Food and Nutrition Board. (2001). *Dietary Reference Intakes for Vitamin A, Vitamin K, Arsenic, Boron, Chromium, Copper, Iodine, Iron, Manganese, Molybdenum, Nickel, Silicon, Vanadium, and Zinc*. Washington, DC: National Academy Press.

Jiang, H. Y., Li, H. S., Carayanniotis, K., & Carayanniotis, G. (2007). Variable inuences of iodine on the T-cell recognition of a single thyroglobulin epitope. *Immunology*, *121*(3), 370–376. doi:10.1111/j.1365-2567.2007.02584.x PMID:17376195

Kaprara, A., & Krassas, G. E. (2006). Selenium and thyroidal function; the role of immunoassays. *Hellenic Journal of Nuclear Medicine*, *9*, 195–203. PMID:17160166

Katagiri, R., Asakura, K., Uechi, K., Masayasu, S., & Sasaki, S. (2016). Iodine excretion in 24-hour urine collection and its dietary determinants in healthy Japanese adults. *Journal of Epidemiology*, *26*(12), 613–621. doi:10.2188/jea.JE20150245 PMID:27374137

Kaukinen, K., Collin, P., Mykkanen, A. H., Partanen, J., Maki, M., & Salmi, J. (1999). Celiac disease and autoimmune endocrinologic disorders. *Digestive Diseases and Sciences*, *44*(7), 1428–1433. doi:10.1023/A:1026612121041 PMID:10489930

Kivity, S., Agmon-Levin, N., Zisappl, M., Shapira, Y., Nagy, E., Danko, K., ... Shoenfeld, Y. (2011). Vitamin D and autoimmune thyroid diseases. *Cellular & Molecular Immunology*, *8*(3), 243–247. doi:10.1038/cmi.2010.73 PMID:21278761

Laurberg, P., Pedersen, I. B., Knudsen, N., Ovesen, L., & Andersen, S. (2001). Environmental iodine intake affects the type of nonmalignant thyroid disease. *Thyroid*, *11*(5), 457–469. doi:10.1089/105072501300176417 PMID:11396704

Laurberg, P., Pedersen, K. M., Hreidarsson, A., Sigfussen, N., Iversen, E., & Knudsen, P. R. (1998). Iodine intake and the pattern of thyroid disorders: A comparative epidemiological study of thyroid abnormalities in the elderly in Iceland and in Jutland, Denmark. *The Journal of Clinical Endocrinology and Metabolism*, *83*(3), 765–769. doi:10.1210/jcem.83.3.4624 PMID:9506723

Li, H. S., Jiang, H. Y., & Carayanniotis, G. (2007). Modifying effects of iodine on the immunogenicity of thyroglobulin peptides. *Journal of Autoimmunity*, *28*(4), 171–176. doi:10.1016/j.jaut.2007.01.001 PMID:17327138

Lieberman, S. (2007). *The Gluten Connection*. New York: Rodale Books.

Liontiris, M. I., & Mazokopakis, E. E. (2017). A concise review of Hashimoto thyroiditis (HT) and the importance of iodine, selenium, vitamin D and gluten on the autoimmunity and dietary management of HT patients; points that need more investigation. *Hellenic Journal of Nuclear Medicine*, *20*(1), 51–56. PMID:28315909

Lundin, K. E., & Wijmenga, C. (2015). Coeliac disease and autoimmune diseasegenetic overlap and screening. *Nature Reviews. Gastroenterology & Hepatology*, *12*(9), 507–515. doi:10.1038/nrgastro.2015.136 PMID:26303674

Markou, K., Georgopoulos, N., Kyriazopoulou, V., & Vagenakis, A. G. (2001). Iodine-Induced hypothyroidism. *Thyroid*, *11*(5), 501–510. doi:10.1089/105072501300176462 PMID:11396709

Markou, K. B., & Koukkou, E. G. (2012). The Greek population is iodine sufficient and not at risk of iodine-induced hyperthyroidism. *The Journal of Nutrition*, *142*(8), 1611–1612. doi:10.3945/jn.112.163980 PMID:22822183

Mazokopakis, E., Papadakis, J. A., Papadomanolaki, M. G., Batistakis, A. G., Giannakopoulos, T. G., Protopapadakis, E. E., & Ganotakis, E. S. (2007). Effects of 12 months treatment with L-selenomethionine on serum anti-TPO levels in patients with Hashimoto's thyroiditis. *Thyroid*, *17*(7), 609–612. doi:10.1089/thy.2007.0040 PMID:17696828

Mazokopakis, E. E., & Chatzipavlidou, V. (2007). Hashimoto's thyroiditis and the role of selenium. Current concepts. *Hellenic Journal of Nuclear Medicine*, *10*, 6–8. PMID:17450242

Mazokopakis, E. E., Giannakopoulos, T. G., & Starakis, K. (2008). Interaction between levothyroxine and calcium carbonate. *Canadian Family Physician Medecin de Famille Canadien*, *54*, 39. PMID:18208953

Mazokopakis, E. E., & Kotsiris, D. A. (2014). Hashimoto's autoimmune thyroiditis and vitamin D deficiency. Current aspects. *Hellenic Journal of Nuclear Medicine*, *17*, 37–40. PMID:24563883

Mazokopakis, E. E., Papadomanolaki, M. G., Tsekouras, K. C., Evangelopoulos, A. D., Kotsiris, D. A., & Tzortzinis, A. A. (2015). Is vitamin D related to pathogenesis and treatment of Hashimoto's thyroiditis? *Hellenic Journal of Nuclear Medicine*, *18*, 222–227. PMID:26637501

Mazokopakis, E. E., & Protopapadakis, E. E. (2007). Recommended dietary selenium intakes and selenium concentrations in nuts. *Hellenic Journal of Nuclear Medicine*, *10*, 34. PMID:17450251

Mazokopakis, E. E., Tzortzinis, A. A., Dalieraki-Ott, E. I., Tsartsalli, A. N., Syros, P. K., Karefilakis, C. M., ... Staraki.s, I. (2010). Coexist. ence of Hashimoto's thyroiditis with papillary thyroid carcinoma A retro. spective study. *Hormones (Athens, Greece)*, *9*(4), 312–317. doi:10.14310/horm.2002.1282 PMID:21112862

Medline Plus. (2018). *Goiter - simple*. U.S. National Library of Medicine.

Messina, M., & Redmond, G. (2006). Effects of soy protein and soy bean isoflavones on thyroid function in healthy adults and hypothyroid patients: A review of the relevant literutare. *Thyroid*, *16*(3), 249–258. doi:10.1089/thy.2006.16.249 PMID:16571087

Michalaki, M., Pylioti, A., Loutas, V., Mamali, I., & Markou, K. B. (2013). Absence of differences in urinary iodine excretion and thyroid function tests in operating room staff members using or not using iodine-containing antiseptic solutions. *Thyroid*, *23*(12), 1659–1660. doi:10.1089/thy.2013.0218 PMID:23724900

Muscogiuri, G., Mari, D., Prolo, S., Fatti, L. M., Cantone, M., Gargnani, P., ... Vitale, G. (2016). 25 Hydroxyvitamin D deficiency and its relationship to autoimmune thyroid disease in the elderly. *International Journal of Environmental Research and Public Health*, *13*(9), 850. doi:10.3390/ijerph13090850 PMID:27571093

Nacamulli, D., Mian, C., Petricca, D., Lazzarotto, F., Barollo, S., Pozza, D., ... Betterle, C. (2010). Influence of physiological dietary selenium supplementation on the natural course of autoimmune thyroiditis. *Clinical Endocrinology*, *73*, 535–539. PMID:20039895

Naiyer, A. J., Shah, J., Hernandez, L., Kim, S. Y., Ciaccio, E. J., Cheng, J., ... Green, P. H. R. (2008). Tissue trans-glutaminase antibodies in individuals with celiac disease bind to thyroid follicles and extracellular matrix and may contribute to thyroid dysfunction. *Thyroid*, *18*(11), 1171–1178. doi:10.1089/thy.2008.0110 PMID:19014325

Parekh, P. P., Khan, A. R., Torres, M. A., & Kitto, M. E. (2008). Concentrations of selenium, barium, and radium in Brazil nuts. *Journal of Food Composition and Analysis*, *21*(4), 332–335. doi:10.1016/j.jfca.2007.12.001

Pearce, E. N., Andersson, M., & Zimmermann, M. B. (2013). Global iodine nutrition: Where do we stand in 2013? *Thyroid*, *23*(5), 523–528. doi:10.1089/thy.2013.0128 PMID:23472655

Pearce, S. H., Brabant, G., Duntas, L. H., Monzani, F., Peeters, R. P., Razvia, S., & Wemeau, J. L. (2013). 2013 ETA guideline: Management of subclinical hypothyroidism. *European Thyroid Journal*, *2*(4), 215–228. doi:10.1159/000356507 PMID:24783053

Pedersen, I. B., Knudsen, N., Carle, A., Vejbjerg, P., Jorgensen, T., Perrild, H., ... Laurberg, P. (2011). A cautious iodization program bringing iodine intake to a low recommended level is associated with an increase in the prevalence of thyroid autoantibodies in the population. *Horumon To Rinsho*, *75*(1), 120–126. doi:10.1111/j.1365-2265.2011.04008.x PMID:21521277

Rayman, M. P. (2000). The importance of selenium to human health. *Lancet*, *356*(9225), 233–241. doi:10.1016/S0140-6736(00)02490-9 PMID:10963212

Rayman, M. P. (2012). Selenium and human health. *Lancet*, *379*(9822), 1256–1268. doi:10.1016/S0140-6736(11)61452-9 PMID:22381456

Robien, K., Oppeneer, S. J., Kelly, J. A., & Hamilton-Reevs, J. M. (2013). Drug-vitamin D interactions: A systematic review of the literature. *Nutrition in Clinical Practice*, *28*(2), 194–208. doi:10.1177/0884533612467824 PMID:23307906

Rohner, F., Zimmermann, M., Jooste, P., Pandav, C., Caldwell, K., Raghavan, R., & Raiten, D. J. (2014). Biomarkers of nutrition for development-iodine review. *The Journal of Nutrition*, *144*(8), 1322S–1342S. doi:10.3945/jn.113.181974 PMID:24966410

Roy, A., Laszkowska, M., Sundström, J., Lebwohl, B., Green, P. H., Kämpe, O., & Ludvigsson, J. F. (2016). Prevalence of celiac disease in patients with autoimmune thyroid disease: A meta-analysis. *Thyroid*, *26*(7), 880–890. doi:10.1089/thy.2016.0108 PMID:27256300

Schomburg, L. (2016). Dietary selenium and human health. *Nutrients*, *9*(1), E22. doi:10.3390/nu9010022 PMID:28042811

Shi, L., Bi, M., Yang, R., Zhou, J., Zhau, S., Fan, C., ... Teng, W. (2014). Defective expression of regulatory B cells in iodine-induced autoimmune thyroiditis in non-obese diabetic H2 (h4) mice. *Journal of Endocrinological Investigation*, *3*(1), 43–50. doi:10.100740618-013-0013-1 PMID:24464449

Sönmezgöz, E., Ozer, S., Yilmaz, R., Onder, Y., Butun, I., & Bilge, S. (2016). Hypovitaminosis D in children with Hashimoto thyroiditis. *Revista Medica de Chile*, *144*(5), 611–616. doi:10.4067/S0034-98872016000500009 PMID:27552012

Stazi, A. V., & Trinti, B. (2008). Selenium deficiency in celiac disease: Risk of autoimmune thyroid diseases. *Minerva Medica*, *99*, 643–653. PMID:19034261

Stazi, A. V., & Trinti, B. (2010). Selenium status and over-expression of interleukin15 in celiac disease and autoimmune thyroid diseases. *Annali dell'Istituto Superiore di Sanita*, *46*, 389–399. PMID:21169670

Sworczak, K., & Wisniewski, P. (2001). The role of vitamins in the prevention and treatment of thyroid disorders. *Endokrynologia Polska*, *62*, 340–344. PMID:21879475

Tonutti, E., & Bizzaro, N. (2014). Diagnosis and classification of celiac disease and gluten sensitivity. *Autoimmunity Reviews*, *13*(4-5), 472–476. doi:10.1016/j.autrev.2014.01.043 PMID:24440147

Topliss, D. J. (2016). Clinical update in aspects of the management of autoimmune thyroid diseases. *Endocrinology and Metabolism (Seoul, Korea)*, *31*(4), 493–499. doi:10.3803/EnM.2016.31.4.493 PMID:28029020

Toulis, K. A., Anastasilakis, A. D., Tzellos, T. G., Carter, B., & Pijl, H. (2010). Selenium supplementation in the treatment of Hashimoto's thyroiditis: A systematic review and a meta-analysis. *Thyroid*, *20*(10), 1163–1173. doi:10.1089/thy.2009.0351 PMID:20883174

Travnicke, J., Herzig, I., Kursa, J., Kroupova, V., & Navratilova, M. (2006). Iodine content in raw milk. *Veterinarni Medicina*, *51*(9), 448–453. doi:10.17221/5574-VETMED

Tuhan, H., Ik, S., Abac, A., Simasek, E., Anik, A., Anal, O., & Bober, E. (2016). Celiac disease in children and adolescents with Hashimoto Thyroiditis. *Turk Pediatri Arsivi*, *51*(2), 100–105. doi:10.5152/TurkPediatriArs.2016.3566 PMID:27489467

U.S. Food and Drug Administration (FDA). (2016). *Food Labeling: Revision of the Nutrition and Supplement Facts Labels, 2016*. Author.

Valentino, R., Savastano, S., Maglio, M., Paparo, F., Ferrara, F., Dorato, M., ... Troncone, R. (2002). Markers of potential coeliac disease in patients with Hashimoto's thyroiditis. *European Journal of Endocrinology*, *146*(4), 479–483. doi:10.1530/eje.0.1460479 PMID:11916614

van der Rhee, H. J., de Vries, E., & Coebergh, J. W. (2016). Regular sun exposure benefits health. *Medical Hypotheses*, *97*, 34–37. doi:10.1016/j.mehy.2016.10.011 PMID:27876126 van Zuuren, E. J., Albusta, A. Y., Fedorowicz, Z., Carter, B., & Pijl, H. (2014). Selenium Supplementation for Hashimoto's thyroiditis: Summary of a Cochrane systematic review. *European Thyroid Journal*, *3*(1), 25–31. doi:10.1159/000356040 PMID:24847462

Vanderpump, M. J. (2011). The epidemiology of thyroid diseases. *British Medical Bulletin*, *99*(1), 39–51. doi:10.1093/bmb/ldr030 PMID:21893493

Vinceti, M., Bonvicini, F., Bergomi, M., & Malagoli, C. (2010). Possible involvement of overexposure to environmental selenium in the etiology of amyotrophic lateral sclerosis: A short review. *Annali dell'Istituto Superiore di Sanita*, *46*, 279–283. PMID:20847461

Vinceti, M., Wei, E. T., Malagoli, C., Bergomi, M., & Vivoli, G. (2001). Adverse health effects of selenium. *Reviews on Environmental Health*, *16*(4), 233–251. doi:10.1515/REVEH.2001.16.4.233 PMID:12041880

Volta, U., De Franceschi, L., Molinaro, N., Tetta, C., & Bianchi, F. B. (1997). Organ-specific autoantibodies in coeliac disease: Do they represent an epiphenomenon or the expression of associated autoimmune disorders? *Italian Journal of Gastroenterology and Hepatology*, *29*, 18–21. PMID:9265573

Wichman, J., Winther, K. H., Bonnema, S. J., & Hegedüs, L. (2016). Selenium supplementation significantly reduces thyroid autoantibody levels in patients with chronic autoimmune thyroiditis: A systematic review and meta-analysis. *Thyroid*, *26*(12), 1681–1692. doi:10.1089/thy.2016.0256 PMID:27702392

Wilde, M. (2018). *How much Iodine is in Seaweed?* Napiers Herbalists Limited.

Wu, Q., Rayman, M. P., Lv, H., Schomburg, L., Cui, B., Gao, C., ... Shi, B. (2015). Low population selenium status is associated with increased prevalence of thyroid disease. *The Journal of Clinical Endocrinology and Metabolism*, *100*(11), 4037–4047. doi:10.1210/jc.2015-2222 PMID:26305620

Xu, C., Wu, F., Mao, C., Wang, X., Zheng, T., Bu, L., ... Xiao, Y. (2016). Excess. iodine promotes apoptosis of thyroid follicular epithelial cells by inducing autophagy suppression and is associated with Hashimoto thyroiditis disease. *Journal of Autoimmunity*, *75*, 50–57. doi:10.1016/j.jaut.2016.07.008 PMID:27448770

Yang, G. Q., Wang, S. Z., Zhou, R. H., & Sun, S. Z. (1983). Endemic selenium intoxication of humans in China. *The American Journal of Clinical Nutrition*, *37*(5), 872–881. doi:10.1093/ajcn/37.5.872 PMID:6846228

Zhao, H., Tian, Y., Liu, Z., Li, X., Feng, M., & Huang, T. (2014). Correlation between iodine intake and thyroid disorders: A cross-sectional study from the South of China. *Biological Trace Element Research*, *162*(1-3), 87–94. doi:10.100712011-014-0102-9 PMID:25161089

Zimmermann, M. B. (2009). Iodine deficiency. *Endocrine Reviews*, *30*(4), 376–408. doi:10.1210/er.2009-0011 PMID:19460960

Zimmermann, M. B., & Boelaert, K. (2015). Iodine deficiency and thyroid disorders. *The Lancet. Diabetes & Endocrinology*, *3*(4), 286–295. doi:10.1016/S2213-8587(14)70225-6 PMID:25591468

Zimmermann, M. B., & Boelaert, K. (2015). Iodine deficiency and thyroid disorders. *The Lancet. Diabetes & Endocrinology*, *3*(4), 286–295. doi:10.1016/S2213-8587(14)70225-6 PMID:25591468

Chapter 16
Prognosis

ABSTRACT

With early diagnosis, timely institution of L-T4 replacement therapy, regular patient follow-up care, and attention to other attendant complications, the prognosis in Hashimoto's thyroiditis (HT) is excellent with patients leading a normal life. Untreated myxedema coma has a poor prognosis and a high mortality rate, particularly in old age. Transient periods of thyrotoxicosis sometimes occur, and rarely full hyperthyroid Graves' disease with active ophthalmopathy. There is an increased prevalence of coronary artery disease in patients with untreated or undertreated HT. The relationship between papillary thyroid carcinoma (PTC) and HT has been controversial. Primary thyroid B-cell lymphoma affects less than one in a thousand persons, and it is more likely to affect those with long-standing autoimmune thyroiditis. Complications of over-replacement with L-T4 should be avoided. This chapter explores the prognosis of Hashimoto's disease.

INTRODUCTION

Morbidity related to Hashimoto's thyroiditis (HT) typically results from failure to reach the diagnosis of hypothyroidism or to institute L-thyroxine (L-T4) replacement therapy in adequate doses on part of the treating physician, or from failure on the part of the patient to take the replacement medication (i.e. non-compliance of the patient).

With early diagnosis, timely institution of L-T4 replacement therapy, informed patient follow-up care, and attention to other attendant complications,

DOI: 10.4018/978-1-5225-9655-4.ch016

the prognosis in HT is excellent, with patients leading a normal life. *Untreated myxedema coma* has a poor prognosis and a high mortality rate. Even with early detection and appropriate treatment, mortality ranges from 30% to 60% (Werner, 2000; Arlot, 1991).

The study by Ono et al reported that, as revealed through multivariable logistic regression, a higher in-hospital mortality rate in myxedema coma was associated with older age and catecholamine use (with or without steroids) (Ono et al., 2017).

Transient periods of *thyrotoxicosis* sometimes occur, and rarely the illness may progress to full hyperthyroid Graves' disease with active orbito-pathy (exophthalmos, inflamed eyes).

The increased prevalence of *lipid disorders* in association with untreated hypothyroidism has the potential to increase morbidity from coronary artery disease in patients with untreated or undertreated HT. A study by Sato et al suggested that in patients with heart failure, those with subclinical hypothyroidism have a worse prognosis, finding a significant increase in the rates of cardiac events and all-cause mortality in heart failure patients in the study with subclinical hypothyroidism compared with those who were euthyroid (Sato et al., 2018).

The relationship between *papillary thyroid carcinoma* (PTC) and HT has been controversial. Some investigations reported that the risk for PTCs is increased in patients with HT (Anand, Singh, Kushwaha, Hussain, & Sonkar, 2014). However, other studies have not observed a positive correlation (Jankovic, Le, & Hershman, 2013). The frequency of the association between PTC and HT ranges from 9% to 58% in a series of studies (Fugazzola, Colombo, Perrino, & Muzza, 2011). Whether HT represents a host immune response to PTC or just a chance occurrence remains unclear. Recently, studies have also focused on the influence of HT on the prognosis of PTC patients associated with HT. Several authors reported that the presence of HT in PTC is associated with smaller tumor size, less tumor invasion, a lower frequency of lymph node metastasis, less advanced TNM stage, and better prognosis (Kim, 2009; Kurukahvecioglu, 2007; Repplinger, 2008; Kiml 2011). In contrast, other studies reported that PTCs that coexist with HT are more likely to be bilateral and multifocal, resulting in a higher frequency of lymph node metastases (Consorti, 2010; Kebebew, 2001; Kim, 2010). Meta-analyses have indicated that HT is present in 26% of multifocal patients compared with 21% of unifocal patients (Lee, Kim, Choi, & Kim, 2003). Zhu et al. (2016) studied 763 PTC patients with and without HT. They reported that PTC patients with HT tended to exhibit multifocality (46.6% *versus* 21.6%,

$P<0.001$) and greater capsular invasion (43.3% *versus* 29.2%, $P<0.001$) as compared to PTC patients without HT.

Primary thyroid *B-cell lymphoma* affects less than one in a thousand persons, and it is more likely to affect those with long-standing autoimmune thyroiditis.

Thyroid-associated orbitopathy (TAO) is usually associated with Graves' disease, affecting approximately 25% of these patients, but can also be associated with Hashimoto thyroiditis occurring in nearly 6% of those patients (Boulos, 2004; Yamada, 2000; Maheshwari, 2012; Dagi, 2010; El-Kaissi, 2004). Kan et al. (2014) studied the prevalence of ophthalmopathy in 110 Hashimoto's thyroiditis for eye signs and reported that the prevalence of eye signs was significantly (p=0.002) higher then that of control subjects (22.7% *versus* 4.0%, respectively) (Kan, Kan, & Ecemis, 2014).

A recent study by Kahaly et al. (2016) indicated that a strong link exists between the presence of TSH receptor-stimulating antibodies (TS-Abs) in patients with Hashimoto thyroiditis and the development of *thyroid-associated orbitopathy* (TAO). The study, which included 700 patients with Hashimoto thyroiditis, found higher serum levels of TS-Abs in those with TAO than in those without this condition, while patients with active and severe TAO had higher TS-Ab levels than did patients with mild and inactive TAO. Healthy controls were negative for TS-Abs.

Therapeutic complications: Complications of over-replacement with L-T4 include accelerated bone loss, reduction in bone mineral density, osteoporosis, tachycardia, increased cardiac wall thickness and contractility, which raise the risk of cardiac arrhythmias (especially atrial fibrillation), particularly in the elderly.

Although it is difficult to predict severity and intractability of Hashimoto's thyroiditis, yet prognosis of this disease is acknowledged to be affected by genes associated with the production or expression of immune regulatory factors. These include interleukin-1beta (1IL-1β), IL-4, IL-5, IL-6, IL-13, interferon-gamma (IFN-γ), transforming growth factor-beta (TGF-β), tumor necrosis factor-alpha (TNF-α), Fox P3, glucocorticoid-induced tumour necrosis factor receptor (GITR), and T-box 21 (TBX21) (Hayashi, 2009; Inoue, 2011; Inoue, 2010; Inoue, 2009; Ito, 2006; Morita, 2012; Nanba, 2008; Tomizawa, 2011).

REFERENCES

Anand, A., Singh, K. R., Kushwaha, J. K., Hussain, N., & Sonkar, A. A. (2014). Papillary Thyroid Cancer and Hashimoto's Thyroiditis: An Association Less Understood. *Indian Journal of Surgical Oncology*, *5*(3), 199–204. doi:10.100713193-014-0325-4 PMID:25419066

Arlot, S., Debussche, X., Lalau, J. D., Mesmacque, A., Tolani, M., Quichard, J., & Fournier, A. (1991). Myxoedema coma: Response of thyroid hormones with oral and intravenous high-dose L-thyroxine treatment. *Intensive Care Medicine*, *17*(1), 16–18. doi:10.1007/BF01708403 PMID:2037720

Boulos, P. R., & Hardy, I. (2004). Thyroid-associated orbitopathy: A clinicopathologic and therapeutic review. *Current Opinion in Ophthalmology*, *15*(5), 389–400. doi:10.1097/01.icu.0000139992.15463.1b PMID:15625899

Consorti, F., Loponte, M., Milazzo, F., Potasso, L., & Antonaci, A. (2010). Risk of malignancy from thyroid nodular disease as an element of clinical management of patients with Hashimoto's thyroiditis. *European Surgical Research*, *45*(3-4), 333–337. doi:10.1159/000320954 PMID:21051899

Dagi, L. R., Elliott, A. T., Roper-Hall, G., & Cruz, O. A. (2010). Thyroid eye disease: Honing your skills to improve outcomes. *Journal of the American Association for Pediatrics Ophthalmology and Strabismus*, *14*(5), 425–431. doi:10.1016/j.jaapos.2010.07.005 PMID:21035070

El-Kaissi, S., Frauman, A. G., & Wall, J. R. (2004). Thyroid-associated ophthalmopathy: A practical guide to classification, natural history and management. *International Medical Journal*, *34*(8), 482–491. doi:10.1111/j.1445-5994.2004.00662.x PMID:15317547

Fugazzola, L., Colombo, C., Perrino, M., & Muzza, M. (2011). Papillary thyroid carcinoma and inflammation. *Frontiers in Endocrinology*, *2*, 88. doi:10.3389/fendo.2011.00088 PMID:22645512

Hayashi, F., Watanabe, M., Nanba, T., Inoue, N., Akamizu, T., & Iwatani, Y. (2009). Association of the -31C/T functional polymorphism in the interleukin-1beta gene with the intractability of Graves' disease and the proportion of T helper type 17 cells. *Clinical and Experimental Immunology*, *158*(3), 281–286. doi:10.1111/j.1365-2249.2009.04034.x PMID:19793334

Inoue, N., Watanabe, M., Morita, M., Tatusmi, K., Hidaka, Y., Akamizu, T., & Iwatani, Y. (2011). Association of functional polymorphisms in promoter regions of IL5, IL6 and IL13 genes with development and prognosis of autoimmune thyroid diseases. *Clinical and Experimental Immunology*, *163*(3), 318–323. doi:10.1111/j.1365-2249.2010.04306.x PMID:21235536

Inoue, N., Watanabe, M., Morita, M., Tomizawa, R., Akamizu, T., Tatsumi, K., ... Iwatani, Y. (2010). Association of functional polymorphisms related to the transcriptional level of FOXP3 with prognosis of autoimmune thyroid diseases. *Clinical and Experimental Immunology*, *162*(3), 402–406. doi:10.1111/j.1365-2249.2010.04229.x PMID:20942809

Inoue, N., Watanabe, M., Nanba, T., Wada, M., Akamizu, T., & Iwatani, Y. (2009). Involvement of functional polymorphisms in the TNFA gene in the pathogenesis of autoimmune thyroid diseases and production of anti-thyrotropin receptor antibody. *Clinical and Experimental Immunology*, *156*(2), 199–204. doi:10.1111/j.1365-2249.2009.03884.x PMID:19250279

Ito, C., Watanabe, M., Okuda, N., Watanabe, C., & Iwatani, Y. (2006). Association between the severity of Hashimoto's disease and the functional +874A/T polymorphism in the interferon-gamma gene. *Endocrine Journal*, *53*(4), 473–478. doi:10.1507/endocrj.K06-015 PMID:16820703

Jankovic, B., Le, K. T., & Hershman, J. M. (2013). Clinical review: Hashimoto's thyroiditis and papillary thyroid carcinoma: is there a correlation? *The Journal of Clinical Endocrinology and Metabolism*, *98*(2), 474–482. doi:10.1210/jc.2012-2978 PMID:23293329

Kahaly, G. J., Diana, T., Glang, J., Kantiz, M., Pitz, S., & Konig, J. (2016). Thyroid Stimulating Antibodies Are Highly Prevalent in Hashimoto's Thyroiditis and Associated Orbitopathy. *The Journal of Clinical Endocrinology and Metabolism*, *101*(5), 1998–2004. doi:10.1210/jc.2016-1220 PMID:26964732

Kan, E., Kan, E. K., & Ecemis, G. (2014). Presence of thyroid-associated ophthalmopathy in Hashimoto's thyroiditis. *International Journal of Ophthalmology*, *7*(4), 644–647. PMID:25161935

Kebebew, E., Treseler, P. A., Ituarte, P. H., & Clark, O. (2001). Coexisting chronic lymphocytic thyroiditis and papillary thyroid cancer revisited. *World Journal of Surgery*, *25*(5), 632–637. doi:10.1007002680020165 PMID:11369991

Kim, E.Y., Kim, W.G., Kim, W.B., Kim, T.Y., Kim, J.M., & Ryu, J., … Shong, Y.K. (2009). Coexistence of chronic lymphocytic thyroiditis is associated with lower recurrence rates in patients with papillary thyroid carcinoma. *Horumon To Rinsho*, *71*, 581–586. PMID:19222495

Kim, H. S., Choi, Y. J., & Yun, J. S. (2010). Features of papillary thyroid microcarcinoma in the presence and absence of lymphocytic thyroiditis. *Endocrine Pathology*, *21*(3), 149–153. doi:10.100712022-010-9124-9 PMID:20506003

Kim, K. W., Park, Y. J., Kim, E. H., Park, D., Ahn, S., Park, D. J., ... Cho, B. Y. (2011). Elevated risk of papillary thyroid cancer in Korean patients with Hashimoto's thyroiditis. *Head & Neck*, *33*(5), 691–695. doi:10.1002/hed.21518 PMID:21484918

Kurukahvecioglu, O., Taneri, F., Yuksel, O., Aydin, A., Tezzel, E., & Onuk, E. (2007). Total thyroidectomy for the treatment of Hashimoto's thyroiditis coexisting with papillary thyroid carcinoma. *Advances in Therapy*, *24*(3), 510–516. doi:10.1007/BF02848773 PMID:17660159

Lee, J. H., Kim, Y., Choi, J. W., & Kim, Y. S. (2003). The association between 15.papillary thyroid carcinoma and histologically proven Hashimoto's thyroiditis: A meta-analysis. *European Journal of Endocrinology*, *168*(3), 343–349. doi:10.1530/EJE-12-0903 PMID:23211578

Maheshwari, R., & Weis, E. (2012). Thyroid associated orbitopathy. *Indian Journal of Ophthalmology*, *60*(2), 87–93. doi:10.4103/0301-4738.94048 PMID:22446901

Morita, M., Watanabe, M., Inoue, N., Inaoka, C., Akamizu, T., Tatsumi, K., ... Iwatani, Y. (2012). Functional polymorphisms in *TBX21* and *HLX* are associated with development and prognosis of Graves' disease. *Autoimmunity*, *145*(2), 129–136. doi:10.3109/08916934.2011.622013 PMID:22014209

Nanba, T., Watanabe, M., Akamizu, T., & Iwatani, Y. (2008). The -590CC genotype in the IL4 gene as a strong predictive factor for the development of hypothyroidism in Hashimoto disease. *Clinical Chemistry*, *54*(3), 621–623. doi:10.1373/clinchem.2007.099739 PMID:18310157

Ono, Y., Ono, S., Yasunaga, H., Matsui, H., Fushimi, K., & Tanaka, Y. (2017). Clinical characteristics and outcomes of myxedema coma: Analysis of a national inpatient database in Japan. *Journal of Epidemiology*, *27*(3), 117–122. doi:10.1016/j.je.2016.04.002 PMID:28142035

Repplinger, D., Bargren, A., Zhang, Y. W., Alder, J., Haymart, M., & Chen, H. (2008). Is Hashimoto's thyroiditis a risk factor for papillary thyroid cancer? *The Journal of Surgical Research*, *150*(1), 49–52. doi:10.1016/j.jss.2007.09.020 PMID:17996901

Sato, Y., Yoshihisa, A., Kimishima, Y., Kiko, T., Watanabe, S., Kanno, Y., ... Takeischi, Y. (2018). Subclinical Hypothyroidism Is Associated With Adverse Prognosis in Heart Failure Patients. *The Canadian Journal of Cardiology*, *34*(1), 80–87. doi:10.1016/j.cjca.2017.10.021 PMID:29275887

Tomizawa, R., Watanabe, M., Inoue, N., Takemura, K., Hidaka, Y., Akamizu, T., ... Iwatani, Y. (2011). Association of functional GITR gene polymorphisms related to expression of glucocorticoid-induced tumour necrosis factor-receptor (GITR) molecules with prognosis of autoimmune thyroid disease. *Clinical and Experimental Immunology*, *165*(2), 141–167. doi:10.1111/j.1365-2249.2011.04414.x PMID:21592113

Werner, S. C., Ingbar, S. H., Braverman, L. E., & Utiger, R. D. (2000). *Werner & Ingbar's The thyroid: a fundamental and clinical text* (8th ed.). Philadelphia, PA: Lipincott Williams &Wilkins.

Yamada, M., Wu Li, A., & Wall, J. (2000). Thyroid-associated ophthalmopathy: Clinical features, pathogenesis, and management. *Critical Reviews in Clinical Laboratory Sciences*, *37*(6), 523–549. doi:10.1080/10408360091174303 PMID:11192331

Zhu, F., Shen, Y. B., Li, F. Q., Fang, Y., Hu, L., & Wu, Y. J. (2016). The effects of Hashimoto thyroiditis on lymph node metastases in unifocal and multifocal papillary thyroid carcinoma: *A Retrospective Chinese Cohort Study. Medicine; Analytical Reviews of General Medicine, Neurology, Psychiatry, Dermatology, and Pediatries*, *95*(6), e2674. doi:10.1097/MD.0000000000002674 PMID:26871795

Related Readings

To continue IGI Global's long-standing tradition of advancing innovation through emerging research, please find below a compiled list of recommended IGI Global book chapters and journal articles in the areas of Hashimoto's disease, disease management, and thyroidism. These related readings will provide additional information and guidance to further enrich your knowledge and assist you with your own research.

Akbar, S., & Prasad, B. V. (2018). Thyroid Disease in Ageing and Risk Factors. In B. Prasad & S. Akbar (Eds.), *Handbook of Research on Geriatric Health, Treatment, and Care* (pp. 339–356). Hershey, PA: IGI Global. doi:10.4018/978-1-5225-3480-8.ch019

Alhaj, O. A. (2017). Functional Properties of Camel Milk. In H. Shekhar, Z. Howlader, & Y. Kabir (Eds.), *Exploring the Nutrition and Health Benefits of Functional Foods* (pp. 147–164). Hershey, PA: IGI Global. doi:10.4018/978-1-5225-0591-4.ch007

Allison, K., & Allison, C. (2017). Mental Illness, Youth, and Lessons from Residential Treatment Centers. In V. Bryan & J. Bird (Eds.), *Healthcare Community Synergism between Patients, Practitioners, and Researchers* (pp. 126–151). Hershey, PA: IGI Global. doi:10.4018/978-1-5225-0640-9.ch007

Alsalamah, S., Alsalamah, H., Gray, A. W., & Hilton, J. (2016). Information Security Threats in Patient-Centred Healthcare. In A. Moumtzoglou (Ed.), *M-Health Innovations for Patient-Centered Care* (pp. 298–318). Hershey, PA: IGI Global. doi:10.4018/978-1-4666-9861-1.ch015

Altinpulluk, H., & Kurubacak, G. (2016). MoBip Project: To Raise Awareness about Bipolar Disorder through an 3D Pop-Up Book. In A. Moumtzoglou (Ed.), *M-Health Innovations for Patient-Centered Care* (pp. 147–169). Hershey, PA: IGI Global. doi:10.4018/978-1-4666-9861-1.ch008

Baumblatt, G. L. (2017). Meeting Patients Where They Are: Using Multimedia and Interactive Voice Technology to Humanize Communication and Engage Patients. In G. Graffigna (Ed.), *Transformative Healthcare Practice through Patient Engagement* (pp. 139–162). Hershey, PA: IGI Global. doi:10.4018/978-1-5225-0663-8.ch006

Bigi, S., & Lamiani, G. (2017). The Power of Words: Deliberation Dialogue as a Model to Favor Patient Engagement in Chronic Care. In G. Graffigna (Ed.), *Transformative Healthcare Practice through Patient Engagement* (pp. 66–92). Hershey, PA: IGI Global. doi:10.4018/978-1-5225-0663-8.ch003

Bird, J. L. (2017). Writing Healing Narratives. In V. Bryan & J. Bird (Eds.), *Healthcare Community Synergism between Patients, Practitioners, and Researchers* (pp. 1–28). Hershey, PA: IGI Global. doi:10.4018/978-1-5225-0640-9.ch001

Buffo, R. (2017). Yerba Mate: Chemistry, Technology, and Biological Properties. In H. Shekhar, Z. Howlader, & Y. Kabir (Eds.), *Exploring the Nutrition and Health Benefits of Functional Foods* (pp. 185–194). Hershey, PA: IGI Global. doi:10.4018/978-1-5225-0591-4.ch009

Castelnuovo, G., Pietrabissa, G., Manzoni, G. M., Corti, S., Novelli, M., Borrello, M., ... Simpson, S. (2017). A Stepped Care mHealth-Based Approach for Promoting Patient Engagement in Chronic Care Management of Obesity with Type 2 Diabetes. In G. Graffigna (Ed.), *Transformative Healthcare Practice through Patient Engagement* (pp. 192–214). Hershey, PA: IGI Global. doi:10.4018/978-1-5225-0663-8.ch008

Chakraborty, C., Gupta, B., & Ghosh, S. K. (2016). Mobile Telemedicine Systems for Remote Patient's Chronic Wound Monitoring. In A. Moumtzoglou (Ed.), *M-Health Innovations for Patient-Centered Care* (pp. 213–239). Hershey, PA: IGI Global. doi:10.4018/978-1-4666-9861-1.ch011

Dotson, E., Hibbler, D. K., & Scott, L. (2017). Culture of Learning Cities: Connecting Leisure and Health for Lifelong Learning Communities. In V. Bryan & J. Bird (Eds.), *Healthcare Community Synergism between Patients, Practitioners, and Researchers* (pp. 152–175). Hershey, PA: IGI Global. doi:10.4018/978-1-5225-0640-9.ch008

Drowos, J. L., & Wood, S. K. (2017). Preparing Future Physicians to Adapt to the Changing Health Care System: Promoting Humanism through Curricular Design. In V. Bryan & J. Bird (Eds.), *Healthcare Community Synergism between Patients, Practitioners, and Researchers* (pp. 106–125). Hershey, PA: IGI Global. doi:10.4018/978-1-5225-0640-9.ch006

Edoh, T. O. (2019). Impact of Patient Health Education on the Screening for Disease Test-Outcomes: The Case of Using Educational Materials From the Internet and Online Health Communities. In T. Edoh, P. Pawar, & S. Mohammad (Eds.), *Pre-Screening Systems for Early Disease Prediction, Detection, and Prevention* (pp. 156–189). Hershey, PA: IGI Global. doi:10.4018/978-1-5225-7131-5.ch006

Edoh, T. O. (2019). Internet-of-Things-Enabled Pre-Screening for Diseases: A Novel Approach for Improving the Conventional Methodology and Paradigm for Screening for Non-Communicable Diseases. In T. Edoh, P. Pawar, & S. Mohammad (Eds.), *Pre-Screening Systems for Early Disease Prediction, Detection, and Prevention* (pp. 1–49). Hershey, PA: IGI Global. doi:10.4018/978-1-5225-7131-5.ch001

Ellington, L., & Bryan, V. C. (2017). Incognito: The Neuroscience of Grief and Grieving. In V. Bryan & J. Bird (Eds.), *Healthcare Community Synergism between Patients, Practitioners, and Researchers* (pp. 272–291). Hershey, PA: IGI Global. doi:10.4018/978-1-5225-0640-9.ch012

Eshiet, E. R., & Smith, E. E. (2017). Herbal Benefits of Tea. In H. Shekhar, Z. Howlader, & Y. Kabir (Eds.), *Exploring the Nutrition and Health Benefits of Functional Foods* (pp. 117–146). Hershey, PA: IGI Global. doi:10.4018/978-1-5225-0591-4.ch006

Faris, M. A., & Attlee, A. (2017). Lentils (Lens culinaris, L.): A Novel Functional Food. In H. Shekhar, Z. Howlader, & Y. Kabir (Eds.), *Exploring the Nutrition and Health Benefits of Functional Foods* (pp. 42–72). Hershey, PA: IGI Global. doi:10.4018/978-1-5225-0591-4.ch003

Freytag, J., & Street, R. L. Jr. (2017). Patient and Family Engagement in THE Conversation: Pathways from Communication to Care Outcomes. In G. Graffigna (Ed.), *Transformative Healthcare Practice through Patient Engagement* (pp. 93–113). Hershey, PA: IGI Global. doi:10.4018/978-1-5225-0663-8.ch004

Gambhir, S., Kumar, Y., Malik, S., Yadav, G., & Malik, A. (2019). Early Diagnostics Model for Dengue Disease Using Decision Tree-Based Approaches. In T. Edoh, P. Pawar, & S. Mohammad (Eds.), *Pre-Screening Systems for Early Disease Prediction, Detection, and Prevention* (pp. 69–87). Hershey, PA: IGI Global. doi:10.4018/978-1-5225-7131-5.ch003

Genova, J., Olson, C. A., & Bender, J. (2017). Using the Communication AssessmenT Checklist in Health to Assess the Communication Quality of Web Based Resources for Prostate Cancer. In G. Graffigna (Ed.), *Transformative Healthcare Practice through Patient Engagement* (pp. 163–191). Hershey, PA: IGI Global. doi:10.4018/978-1-5225-0663-8.ch007

Giokas, K., Costarides, V., & Koutsouris, D. (2016). Integrated Platform for the Lifestyle Change and Holistic Approach to Personalized Prevention and Self-Management of Patients with High Blood Pressure. In A. Moumtzoglou (Ed.), *M-Health Innovations for Patient-Centered Care* (pp. 72–90). Hershey, PA: IGI Global. doi:10.4018/978-1-4666-9861-1.ch004

Giokas, K., Katrakazas, P., & Koutsouris, D. (2016). A Collaborative m-Health Platform for Evidence-Based Self-Management and Detection of Chronic Multimorbidity Development and Progression. In A. Moumtzoglou (Ed.), *M-Health Innovations for Patient-Centered Care* (pp. 52–71). Hershey, PA: IGI Global. doi:10.4018/978-1-4666-9861-1.ch003

Gupta, A. (2017). Functional Foods in Hypertension: Functional Foods in Cardiovascular Diseases. In H. Shekhar, Z. Howlader, & Y. Kabir (Eds.), *Exploring the Nutrition and Health Benefits of Functional Foods* (pp. 376–396). Hershey, PA: IGI Global. doi:10.4018/978-1-5225-0591-4.ch017

Hartman, A., & Brown, S. (2017). Synergism through Therapeutic Visual Arts. In V. Bryan & J. Bird (Eds.), *Healthcare Community Synergism between Patients, Practitioners, and Researchers* (pp. 29–48). Hershey, PA: IGI Global. doi:10.4018/978-1-5225-0640-9.ch002

Hiwale, S., Ulman, S., & Subbaraman, K. (2019). Barriers to Adoptions of IoT-Based Solutions for Disease Screening. In T. Edoh, P. Pawar, & S. Mohammad (Eds.), *Pre-Screening Systems for Early Disease Prediction, Detection, and Prevention* (pp. 50–68). Hershey, PA: IGI Global. doi:10.4018/978-1-5225-7131-5.ch002

Howlader, M. Z., & Shekhar, H. U. (2017). Health Benefits and Risks of Rice. In H. Shekhar, Z. Howlader, & Y. Kabir (Eds.), *Exploring the Nutrition and Health Benefits of Functional Foods* (pp. 195–222). Hershey, PA: IGI Global. doi:10.4018/978-1-5225-0591-4.ch010

Iltchev, P., Śliwczyński, A., Szynkiewicz, P., & Marczak, M. (2016). Mobile Health Applications Assisting Patients with Chronic Diseases: Examples from Asthma Care. In A. Moumtzoglou (Ed.), *M-Health Innovations for Patient-Centered Care* (pp. 170–196). Hershey, PA: IGI Global. doi:10.4018/978-1-4666-9861-1.ch009

Ismail, T., Akhtar, S., & Riaz, M. (2017). Pomegranate Peel and Fruit Extracts: A Novel Approach to Avert Degenerative Disorders – Pomegranate and Degenerative Diseases. In H. Shekhar, Z. Howlader, & Y. Kabir (Eds.), *Exploring the Nutrition and Health Benefits of Functional Foods* (pp. 165–184). Hershey, PA: IGI Global. doi:10.4018/978-1-5225-0591-4.ch008

Jain, A., & Rani, V. (2017). Food and Cardiac Health: Protective Effects of Food on Cardiovascular System. In H. Shekhar, Z. Howlader, & Y. Kabir (Eds.), *Exploring the Nutrition and Health Benefits of Functional Foods* (pp. 1–15). Hershey, PA: IGI Global. doi:10.4018/978-1-5225-0591-4.ch001

Janzek-Hawlat, S., & Tellioğlu, H. (2017). Waiting for Health Care Services. In G. Graffigna (Ed.), *Transformative Healthcare Practice through Patient Engagement* (pp. 276–301). Hershey, PA: IGI Global. doi:10.4018/978-1-5225-0663-8.ch011

Ju, K. H., & Eung-Soo, H. (2017). Health Promoting Effects of Kimchi. In H. Shekhar, Z. Howlader, & Y. Kabir (Eds.), *Exploring the Nutrition and Health Benefits of Functional Foods* (pp. 73–98). Hershey, PA: IGI Global. doi:10.4018/978-1-5225-0591-4.ch004

Kakulapati, V., Balaram, V., & Krishna, P. V. (2018). Improved Health Monitoring Informatics by New Similarity Measures. In B. Mishra & R. Kumar (Eds.), *Big Data Management and the Internet of Things for Improved Health Systems* (pp. 212–229). Hershey, PA: IGI Global. doi:10.4018/978-1-5225-5222-2.ch012

Kakulapati, V., Vasumathi, D., Mahender Reddy, S., & Deepthi, B. S. (2019). Fuzzy-Based Predictive Analytics for Early Detection of Diabetes. In T. Edoh, P. Pawar, & S. Mohammad (Eds.), *Pre-Screening Systems for Early Disease Prediction, Detection, and Prevention* (pp. 219–247). Hershey, PA: IGI Global. doi:10.4018/978-1-5225-7131-5.ch008

Kenski, C. M., & Falcone, J. N. (2017). Humane Education: A Call to Action for Elementary School Students. In V. Bryan & J. Bird (Eds.), *Healthcare Community Synergism between Patients, Practitioners, and Researchers* (pp. 88–105). Hershey, PA: IGI Global. doi:10.4018/978-1-5225-0640-9.ch005

King, B. M., Barry, C. D., Bamdas, J. A., Bronner, K., & Edwards, K. A. (2017). HeartMath®: A University Initiative. In V. Bryan & J. Bird (Eds.), *Healthcare Community Synergism between Patients, Practitioners, and Researchers* (pp. 49–64). Hershey, PA: IGI Global. doi:10.4018/978-1-5225-0640-9.ch003

Koumpouros, Y., & Georgoulas, A. (2016). mHealth R&D Activities in Europe. In A. Moumtzoglou (Ed.), M-Health Innovations for Patient-Centered Care (pp. 20-51). Hershey, PA: IGI Global. doi:10.4018/978-1-4666-9861-1.ch002

Kumar, U. (2019). Applications of Machine Learning in Disease Pre-screening. In T. Edoh, P. Pawar, & S. Mohammad (Eds.), *Pre-Screening Systems for Early Disease Prediction, Detection, and Prevention* (pp. 278–320). Hershey, PA: IGI Global. doi:10.4018/978-1-5225-7131-5.ch010

Lee, C. (2017). Application of the Dietary Processed Sulfur Supplementation for Enhancing Nutritional and Functional Properties of Meat Products. In H. Shekhar, Z. Howlader, & Y. Kabir (Eds.), *Exploring the Nutrition and Health Benefits of Functional Foods* (pp. 254–264). Hershey, PA: IGI Global. doi:10.4018/978-1-5225-0591-4.ch012

Mayo, B., Guadamuro, L., Flórez, A. B., & Delgado, S. (2017). Soy and Soy Products, Isoflavones, Equol, and Health. In H. Shekhar, Z. Howlader, & Y. Kabir (Eds.), *Exploring the Nutrition and Health Benefits of Functional Foods* (pp. 223–253). Hershey, PA: IGI Global. doi:10.4018/978-1-5225-0591-4.ch011

Mehta, P. (2017). Framework of Indian Healthcare System and its Challenges: An Insight. In V. Bryan & J. Bird (Eds.), *Healthcare Community Synergism between Patients, Practitioners, and Researchers* (pp. 247–271). Hershey, PA: IGI Global. doi:10.4018/978-1-5225-0640-9.ch011

Metelmann, B., & Metelmann, C. (2016). M-Health in Prehospital Emergency Medicine: Experiences from the EU funded Project LiveCity. In A. Moumtzoglou (Ed.), *M-Health Innovations for Patient-Centered Care* (pp. 197–212). Hershey, PA: IGI Global. doi:10.4018/978-1-4666-9861-1.ch010

Mitra, S., & Khandelwal, S. (2017). Health Benefits of Tea: Beneficial Effects of Tea on Human Health. In H. Shekhar, Z. Howlader, & Y. Kabir (Eds.), *Exploring the Nutrition and Health Benefits of Functional Foods* (pp. 99–116). Hershey, PA: IGI Global. doi:10.4018/978-1-5225-0591-4.ch005

Mohammad, S. (2019). Safety and Regulatory Aspects of Systems for Disease Pre-Screening. In T. Edoh, P. Pawar, & S. Mohammad (Eds.), *Pre-Screening Systems for Early Disease Prediction, Detection, and Prevention* (pp. 321–344). Hershey, PA: IGI Global. doi:10.4018/978-1-5225-7131-5.ch011

Moumtzoglou, A. S. (2016). Tailored M-Health Communication in Patient-Centered Care. In A. Moumtzoglou (Ed.), *M-Health Innovations for Patient-Centered Care* (pp. 319–340). Hershey, PA: IGI Global. doi:10.4018/978-1-4666-9861-1.ch016

Moumtzoglou, A. S. (2016). The Nexus of M-Health and Self-Efficacy. In A. Moumtzoglou (Ed.), *M-Health Innovations for Patient-Centered Care* (pp. 341–365). Hershey, PA: IGI Global. doi:10.4018/978-1-4666-9861-1.ch017

Muyonga, J. H., Nansereko, S., Steenkamp, I., Manley, M., & Okoth, J. K. (2017). Traditional African Foods and Their Potential to Contribute to Health and Nutrition: Traditional African Foods. In H. Shekhar, Z. Howlader, & Y. Kabir (Eds.), *Exploring the Nutrition and Health Benefits of Functional Foods* (pp. 320–346). Hershey, PA: IGI Global. doi:10.4018/978-1-5225-0591-4.ch015

Paliwal, G., & Bunglowala, A. (2019). Ubiquitous Wearable Healthcare Monitoring System Architectural Design for Prevention, Detection, and Monitoring of Chronic Diseases. In T. Edoh, P. Pawar, & S. Mohammad (Eds.), *Pre-Screening Systems for Early Disease Prediction, Detection, and Prevention* (pp. 190–218). Hershey, PA: IGI Global. doi:10.4018/978-1-5225-7131-5.ch007

Passi, S. J. (2017). Functional Foods and Cardiac Health. In H. Shekhar, Z. Howlader, & Y. Kabir (Eds.), *Exploring the Nutrition and Health Benefits of Functional Foods* (pp. 16–41). Hershey, PA: IGI Global. doi:10.4018/978-1-5225-0591-4.ch002

Perroti, R., Pouliakis, A., Margari, N., Panopoulou, E., Karakitsou, E., Iliopoulou, D., ... Koutsouris, D. D. (2018). CytoNet, A Versatile Web-Based System for Accessing Advisory Cytology Services: Application of Artificial Intelligence. *International Journal of Reliable and Quality E-Healthcare, 7*(3), 37–56. doi:10.4018/IJRQEH.2018070103

Poonia, A. (2017). Antimicrobial Edible Films and Coatings for Fruits and Vegetables. In H. Shekhar, Z. Howlader, & Y. Kabir (Eds.), *Exploring the Nutrition and Health Benefits of Functional Foods* (pp. 301–319). Hershey, PA: IGI Global. doi:10.4018/978-1-5225-0591-4.ch014

Postolache, G., Oliveira, R., Moreira, I., & Postolache, O. (2017). Why, What and When in-Home Physiotherapy? In G. Graffigna (Ed.), *Transformative Healthcare Practice through Patient Engagement* (pp. 215–246). Hershey, PA: IGI Global. doi:10.4018/978-1-5225-0663-8.ch009

Pouliakis, A., Archondakis, S., Margari, N., & Karakitsos, P. (2016). From Telecytology to Mobile Cytopathology: Past, Present, and Future. In A. Moumtzoglou (Ed.), *M-Health Innovations for Patient-Centered Care* (pp. 240–261). Hershey, PA: IGI Global. doi:10.4018/978-1-4666-9861-1.ch012

Recchia, V., Dodaro, A., Maglie, R. B., & Leo, C. G. (2017). Communication and Education Processes Involved in COPD Patient Engagement within the Italian Health System. In G. Graffigna (Ed.), *Transformative Healthcare Practice through Patient Engagement* (pp. 29–65). Hershey, PA: IGI Global. doi:10.4018/978-1-5225-0663-8.ch002

Ross, D. B., Exposito, J. A., & Kennedy, T. (2017). Stress and Its Relationship to Leadership and a Healthy Workplace Culture. In V. Bryan & J. Bird (Eds.), *Healthcare Community Synergism between Patients, Practitioners, and Researchers* (pp. 213–246). Hershey, PA: IGI Global. doi:10.4018/978-1-5225-0640-9.ch010

Sagahyroon, A. (2016). mHealth: Sleeping Disorders Diagnosis. In A. Moumtzoglou (Ed.), M-Health Innovations for Patient-Centered Care (pp. 115-125). Hershey, PA: IGI Global. doi:10.4018/978-1-4666-9861-1.ch006

Saita, E., Zanini, S., Minetti, E., & Acquati, C. (2017). Best Practices to Promote Patient and Donor Engagement to Care in Living Donor Transplant. In G. Graffigna (Ed.), *Transformative Healthcare Practice through Patient Engagement* (pp. 1–28). Hershey, PA: IGI Global. doi:10.4018/978-1-5225-0663-8.ch001

Sen, S., & Chakraborty, R. (2017). Food in Health Preservation and Promotion: A Special Focus on the Interplay between Oxidative Stress and Pro-Oxidant/Antioxidant. In H. Shekhar, Z. Howlader, & Y. Kabir (Eds.), *Exploring the Nutrition and Health Benefits of Functional Foods* (pp. 265–300). Hershey, PA: IGI Global. doi:10.4018/978-1-5225-0591-4.ch013

Sharma, A., & Patidar, S. (2019). A Fourier-Bessel Expansion-Based Method for Automated Detection of Atrial Fibrillation From Electrocardiogram Signals. In T. Edoh, P. Pawar, & S. Mohammad (Eds.), *Pre-Screening Systems for Early Disease Prediction, Detection, and Prevention* (pp. 248–277). Hershey, PA: IGI Global. doi:10.4018/978-1-5225-7131-5.ch009

Shiva, A., Sai, V. T., Siva, S. V., Rajamani, K. T., & Siva, S. S. (2016). Development of an Interactive GUI Tool for Thyroid Uptake Studies using Gamma Camera. *International Journal of Biomedical and Clinical Engineering*, *5*(1), 1–8. doi:10.4018/IJBCE.2016010101

Sidhu, J. S., & Zafar, T. A. (2017). Functional Foods of the Indian Subcontinent. In H. Shekhar, Z. Howlader, & Y. Kabir (Eds.), *Exploring the Nutrition and Health Benefits of Functional Foods* (pp. 347–375). Hershey, PA: IGI Global. doi:10.4018/978-1-5225-0591-4.ch016

Singh, D., Purkait, G., Banerjee, A., & Chatterjee, P. (2019). Innovative Approaches for Pre-Screening and Sensing of Diseases. In T. Edoh, P. Pawar, & S. Mohammad (Eds.), *Pre-Screening Systems for Early Disease Prediction, Detection, and Prevention* (pp. 88–107). Hershey, PA: IGI Global. doi:10.4018/978-1-5225-7131-5.ch004

Sourial, M., Bamdas, J. A., Constanzo, A., & Ishak, M. E. (2017). A Need for Greater Collaboration: Initiatives to Improve Transitions of Care. In V. Bryan & J. Bird (Eds.), *Healthcare Community Synergism between Patients, Practitioners, and Researchers* (pp. 65–87). Hershey, PA: IGI Global. doi:10.4018/978-1-5225-0640-9.ch004

Stavros, A., Vavoulidis, E., & Nasioutziki, M. (2016). The Use of Mobile Health Applications for Quality Control and Accreditational Purposes in a Cytopathology Laboratory. In A. Moumtzoglou (Ed.), *M-Health Innovations for Patient-Centered Care* (pp. 262–283). Hershey, PA: IGI Global. doi:10.4018/978-1-4666-9861-1.ch013

Tamposis, I., Pouliakis, A., Fezoulidis, I., & Karakitsos, P. (2016). Mobile Platforms Supporting Health Professionals: Need, Technical Requirements, and Applications. In A. Moumtzoglou (Ed.), *M-Health Innovations for Patient-Centered Care* (pp. 91–114). Hershey, PA: IGI Global. doi:10.4018/978-1-4666-9861-1.ch005

Thomas, L. M. V., M. K., & B., A. (2019). Clinical Decision Support System for Early Disease Detection and Management: Statistics-Based Early Disease Detection. In T. Edoh, P. Pawar, & S. Mohammad (Eds.), Pre-Screening Systems for Early Disease Prediction, Detection, and Prevention (pp. 108-155). Hershey, PA: IGI Global. doi:10.4018/978-1-5225-7131-5.ch005

Tiwari, M., Agrawal, D. S., & Mitra, S. (2017). Abnormal Uterine Bleeding (AUB) and Thyroid Function in Chhattisgarh. *International Journal of User-Driven Healthcare*, *7*(2), 29–41. doi:10.4018/IJUDH.2017070103

Triberti, S., & Chirico, A. (2017). Healthy Avatars, Healthy People: Care Engagement Through the Shared Experience of Virtual Worlds. In G. Graffigna (Ed.), *Transformative Healthcare Practice through Patient Engagement* (pp. 247–275). Hershey, PA: IGI Global. doi:10.4018/978-1-5225-0663-8.ch010

Vlachopapadopoulou, E., & Fotiadis, D. I. (2016). The Contribution of mHealth in the Care of Obese Pediatric Patients. In A. Moumtzoglou (Ed.), *M-Health Innovations for Patient-Centered Care* (pp. 126–146). Hershey, PA: IGI Global. doi:10.4018/978-1-4666-9861-1.ch007

Waegemann, C. P. (2016). mHealth: History, Analysis, and Implementation. In A. Moumtzoglou (Ed.), M-Health Innovations for Patient-Centered Care (pp. 1-19). Hershey, PA: IGI Global. doi:10.4018/978-1-4666-9861-1.ch001

Wambuguh, O. J. (2019). *Examining the Causal Relationship Between Genes, Epigenetics, and Human Health* (pp. 1–603). Hershey, PA: IGI Global. doi:10.4018/978-1-5225-8066-9

Weiss-Randall, D. N. (2017). The Role of Self-Efficacy and Aging in Managing Disease. In V. Bryan & J. Bird (Eds.), *Healthcare Community Synergism between Patients, Practitioners, and Researchers* (pp. 176–212). Hershey, PA: IGI Global. doi:10.4018/978-1-5225-0640-9.ch009

Zimeras, S. (2016). Computer Virus Models and Analysis in M-Health IT Systems: Computer Virus Models. In A. Moumtzoglou (Ed.), *M-Health Innovations for Patient-Centered Care* (pp. 284–297). Hershey, PA: IGI Global. doi:10.4018/978-1-4666-9861-1.ch014

Zordich, T., & Menichetti, J. (2017). Engaging Patients and Lowering Costs: Technology to the Rescue. In G. Graffigna (Ed.), *Transformative Healthcare Practice through Patient Engagement* (pp. 115–138). Hershey, PA: IGI Global. doi:10.4018/978-1-5225-0663-8.ch005

About the Author

Mahmoud Sakr, MD, PhD, FACS, Professor of Surgery, graduated in 1981 and had his Master (MS) and Doctorate Degree (PhD) at Alexandria University, Egypt. He had his fellowship in Surgery and Organ Transplantation at University of Pittsburgh School of Medicine, PA, USA. He published 18 books and 105 articles in esteemed journals and is an editorial board member of repute in many international journals.

Index

G

H

I

J

L

M

N

O

P

Z

www.ingramcontent.com/pod-product-compliance
Lightning Source LLC
LaVergne TN
LVHW080854300926
849162LV00003B/419